Additional Praise for
The Power Nutrient Solution

"Being deficient in your essential micronutrients causes long-latency diseases such as osteoporosis, cancer, diabetes, heart disease, dementia, obesity, and more. The Caltons have properly identified the problem and offer us a powerful solution that will help you lose weight, increase energy, and reverse disease faster than you may have ever thought possible."

—MARK HYMAN, MD, author of the #1 New York Times bestseller *The Blood Sugar Solution 10-Day Detox Diet*

"It took 100 countries, 7 continents, and 6 years for the Caltons to discover the Fountain of Youth. It only took them one book to share it with you. *The Power Nutrient Solution* is your guide to longevity, radiant health, and an excuse to eat more delicious food. Today is the day for you to start your plan!"

—GEORGE BRYANT, coauthor of the *New York Times* bestseller *The Paleo Kitchen*

"Micronutrients often become the missing link for fast, lasting fat loss and optimal health. In their groundbreaking new book, Mira and Jayson Calton connect the dots to provide a powerfully effective, easy-to-implement plan that helps you become lean, toned, and vibrantly healthy. Don't miss this one!"

—JJ VIRGIN, author of the *New York Times* bestseller, *JJ Virgin's The Sugar Impact Diet*

"Nutrient deficiencies are often at the root cause of many chronic health conditions. Dr. Jayson and Mira Calton draw on their many years of working in the field of nutrition and dietary supplement science to show us how to reverse disease though micronutrient therapy. A must-read for anyone wanting to reverse a chronic health condition or struggling with energy levels, weight, or feeling unwell."

—IZABELLA WENTZ, PharmD, FASCP, *New York Times* bestselling author *Hashimoto's Thyroiditis*

"The Caltons have outdone themselves with *The Power Nutrient Solution*. This nutritional masterpiece offers exceptional information, guidance, and most important, hope for healing. *The Power Nutrient Solution* is truly an enjoyable, eye-opening read…and makes a great gift for someone you want to give the gift of healing."

—TANA AMEN, BSN, RN, Amen Clinics, vice president, and New York Times bestselling author of *The Omni Diet*

"*The Power Nutrient Solution* isn't your average 'diet' book. On the contrary, it's a true strategy book teaching you how to regain your health and optimize your life through nutrition! I don't say this lightly when I say micronutrients are one of the most powerful truths in nutrition today and the Caltons have nailed it in this great book. They've lived it themselves and proven it out in their own lives and now you have their secret in your hands. Highly recommended!"

—LEANNE ELY, CNC, *New York Times* bestselling author and founder of SavingDinner.com

"If you are stressed, overweight, exhausted, or suffering from any health condition, then read this book."

—SARA GOTTFRIED, MD, *New York Times* **bestselling author of** *The Hormone Reset Diet*

"A huge variety of micronutrient deficiencies increase risk of chronic illness, and it's easy to understand why: If you don't have all the nutrients your body needs to be healthy, you won't be healthy. *The Power Nutrient Solution* is a thorough guide to preventing or reversing disease by embracing more nutrient-dense foods. Mira and Jayson will show you just how widespread micronutrient deficiencies are and how to increase the nutrient density of your diet whether you prefer to eat Paleo, vegetarian, or whatever you want. They'll also coach you through cravings, purging the pantry, managing stress, exercising, reducing environmental toxins, getting off medications, when to supplement, and how to shop for the best produce, animal products, and even condiments without breaking the bank. With a 28-day menu plan and tons of customization options depending on your specific health condition, *The Power Nutrient Solution* has everything you need to get started as a nutrivore!"

—SARAH BALLANTYNE, PhD, *New York Times* **bestselling author of** *The Paleo Approach* **and** *The Paleo Approach Cookbook*

"We know today that getting *all* of the nutrition we need from our food is tricky, but do you know why? From depleted soils, to nonorganic and GMO foods, to foods and activities that deplete our body's nutrient stores on a daily basis, the list of violations against our health goes on and on. In *The Power Nutrient Solution*, the Caltons not only explain the *causes* of widespread nutrient deficiencies, but they also outline a clear plan for everyone to become sufficient, as well."

—DIANE SANFILIPPO, *New York Times* **bestselling author of** *Practical Paleo*

THE
POWER NUTRIENT
SOLUTION

The **28-DAY MICRONUTRIENT MIRACLE PLAN** to Lose Weight, Boost Energy, and Reverse Disease

JAYSON CALTON, PhD, AND MIRA CALTON, CN

RODALE.

We dedicate this book to all those who have experienced, and are about to experience, the miraculous power of micronutrient sufficiency.

Contents

Introduction

How *The Power Nutrient Solution* Will Change Your Life

Have you ever found that the hardest people to convince of *anything* are often your own family? No matter how many degrees or years of experience you have in your particular field, family members always seem to seek advice from everyone else except you. So you can imagine our surprise when our brother-in-law, Craig, a 44-year-old television executive, called us one Saturday afternoon to talk about how to get rid of his high blood pressure. Craig explained that he had been struggling with high blood pressure for more than 10 years and that he had tried to lower it on his own by eating a little better and exercising when he could, but with his busy schedule, sadly his condition remained unchanged. In fact, his doctor had told him that his high blood pressure was most likely genetic and that if he hadn't been able to bring his numbers down over the last 10 years, really no amount of dietary changes or exercise were likely going to help. "Yesterday he told me that he wants me to start taking prescription medication immediately," said Craig. "I don't want to start taking medication at 44. Is there anything you guys can do to help?"

Help? We were going to do more than help. We were bursting at the seams with excitement over the thought of putting Craig on our Power Nutrient Solution Protocol (otherwise known as our Micronutrient Miracle plan), especially since he was the new father of our two adorable little nieces, Chloe and Halle. We explained to Craig that his high blood pressure was likely being caused by a deficiency in specific micronutrients and that he would have to become sufficient in those essential micronutrients in order to reverse his condition. We quickly e-mailed him a detailed outline of exactly what we wanted him to do for the next 28 days, and then we waited.

We didn't hear from him again for several weeks. When the phone rang one Friday afternoon, we both ran over and looked at the caller ID to see if it was Craig—and it was. "You were right," he said, "and my doctor can't believe it!" "What happened?" we exclaimed. "I did exactly what you told me to do for the last 4 weeks, and just now at the doctor's office, my blood pressure was perfect—120/80 on the nose," he replied. "The nurse even checked it twice. I'm a believer; those micronutrients of yours really are powerful." We congratulated Craig and told him to continue doing exactly what he had been doing so that he would maintain his newfound micronutrient sufficiency and keep his blood pressure in check. We are very happy to report that Craig did just that, and his blood pressure is still picture-perfect 4 years later.

Do you have high blood pressure or know someone who does? According to the Centers for Disease Control and Prevention, 67 million Americans,[1] or 1 out of every 3 adults, are affected by high blood pressure, which is often referred to as the "silent killer." This is because it usually has no warning signs or symptoms and greatly increases the risk of developing heart disease or having a stroke, the first and third leading causes of death in the United States. Additionally, high blood pressure is estimated to cost the United States nearly $100 billion in health-care services, medications, and missed workdays. The good news is, both medical and nutritional science have proven that high blood pressure is completely preventable and reversible, as Craig and so many others have proven to themselves.

Craig did not have to change his diet, give up his favorite foods, or force himself to exercise every day to achieve his results. He simply followed the food and supplement plan we provided to him and incorporated the core philosophies of our Micronutrient Miracle plan into his current lifestyle, and he was able to quickly and almost effortlessly take back control of his health.

A Personal Beginning

People always ask us how we became so impassioned about micronutrients. After all, it isn't the sexiest topic on the planet. The truth is that the story of how we ended up in our current position, teaching the miraculous benefits of becoming micronutrient sufficient, is one of tragedy, true love, mystical adventure, and ultimately, service. And it all started one cold Manhattan morning in 2001.

Mira's Story

Hi, my name is Mira Calton. When I turned 30, everything in my life changed. Up until that point, you would have thought I was on top of the world. I ran my own public relations firm from my high-rise apartment in New York City. Dressed to the nines by my fashion designer clients, I spent my days writing press releases, contacting magazine editors, and running from television studio to film set throughout the city. I spent my evenings at restaurant openings and film premieres generating buzz for those I represented.

But that all came to a screeching halt when I could no longer hide what was going on with my body. You see, I had ignored the pain in my hips and lower back for almost a year. I blamed the intermittent bouts of discomfort on my hectic lifestyle and long hours in stilettos. However, now in the darkness of winter, I had to face the facts. I had been working from home for more than a month—no longer able to visit clients and making excuses for not attending functions—because the pain had completely overwhelmed me.

I made an appointment with my doctor—an event I had tried hard to put off—and that day in his office, it felt like my life had ended. Honestly, I don't know who was more stunned, my doctor or me. We both repeated the same phrase in disbelief: "How could this even be possible?" Sitting in a paper cape on the examination table, I was diagnosed with advanced osteoporosis. My bones had deteriorated to those of an 80-year-old woman. And the worst part of all was that my doctor didn't think they would get any better. It seemed I was fated to live a life filled with prescription medications with a host of detrimental side effects that at best would keep my bones from getting worse.

No longer able to perform my job or take care of myself, I was forced to sell the company I had worked so hard to build. I moved to Florida to live with my sister, and if you know me, then you know that being reliant on others has never been easy for me. But being nearly bedridden gives you a lot of time to reflect. *What had I done for this to happen to my body? What could I do now to change my fate? Was there anything I could do that could possibly make me healthy and strong and reverse my advanced osteoporosis?*

After spending many months thoroughly researching the negative side effects of the medications I had been prescribed, I decided *not* to follow the advice of my physician and chose to forgo taking medication. Instead, I took my health into my own hands and began to search for an alternative, natural treatment. I pledged to find a healthier diet, be more active, sleep longer hours, and find alternate theories on the reversal of osteoporosis. However, after several years, I realized that my efforts were not proving successful.

That's when fate stepped in. My path was blessed when I met a doctor of nutrition with more than a decade of clinical experience who was willing to look at my bone health from a completely new angle.

Jayson's Story

Hi, my name is Dr. Jayson Calton. When I first met Mira, I was shocked to find out that such a young, vibrant woman was suffering from such an advanced form of osteoporosis. When she told me that she had refused to take the medication her doctor had prescribed and instead was looking for an alternative, natural treatment for her condition, I was immediately intrigued.

I informed Mira that I had been working in the field of nutritional medicine for 14 years and had helped thousands of clients suffering from a wide variety of health conditions and diseases using my unique low-carbohydrate (ketogenic) diet program focused on whole foods and supplementation with micronutrients (vitamins and minerals). Although much of my work had been focused on weight loss in the beginning, once in a while clients would report back to me that the program had lowered their high cholesterol or that their chronic headaches were gone. By the time I met Mira, thousands of clients had reported that the diet had either alleviated or reversed more than 20 different health conditions beyond weight loss. In fact, nearly every client was experiencing this effect to some extent. Because of this, I believed I could help her find a way to reverse her condition.

Although my successful diet and exercise programs were part of my initial recommendation for Mira, I knew that this protocol would not be enough on its own. Mira was a special case; severe micronutrient deficiencies had played a central role in the development of her advanced osteoporosis, so we needed to determine the cause of her deficiencies and then get her body to absorb the vitamins and minerals necessary to rebuild her bones. This forced me to shift my attention away from the macronutrient side of food (carbohydrates, fats, and proteins), which I had been focusing on for most of my career, and take a much deeper look at the essential micronutrients themselves.

Together we pinpointed specific diet and lifestyle habits that may have contributed to her disease. Mira was shocked to learn that her daily low-fat muffin and black coffee for breakfast, spinach salad for lunch, and Chinese takeout for dinner had all, in their own ways, contributed to her micronutrient deficiencies. In fact, the majority of the foods she was eating were micronutrient-poor, filled with what we call *naked calories*—foods that have been stripped of their essential, health-promoting vitamins and minerals and are therefore "naked." She was getting plenty of these naked calories but very few of the vitamins and minerals her body needed.

Her life in the big city didn't help matters either. Like many urban dwellers, her days had been filled with stress, excessive caffeine and alcohol consumption, carbon monoxide inhalation, poor sleep patterns, excessive exercise, and frequent dieting. This was a lifestyle and environment that further sabotaged her body's ability to absorb the micronutrients necessary for health and vitality.

We changed Mira's eating habits to replace micronutrient-poor foods with more micronutrient-rich alternatives. We eliminated many of her poor lifestyle habits and began a program of weight-bearing exercise, and, perhaps most important, we developed and implemented a very specific micronutrient therapy protocol. Slowly, Mira began to feel better. However, we knew that only a new DEXA scan, the common test given to measure bone mineral density, would give us the information and the proof we were praying for. I joined Mira on her return visit to her doctor's office to hear the test results. The news couldn't have been any better. Within 2 years, Mira's advanced osteoporosis was completely reversed.

Our Success Spawns New Questions

As you can imagine, we were elated. Our years of searching through scientific research looking for any information we could find on the roles that nutrition and lifestyle habits had in the causation, prevention, and reversal of disease, specifically as they related to micronutrient deficiency, had paid off. Hundreds of studies conducted at acclaimed universities and research papers from established foundations and government agencies all seemed to point more toward nutritional and lifestyle factors as the main culprits of disease prevalence in modernized societies and less often to genetic components. It seemed to us that we had discovered something very important, and we were eager to explore this idea further to see where it would lead us. Our intense research and mutual respect had also given us something beyond the reversal of osteoporosis to celebrate. After many months of working so closely together, we had also fallen in love. (See? We told you this was a love story!)

Now working as a couple and inspired by our success in reversing Mira's osteoporosis, we turned our complete attention to the investigation of micronutrient deficiency. We wanted to know everything about it—how prevalent it was, both in the United States and around the world; the specific dietary and lifestyle habits that could increase the risk of becoming deficient; and, perhaps most important, which common health conditions and diseases beyond osteoporosis had medical science identified as having micronutrient deficiency as a causative factor.

Could the dietary, lifestyle, and supplementation protocols we had used to improve Mira's health also be instrumental in the prevention or reversal of other conditions?

Could others suffering from osteoporosis or osteopenia go from frail-boned individuals living in pain and limited by disease to pain-free, strong-boned individuals through proper nutrition, lifestyle, and supplementation alone? Could a person delay, prevent, or even reverse advanced stages of a disease without medications? Our investigation into micronutrient deficiency led us on an incredible journey, a quest for knowledge that spanned both many years and many miles.

Digging Deeper: The Calton Project

In 2005, we were married and set off on a 6-year around-the-world expedition with one goal in mind: to observe cultures around the globe, both urban and remote, to discover how different dietary and lifestyle habits affect overall health. We were no longer satisfied by simply reading research studies performed at acclaimed institutions and universities concerning the relationship between dietary patterns and health. Instead, we wanted to sit with, eat with, and ask questions of people from diverse cultures in an attempt to relearn what modern man had forgotten about the healing power of proper nutrition, as well as the disease-producing power of nutritional deficiencies. We would follow in the tradition of Weston A. Price, who had explored the diets and health of native peoples back in the 1930s. For us, the knowledge would be in the discovery, and we would use that knowledge to rethink how we eat in America and around the world to achieve optimal health.

We called this mystical adventure to more than 135 countries on all seven continents The Calton Project. And our quest for a fresh perspective on nutrition sent us traveling from the low-lying Sepik River in Papua New Guinea to the heights of the Andes in Peru and the Himalayas in Tibet. Our observations and interviews with such diverse cultures led us to a unique global understanding of nutrition and its ability to both prevent and cause disease.

Our discoveries on The Calton Project, together with our continuous, diligent exploration of mainstream research studies, have driven us to one final conclusion: *The primary causative factor of almost every one of today's most debilitating health conditions and diseases lies in a preventable "hidden" pandemic.* We're talking about diseases like cancer, osteoporosis, heart disease, diabetes, Alzheimer's, and obesity, to name but a few. It was this same pandemic that gave Craig his high blood pressure and Mira her advanced osteoporosis. *It is called micronutrient deficiency, and we believe that it is the most widespread and dangerous health condition of the 21st century.*

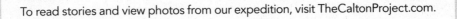

To read stories and view photos from our expedition, visit TheCaltonProject.com.

What Is the Micronutrient Miracle?

If you wanted to be the healthiest you have ever been, free of disease, loaded with energy, and fated for a long and vibrant life, what would you eat? It's a good question, right? Would you follow, let's say, a low-fat, plant-based diet? How about a Paleo or Primal diet filled with the foods of your ancestors? Or would you perhaps follow a ketogenic diet and eat high-fat, low-carbohydrate foods? What if we told you that the diet you choose doesn't matter, that the key to living a long, healthy, energy-packed life is something else completely?

What we are about to reveal to you is going to change the way that you look at food forever, so make sure you pay close attention. The information that we are about to share here with you is the exact same information we provide to our private clients.

The secret doesn't lie in your carbohydrate, fat, or protein ratios.

Nor is it determined by the dietary profile you follow.

In fact, there is no one dietary philosophy or magic ratio of foods that will keep you healthy.

In our travels, we observed groups from vastly different regions of the world who were thriving and eating vastly different diets. Some were eating low-carbohydrate diets, while others were eating high-carbohydrate diets. Some ate more of a plant-based diet and only included meat once or twice a week, and others ate diets almost entirely based on meat, with very little plant nutrition. Sure, different diets can and do influence your health in different ways, and this can be a powerful tool, but simply following a specific diet is not enough to produce optimal health; there is something else—a missing piece of the puzzle that changes everything.

By now you have probably guessed that we are talking about micronutrients. The word *micronutrients* may sound complicated, but it's really just an all-encompassing term for things you are already familiar with—vitamins, minerals, essential fatty acids, and amino acids. You can think of them as the "good stuff" in food that our bodies require every day to obtain and sustain optimal health. They are called *micro*nutrients because your body only needs them in *micro*, or very small, quantities. This is in contrast to *macro*nutrients— such as carbohydrates, fats, and proteins—which your body uses as energy in the form of calories. They are required in *macro*, or much larger, quantities.

Basically, you can think of macronutrients as the components in food that provide the energy and building materials for our bodies and micronutrients as completely different components in that same food that provide the "workers" to make the body function. For example, the mineral magnesium is involved in over 300 essential metabolic reactions in the body. It is necessary for the transmission of muscular activity and nerve impulses, temperature regulation,

Is Micronutrient Deficiency Affecting Your Health?

Micronutrient deficiency can cause a wide variety of health conditions and diseases. Examine the short list of questions below to see if deficiency is a factor in your life.

- Do you suffer from food cravings, restless sleep, headaches, or low energy?
- Have you experienced stubborn weight loss or unexpected weight gain even though you haven't changed anything about your diet?
- Has a physician recently diagnosed you with osteoporosis, heart disease, high blood pressure, diabetes, or cancer?
- Do you have digestive issues or leaky gut, or have you been told you have an autoimmune condition?
- Do you find that your nails are brittle, your hair is not as healthy as you would like, or your skin complexion is not what you dream of?
- Are you dissatisfied with your current physical and mental performance, and do you feel you could be functioning at a much higher level?
- Have you noticed hormonal changes in your body, such as lowered sex drive, hot flashes, or PMS?
- Are you noticing memory loss, brain fog, or depression, or have you been diagnosed with age-related macular degeneration?

If you answered yes to any of these questions, you likely have a deficiency in one or more essential micronutrients. Read on to learn how you can reverse this deficiency on the 28-day Micronutrient Miracle plan.

detoxification reactions, and the formation of healthy bones and teeth. It is also involved in the synthesis of DNA and RNA and in energy production. So you can see how many different things could go wrong if you were deficient in even just one micronutrient.

In our practice as celebrity nutrition and lifestyle medicine experts, the amazing results our clients experience are not true miracles. In fact, the powers of the essential micronutrients are very well documented in scientific journals. It is the human body's ability to use these micronutrients to prevent and reverse nearly all the health conditions and lifestyle diseases currently plaguing billions of people across the globe that we find truly miraculous.

Hidden Hunger: The Cause of Today's Lifestyle Conditions and Diseases

Did you know that there are two types of hunger your body can experience? Most of us are familiar with the first type, which occurs when you have not eaten enough food or have not eaten for a long period of time. Your body usually lets you know that you are experiencing this form of *obvious hunger* with stomach grumbling and hunger pangs. The second type of hunger is not so obvious; it is known as "hidden hunger," and it occurs when you have not ingested enough essential micronutrients. In the past, eating more food would alleviate both forms of hunger. That's because the food of our ancestors delivered both caloric value and abundant micronutrient value. However, in modern times, simply eating more food will not necessarily reverse hidden hunger because many of today's foods have become increasingly devoid of their essential vitamins and minerals. Because of this, hidden hunger now affects billions of people around the globe both in impoverished third world countries as well as in wealthy industrialized nations, and it is currently the world's most widespread nutritional disorder.

Stop Putting the Cart Before the Horse

You may be noticing that the Micronutrient Miracle plan is completely different from other diet plans you may have tried in the past. That's because our philosophy of how to achieve and sustain optimal health is a 180-degree shift from conventional thinking. Let's face it: Most health professionals are caught up in something we refer to as the "macronutrient wars." They fight about whether a low-carbohydrate diet is better than a low-fat one, whether you should eat more protein, whether you should eat more or fewer meals, or whether or not calories matter. And sometimes they even fight about choosing the foods you eat based on your blood type.

It is a sea of confusion that is easy to get lost in, leaving you both confused and frustrated. It's a war that I (Jayson) know all too well, and it's one that I was actively caught up in when I first met Mira. But, as we stated earlier, what we have come to learn is that the diet you choose, the number of calories you eat, and whether you have type O or type B blood really are not the most important factors in determining your health. In fact, we always say that putting your dietary preferences before micronutrient sufficiency is like putting the proverbial cart before the horse.

The fact is that deficiencies in specific micronutrients lead to specific health conditions and diseases. Take osteoporosis, for example; it comes from being deficient in a very specific list of vitamins and minerals that everyone must have to build and maintain strong bones. So, if an individual was following a Paleo diet and was deficient in the bone-builders calcium, magnesium, and vitamins D and K, that person would be at risk for developing osteoporosis. Similarly, if a completely different individual adhered to a vegan diet and was deficient in the same micronutrients, that person would also be opening the door to osteoporosis. Dietary philosophy is completely irrelevant.

The bottom line is that no diet can protect you from any micronutrient deficiency disease in and of itself. If you are deficient in any of the essential

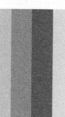

Kym Hermann,
NC (Nutritional Consultant) and
CMS (Certified Micronutrient Specialist),
Tells It Like It Is.

"One of the things I notice is that many people spend so much time worrying about macronutrients that they fail to realize that the quality of their food matters, too. I've seen too many clients come in focused on the perfect balance of calories and macronutrients—completely ignoring what really counts—so they are extremely deficient in micronutrients. The result? Illness, autoimmune disorders, thyroid dysfunction, depression, and the inability to lose weight. I want to jump on top of a mountain and shout out to people, 'Wake up! It is the micronutrients that count!'"

micronutrients, regardless of your dietary profile, you are at risk. So it makes no sense to have the diet you choose be the basis of your nutritional philosophy. But if you turn the nutritional equation around and make micronutrient sufficiency your main dietary objective, then everything changes. By adopting our Micronutrient Miracle protocol and putting the proverbial horse (micronutrient sufficiency) in front of the proverbial cart (dietary preference), where it belongs, you can shut the door on micronutrient deficiency–based diseases while enjoying any type of diet your heart desires.

All Roads Lead to Rome

You read that right. The Micronutrient Miracle plan allows you to follow any type of diet your heart desires. We aren't going to tell you to eat a bland grilled chicken breast with steamed vegetables if what you really want is a juicy cheeseburger and fries. Great news, right? You may be asking yourself how this is possible. Let's think about it like this: You have no doubt heard the phrase "All roads lead to Rome," right? Well, the Romans were smart to strategically build all their roads like wagon wheel spokes coming out of Rome in all directions. This guaranteed that if a person continued down any of the roads long enough, eventually they would end up in Rome, where Roman tax collectors could collect an entrance fee.

Now think of Rome as optimal health—a place we are all trying to get to—and all the different dietary philosophies as the various roads surrounding it. To the north there is Vegetarian Street, to the south, Paleo Street, and so on. While all the diets can bring you to optimal health, before you are let inside, you must pay a tax, and the only currency your body will accept is micronutrient sufficiency. If you don't have your little piece of paper that says you are micronutrient sufficient, you are not getting in.

To help you meet your goal of optimal health, we have identified three steps you must take. These three steps are the same regardless of which dietary philosophy (spoke on the wheel) you are following on your quest. The Micronutrient Miracle plan will guide you on your journey by:

1. **Teaching you to switch to rich.** This essential first step will fill your body with the vitamins and minerals it needs to function at its best. Often, the spoke you are traveling on will determine the spectrum of foods you will be picking from. For example, those on a vegan road will not be choosing beef as their source of vitamin A, nor will a Paleo

dieter be choosing dairy as a source of vitamin D; these foods do not fit into the dietary guidelines of these particular spokes. Regardless of your dietary profile, in this important first step, we will help you identify the foods that contain the highest levels of micronutrients.

2. **Helping you to drive down your own micronutrient depletion.** Would you be surprised to learn that you may unknowingly be causing your own micronutrient depletion? It's true. Some of your everyday dietary and lifestyle habits may either cause you to use your vitamins and minerals faster, leaving you running on low, or make it so that you can't absorb the micronutrients you are getting through your food. In this second step, you will learn to identify these micronutrient thieves robbing you of the extraordinary health you deserve.

3. **Instructing you on the ABCs.** No, we aren't talking about the alphabet. We are talking about smart supplementation practices and how avoiding the four major flaws common to most supplements today is the third and final step to guaranteeing micronutrient sufficiency is met and exceptional health transformations occur.

Sounds pretty simple, doesn't it? Your path is your own. Your food options are up to you. You are simply taking three giant steps down whichever spoke you already enjoy. And the plan is even more personalized than that. We will give you the tools necessary to tailor the plan to speak directly to your health concerns. You can choose to focus on reaching a desired weight, getting your blood pressure under control, increasing your bone density, or improving any one of a long list of other conditions and diseases. And because no two people are exactly alike, your Micronutrient Miracle plan will be uniquely your own.

Reversing Disease, Preventing Disease, and the Other Miraculous Benefits

Most medical and nutritional professionals agree that genetics play a very small role in determining your overall health. Even when it comes to cancer, one of the deadliest diseases in the world, only 5 to 10 percent of all cases can be attributed to genetic defects.[2] This is fantastic news because it means that the remaining 90 to 95 percent of cases are rooted in environmental and lifestyle factors, such as diet, pollution, stress, smoking, and alcohol consumption—all of which directly affect your micronutrient levels, as you will learn in the Micronutrient Miracle plan. This means that of the approximately 1 million

Americans and more than 10 million people worldwide that will be diagnosed with cancer this year, as many as 950,000 Americans and 9.5 million people worldwide could prevent this horrifying reality with just a few simple lifestyle and dietary changes—and we are going to show you how to make them.

You are what you eat, and every day science is proving the validity of this simple yet powerful statement. We cannot overstate the true power you have over your own health. One's health is not like one's age. Your age continues in one direction from the time you are born to the time you die. Your health is more like a wave; you can be young and in good health, or you can be young and in poor health. Similarly, one can be a healthy 65 or an unhealthy 65. You can't change your age (although a little fib now and then won't hurt anything), but you can control whether you are going to live with a strong, healthy body and mind, riding high on the crest of the wave, or a frail, medicated one, being dragged under by the deadly current.

Another thing to keep in mind is that disease prevention is just as important as disease reversal. We tend to highlight stories of clients who underwent miraculous changes and reversed a debilitating or deadly health condition or disease, but in truth, the thousands of clients out there who used the Micronutrient Miracle plan as a way to prevent getting those health conditions and diseases in the first place deserve just as much praise and attention.

How much would it be worth to you to live your whole life disease-free, to not be diagnosed with cancer or heart disease, to maintain a sharp, clear mind and strong body, to not fall victim to diabetes and have to deal with daily insulin shots? What are your plans for the future? Perhaps you dream of one day retiring and finally traveling to that European city you have always wanted to visit or taking an around-the-world cruise? Have you thought about how your health will affect those plans? Will you be healthy enough to walk the streets of that city or take that long journey by boat? We don't often think about what an incredible gift good health truly is, but ultimately it may just be the greatest gift you can give to both yourself and your loved ones.

You can take control of your health—and the 28-day Micronutrient Miracle plan will show you exactly how, every step of the way. By working toward becoming micronutrient sufficient, you will be shutting the door on dozens of potential health-hindering conditions and diseases that could put your dreams at risk. So as you can see, this plan can literally stop disease before it starts. But that's not all. Not only will you have naturally increased energy, but you will also have a more alert mind and look and feel better than ever before. Turn to the following page where there are three additional benefits listed that you may not have considered.

The Micronutrient Miracle plan will help you:

1. **Live an extraordinary life, not an ordinary one—and live it longer.** Micronutrient sufficiency can help you to thrive, not merely survive, as you age. Don't you want to be that 70-year-old, playing soccer with your grandkids or the 80-year-old dancing the night away on that Mediterranean cruise? We know we sure do! Not only will staying healthy and strong make it so that you can take advantage of all that life has to offer, but studies suggest that taking micronutrient supplementation might actually add years to your life, as well. In a 2009 study published in the *American Journal of Clinical Nutrition*, researchers determined that those who took multivitamins had younger DNA, which equated to living approximately 9.8 years longer.[3] Wow!

2. **Live without the crippling burden of medical bills.** Let's face it: Not only is being ill unpleasant, but it's also expensive. In a 2013 study, researchers determined that "significant cost savings can be realized by health care payers, such as insurance companies, and consumers through the use of dietary supplements that have a demonstrable and substantial effect on the risk of costly disease-related events."[4] They proved that supplementation with only three micronutrients—B_6, B_9 (folate), and B_{12}— by those who have or have the potential for coronary heart disease would prevent thousands upon thousands of hospital stays and surgeries. After crunching the numbers, the researchers determined that this would yield a savings of $1.52 billion per year—a cumulative cost avoidance to health-care payers of $12.12 billion from 2013 to 2020 in the United States alone. Just imagine how much money you might save if we harnessed the disease-preventing power of all of the essential micronutrients.

3. **Set a good example for the next generation.** Children are always looking to their parents and grandparents for guidance on how to live their lives— although they don't often admit it. Your healthy habits can speak volumes. Show the next generation, through your actions, that health is a priority.

So what are you waiting for? It is time that you find out what your miracle will be. By following the Micronutrient Miracle plan, you can create the health that you deserve. Like Craig, whose blood pressure was naturally regulated, or Mira, whose osteoporosis was reversed, you too can experience a transformation that is unique to you. We know that the program will work for you and look forward to guiding you along your journey to extraordinary health. So let's get started!

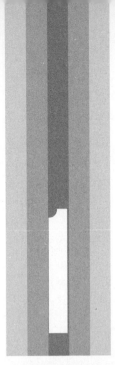

MICRONUTRIENT DEFICIENCY: The Hidden Pandemic Keeping Us Tired, Fat, and Sick

MICRONUTRIENT DEFICIENCY is the most widespread and dangerous health condition of the 21st century. This statement is the foundation of our nutritional philosophy. It's pretty shocking, right? It isn't just a theory, either. In this chapter, we will systematically prove this statement to be true. We will start by revealing published statistics that substantiate our claim that micronutrient deficiency is the most widespread health condition of the 21st century and should be considered a global pandemic. Then we will explore the factors that contributed to the world's population becoming so deficient. We will also show you just how far we have strayed from the diets and lifestyles of our ancestors and how this divergence has left us with a diet that no longer can sustain health. Finally, you will learn the dangerous ramifications of this widespread deficiency.

While this chapter may seem depressing as you read through it, stay with us and keep reading. It will be worth it. You can't fully understand the importance of this program and the scientifically proven health benefits you can achieve by becoming sufficient in micronutrients until you fully understand the micronutrient-depleted state you are likely in and how it may be negatively affecting your health.

The Most Widespread Condition
of the 21st Century

We will begin proving the statement that micronutrient deficiency is the most widespread and dangerous health condition of the 21st century by taking a look at the facts that led us to conclude that it is the most *widespread* health condition. (We will cover the most *dangerous* part later in the chapter.) Let's start with this fact: According to USDA published statistics, more than 96 percent of Americans are not reaching adequate intakes of micronutrients from food alone, based on the government's average requirement standard.[1] Put another way, less than 4 percent of all Americans ages 2 and over eat a diet that meets the minimum adequacy requirements for the essential vitamins and minerals needed to maintain basic health. With approximately 317 million people in the United States, this means that there are more than 304 million men, women, and children suffering from a micronutrient deficiency of some kind right now.

Let that number sink in for a minute: 304 million people. While this statistic alone is disturbing to say the least, believe it or not, it gets worse! Before we show you just how much worse, let's get a little perspective on the sheer magnitude of this number by comparing the 304 million people suffering from a micronutrient deficiency with the statistics on other serious health conditions, such as heart disease, cancer, osteoporosis, and diabetes. Surely these well-known diseases affect more people than micronutrient deficiency, a condition that most people don't even know exists.

Let's start with heart disease. It turns out that heart disease is the leading cause of death in the United States for both men and women, claiming a life every 33 seconds, and it is estimated that this deadly disease affects just over 80 million Americans.[2] While we are in no way trying to downplay this devastating statistic, it does mean that *nearly four times more people* are affected by micronutrient deficiency than heart disease.

Cancer is another disease that is constantly in the news, and rightfully so. Statistics show that there are approximately 1.7 million new cancer cases each year in America and that we have a 40.8 percent chance of developing this horrifying disease over our lifetime. However, in total, according to the National Institutes of Health's National Cancer Institute, fewer than 13.5 million Americans are living with cancer.[3]

Osteoporosis, the disease that ended Mira's PR career and could have crippled her for life, is on the rise in both women and men. However, the number of Americans that currently have osteoporosis or are at risk for it due to low bone mass is estimated at 40 million.[4] Lastly, diabetes, the seventh leading cause of death in the United States, is estimated by the American Diabetes Association to affect just over 29 million Americans.[5]

Most of us know at least one person who is affected by one of these debilitating and life-threatening diseases. Perhaps you have even donated to or joined an organization formed to help end one of these devastating conditions (we have). However, when you look at the number of people who currently have heart disease, cancer, osteoporosis, and diabetes—*combined*—it totals up to 162.5 million people. To put that in perspective, when you combine the number of people who are currently diagnosed with today's most prevalent and deadly diseases—including all forms of heart disease, all types of cancer, osteoporosis (including those at risk for osteoporosis), and both classes of diabetes—the total is just more than half (53 percent) of the 304 million who are currently affected by micronutrient deficiency. This makes micronutrient deficiency the most widespread health condition of the 21st century.

From Bad News to Worse

Take a moment now to examine the US vitamin and mineral adequacy statistics in the table below.

TABLE 1.1
PERCENTAGE OF THE US POPULATION AGES 2 AND UP WITH ADEQUATE MICRONUTRIENT INTAKES, BASED ON THE ESTIMATED AVERAGE REQUIREMENTS

MICRONUTRIENT	PERCENTAGE	MICRONUTRIENT	PERCENTAGE
Vitamin A	46.0	Vitamin B_{12}	79.7
Vitamin C	51.0	Phosphorus	87.2
Vitamin D	4.0*	Magnesium	43
Vitamin E	13.6	Iron	89.5
Thiamine	81.6	Selenium	91.5
Riboflavin	89.1	Zinc	70.8
Niacin	87.2	Copper	84.2
Vitamin B_6	73.9	Calcium	30.9
Folate	59.7	Potassium	7.6

Source: NHANES 1999–2004

*Vitamin D data from NHANES 2003–2006

So, what did you think? Perhaps, at first glance, the percentages were not as bad as you thought they were going to be. However, as you start to look closer, things go downhill fast. Do you remember that statistic we shared with you earlier in this chapter, the one about 96 percent of Americans not being able to get the essential micronutrients they need to maintain basic health from their food? Well, look at vitamin D: According to the USDA, the government agency responsible for reporting NHANES statistical findings, only 4 percent of the entire US population over the age of 2 has an adequate intake of vitamin D, an essential fat-soluble vitamin whose deficiency has been shown to greatly increase the risk of cancer, Alzheimer's disease, diabetes, multiple sclerosis, and osteoporosis, to name but a few conditions. Additionally, the chart shows that only 7.6 percent of the population has an adequate intake of potassium, an essential mineral that, when deficient, has been shown to increase the risk for hypertension, osteoporosis, kidney stones, and stroke. And did you notice vitamin E? This essential vitamin and powerful antioxidant only has an adequacy rate of 13.6 percent. So, 96 percent of the US population is deficient in vitamin D, more than 92 percent is deficient in potassium, and nearly 9 out of 10 Americans are deficient in vitamin E. The USDA data also reveals that more than 7 out of 10 Americans are deficient in calcium, an important mineral essential for the maintenance of bones and teeth, blood clotting, muscle contraction, and nerve function. And it shows that approximately 5 out of 10 are deficient in vitamin A, vitamin C, and magnesium, all of which are absolutely mandatory in adequate amounts to maintain basic health. Out of the 18 essential micronutrients on this chart, *all* of them were found to be deficient to some extent, meaning that there wasn't a single micronutrient for which all Americans met the government's minimum standards. Why? Could it be because the standards are set too high? Let's see.

While the fact that 96 percent of Americans (304 million) are not able to meet minimum adequacy requirements for the essential micronutrients already seems pretty bad, we are about to follow through on the promise that we made to you earlier: We will share with you now how the statistics are really far worse. It's about time to jump down the rabbit hole and see just how deep America's micronutrient deficiency really goes. In order to do so, we need to bring you up to speed on how micronutrients are measured by introducing you to the often-confusing dietary guideline reference intake acronyms and abbreviations. (Say that ten times fast.) The USDA based the adequacy rates shown in Table 1.1, page 3, on something it calls the Estimated Average Requirement, or EAR. The EAR is defined as the amount of a micronutrient that would be expected to satisfy the requirement needs of 50 percent of people age 2 and up.

Hmm. Why would the government want to use data that only showed the adequacy rates of half of the population? Wouldn't it make more sense to base the adequacy rates on the amount of each micronutrient that would satisfy the basic requirements for all of us? In fact, there is a government intake acronym that does just that. It's called the Reference Daily Intake, or RDI, and it's defined as the daily dietary intake level of a micronutrient designed to be sufficient to prevent micronutrient deficiency diseases by meeting the requirements of nearly all (97 to 98 percent) healthy individuals in each life-stage and sex group. At first this may seem like an inconsequential detail, but let's look at how swapping the EAR with the RDI affects *actual adequacy intake rates* for a specific micronutrient.

WHAT A DIFFERENCE AN ACRONYM CAN MAKE

To see how changing the EAR to the RDI really affects adequacy rates, we are going to do a small experiment. Take a look back at the USDA adequacy rate for B_{12} in Table 1.1, page 3. Let's round it up from 79.7 to 80 percent just to keep the math easy. You will also need three key pieces of information to conduct this experiment.

1. The EAR for B_{12} is 2 micrograms.
2. The RDI for B_{12} is 6 micrograms.
3. The mean, or average, level of B_{12} ingested by the NHANES participants was approximately 5.1 micrograms.

Notice that the amount to achieve EAR sufficiency is far lower than that for RDI sufficiency. If the adequacy rates were calculated using the RDIs as the baseline—the amount considered sufficient to meet the requirements of nearly all (97 to 98 percent) of healthy individuals—the rates would be much different. To see just how different, let's draw out the data.

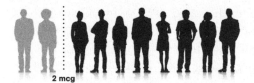

1▸ 2 out of every 10 people (20%) did not reach EAR sufficiency (2 mcg) of B_{12}.

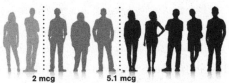

2▸ The mean, or average, level of B_{12} ingested by the study participants was 5.1 mcg. We can see that, given even distribution, approximately 5 of the 10 people ingested less than 5.1 mcg of B_{12}.

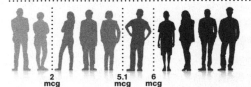

3▸ If 2 out of every 10 of the study participants were deficient at meeting the 2 mcg EAR requirement for B_{12}, then when we adjust the diagram to include the 6 mcg requirement of the RDI, we can see that 6 out of the 10 people (60%) would not meet RDI sufficiency (6 mcg) of B_{12}. This would leave only 4 out of 10 individuals (40%) of the US population sufficient in B_{12}.

Is this starting to make sense? It's shocking, right? The USDA statistics using the low EAR standard may have lulled us into a false sense of security by reporting that 80 percent of us are getting adequate amounts of B_{12} from our diets, but when we use the higher RDI requirements for B_{12} intake, which include nearly all Americans, the adequacy rate quickly falls to an unimpressive 40 percent. While our simple experiment can in no way determine actual sufficiency rates without more information, we believe these numbers are a fair estimate. In fact, because the RDI only covers 97 to 98 percent of the population, the adequacy rates could be a few percentage points worse. Even when a margin of error of 10 to 20 percent is taken into account, it still leaves more than 50 percent of the population who are not meeting minimum RDI intake, a level that many health care professionals consider the nutritional equivalent of minimum wage. Although RDI levels may be enough to prevent a micronutrient deficiency condition, they are a long way from the amount needed to achieve optimal health.

TABLE 1.2
A COMPARISON OF ADEQUACY RATES FOR VITAMIN B$_{12}$

B_{12} adequacy rate using the EAR	80%
B_{12} adequacy rate using the RDI	40%
Adequacy rate accounting for a 10–20% margin of error using the RDI	32–48%

Additionally, while the USDA adequacy chart shows that 7.6 percent of us are sufficient in potassium, 46 percent of us are sufficient in vitamin A, and 79.7 percent are sufficient in B_{12}, where does it show how many of us are sufficient in all three, or all 18, for that matter? This vital information is not there, and one would have to think the percentages go way down. The bottom line is, once you realize just how micronutrient deficient we really are, the desperate reality of our situation becomes disturbingly clear. We are in the middle of a micronutrient deficiency pandemic, and the vast majority of the general public is unaware of it. Now, just in case you are still not convinced, here are what some other health professionals have to say on the subject.

According to *New York Times* bestselling author Mark Hyman, MD, "A whopping 92 percent of us are deficient in one or more nutrients at the Recommended Daily Allowance (RDA) level. . . . The RDA [similar to RDI] standards do not necessarily outline the amount needed for optimal health."[6]

Additionally, Mehmet Oz, MD, of *The Dr. Oz Show*, reported these statistics concerning the prevalence of micronutrient deficiency: "A study of 3 million people revealed that less than 1 percent of the participants got enough essential vitamins from diet alone. That's why you must take a multivitamin; it also helps prevent heart disease, breast cancer, and colon cancer."[7]

So here is the take-home message: Regardless of which acronym you use, the EAR or the RDI, and according to today's most respected physicians, nearly everyone in America is now living with micronutrient deficiency, which is the root cause of nearly every major health condition and disease today.

Micronutrient Deficiency—A Global Issue

Micronutrient deficiency is not just a problem in the United States. According to the World Health Organization (WHO), more than 2 billion people in both developing and developed countries suffer from micronutrient deficiencies.[8] According to a 2010 study in the journal *Public Health Reviews*, "These are silent epidemics of vitamin and mineral deficiencies affecting people of all genders and ages, as well as certain risk groups. They not only cause specific diseases, but they act as exacerbating factors in infectious and chronic diseases, greatly impacting morbidity, mortality, and quality of life. . . . Micronutrient deficiency conditions relate to many chronic diseases, such as osteoporosis, osteomalacia, thyroid deficiency, colorectal cancer, and cardiovascular diseases."[9]

In Great Britain, researchers conducting the National Diet and Nutrition Survey, on behalf of the Food Standards Agency, observed UK residents to determine if they were taking in enough essential micronutrients from food alone to maintain basic health. They determined that *every person* was at risk for micronutrient deficiency to some degree. The study found that 60 percent of the subjects were deficient in zinc and 30 percent were deficient in calcium. It also found that the average intake of selenium, a micronutrient shown to have anticancer, fertility, and detoxification benefits, was only at 50 percent of the Reference Nutrient Intake (RNI)—the UK's equivalent to the RDI. Additionally, more than half (51 percent) of the women in the study were also found to be deficient in vitamin B_9 (folate)—an essential vitamin that reduces the risk of spina bifida, a neural tube defect in newborns. Teenage females were shown to have the greatest deficiencies—97 percent were deficient in magnesium, 76 percent in calcium, 72 percent in zinc, and 52 percent in vitamin B_9.[10]

In China, even in areas that offer subtropical latitude and abundant sunshine, such as Shanghai, vitamin D deficiency is becoming a major concern. In fact, 2012 research shows that 84 percent of men and 89 percent of women have vitamin D levels that are insufficient to meet minimum requirements. According to the researchers, this may leave a large percentage of the population at risk not only for bone-related conditions but also for diabetes, cancer, multiple sclerosis and other autoimmune disorders, cardiovascular diseases, and infectious diseases.[11] Similarly, although they live in one of the sunniest regions in the world, 90 percent of United Arab Emirates (UAE) residents are deficient in vitamin D, according to the International Osteoporosis Foundation (IOF).[12]

And deficiency rates around the world continue to climb. In 1987, the WHO estimated that vitamin A deficiency affected only 39 countries. That number rose to 45 countries in 1995 and again in 2005 to 122 countries. This means that while more countries around the world are becoming developed, the number of countries with a vitamin A deficiency of public health significance nearly tripled over 18 years.[13]

Additionally, rickets, the childhood disease that caused an epidemic of bowed legs and curved spines during the Victorian era, is making a shocking comeback in 21st-century Britain. According to Britain's National Health Service, because of vitamin D deficiency, the number of children diagnosed with rickets is soaring, with figures quadrupling in the last 10 years. To combat this problem, it was announced "that the Chief Medical Officer has now advised that all children from the age of 6 months to 5 years should take vitamin D supplements in order to prevent deficiency and its effect on later health issues."[14]

All these statistics point to the fact that America is not alone in this micronutrient deficiency pandemic. We are not trying to be alarmists; however, we can't stress enough how serious this situation is. Think about it for a second. This means that regardless of which country you live in, there is a huge likelihood that you are micronutrient deficient. Consider now your family and friends. They too are likely deficient. It is imperative that we, as a global community, recognize micronutrient deficiency as the silent global pandemic that it is. Our hope is that by shining a light on the reality of this deficiency, people will be able to recognize the factors that are causing this depletion and take steps to reverse it—before it is too late.

Good Food, Gone Bad

So, how did we all get into this situation in the first place? What happened to just eating a balanced diet and getting all the essential micronutrients we need from the foods we eat? After all, isn't that what our ancestors did? These are good questions and ones that are becoming more relevant each year. The truth is that throughout most of history, our ancestors survived and thrived by simply eating the foods nature provided, allowing nature, in her infinite wisdom, to nourish and sustain them. Fresh, unadulterated local vegetables, meats, fish, fruits, eggs, dairy products, and naturally pressed oils were able to provide the essential nutrition our ancestors needed to maintain their health and protect them from the barrage of health conditions and diseases we are now suffering from on a daily basis.

Then something changed. Small groups, or tribes, of people that only hunted or foraged for the limited amount of food needed to sustain a few people started to grow. More food was needed, so approximately 10,000 years ago, people started farming to increase the production of food. More food equaled more people, and both the farms and the population kept growing. Three hundred years ago (approximately AD 1700), there were roughly 610 million people on the planet; today there are more than 7 billion hungry mouths to feed every day.[15] And with five babies born every second and only two people dying every second, there will be 8.5 billion mouths to feed in approximately 10 years. Because of this, farmers around the world must employ every resource available to them to push their crop yields to the absolute limits, which has led to more food being produced now than ever before. However, this food has very little in common with the food that nourished our ancestors just 300 years ago, especially when it comes to micronutrient content.

The simple fact is that sick soil equals sick plants, sick animals, and sick people. And make no mistake about it, not only is the world's soil on its deathbed, but we may also be on the verge of literally running out of it. "A rough calculation of current rates of soil degradation suggests we have about 60 years of topsoil left," according to John Crawford, PhD, soil expert and University of Sydney professor. "Some 40 percent of soil used for agriculture around the world is classed as either degraded or seriously degraded—the latter means that 70 percent of the topsoil, the layer allowing plants to grow, is gone. Because of various farming methods that strip the soil of carbon and make it less robust as well as weaker in nutrients, soil is being lost at between 10 and 40 times the rate at which it can be naturally replenished. Even the well-maintained farming land in Europe, which may look idyllic, is being lost at unsustainable rates."[16]

No, this is not a *War of the Worlds*–type prank. Credible scientists from around the world agree that our soil is in big trouble, and perhaps one of the biggest problems is mineral deficiency. While the human body can manufacture certain vitamins, like vitamin K and vitamin D, no organism—human or animal—can synthesize any amount of any mineral! **The bottom line is that we either get our essential minerals from our food or a supplement or we don't get them at all.**

Over the past 100 years, the level of minerals in soil throughout the world has been on the decline. At the United Nations Conference on Environment and Development in 1992, it was revealed in the Earth Summit report that farmlands in North America, South America, Asia, Africa, and Europe have become depleted of minerals on an alarming scale in the past 100 years. Researchers found that soils in Asia and Europe have suffered a 76 percent and 72 percent reduction in mineral content, respectively, while North America's farms and rangelands showed the greatest amount, with a startling mineral depletion of 85 percent.[17]

And the shocking part of these statistics is that our government has known about this issue for nearly 80 years. Take a look at this statement from an article presented by Senator Duncan Fletcher to Congress in 1936.

> *"The alarming fact is that foods—fruits and vegetables and grains—now being raised on millions of acres of land that no longer contains enough of certain needed minerals are starving us—no matter how much of them we eat! . . . Ninety-nine percent of the American people are deficient in these minerals, and that a marked deficiency in any one of the more important minerals actually results in disease. . . . We know that vitamins are complex chemical substances, which are indispensable to nutrition, and that each of them is of importance for the normal function of some special structure of the body. Disorder and disease result from any vitamin deficiency. It is not commonly realized, however, that vitamins control the body's appropriation of minerals, and in the absence of minerals they have no function to perform. Lacking vitamins, the system can make some use of minerals, but lacking minerals, vita-mins are useless."[18]*

We are not suggesting a conspiracy theory that farmers or government agencies are purposely depleting our soil in order to make us sick. This is not what we believe. What we do know, though, is that farmers are being paid to produce maximum yield per acre, not maximum nutritional value. In the 1930s, corn yields of 50 bushels an acre were considered quite good, but today, some farmers are pushing their land to produce corn yields greater than 200 bushels an acre. Farmers are forced, for economic reasons, to grow crops faster and are not financially rewarded for increasing a crop's micronutrient value. "The focus has been on breeding high-yield crops which can survive on degraded soil, so it's hardly surprising that 60 percent of the world's population is deficient in nutrients like iron. If it's not in the soil, it's not in our food," stated Dr. Crawford. "Modern wheat varieties, for example, have half the micronutrients of older strains, and it's pretty much the same for fruit and vegetables."

For example, in 1914 an apple would have contained 13.5 milligrams of calcium, 28.9 milligrams of magnesium, and 4.6 milligrams of iron. However, according to measurements taken by the USDA back in 1992, our depleted soil only yielded apples that contained 7 milligrams of calcium (48.15 percent less), 5 milligrams of magnesium (82.7 percent less), and 0.18 milligrams of iron (96 percent less). And that was back in 1992. If we consider that it has been more than 20 years since those measurements were taken, our apple today, if depletion rates remained the same, would now have lost 61 percent of its calcium, 100 percent of its magnesium, and 100 percent of its iron.[19]

IT SEEMS EVEN THE ATMOSPHERE IS AGAINST US

While the mineral loss in our soil is bad, we are sorry to report that the story gets worse here, too. In a ground-shaking study published in 2014, it was revealed that elevated concentrations of atmospheric carbon dioxide have been found to negatively affect C3 plants (which include rice, wheat, soybean, rye, oats, millet, barley, and potato) by increasing carbohydrate concentrations and decreasing protein and mineral concentrations. Like other plants, these crops, which provide more than 2 out of every 5 calories humans consume, convert carbon dioxide (or CO_2) from the air into sugars and other carbohydrates. In fact, since the Industrial Revolution, the increase in atmospheric CO_2 has increased the production of sugars and carbohydrates in C3 plants by as much as 46 percent. Higher CO_2 levels are also known to lower protein concentrations in C3 plants, but the effect CO_2 had on the concentrations of minerals was largely unknown. However, the study's lead researcher, Irakli Loladze, found that elevated CO_2 levels indeed reduce the overall concentrations of 25 minerals in C3 plants by 8 percent on average.[20] He argues, "This reduction in the nutritional value of plants could have profound impacts on human health: A diet that is deficient in minerals and other nutrients can cause malnutrition, even if a person consumes enough calories. . . . Diets that are poor in minerals . . . lead to reduced growth in childhood, to a reduced ability to fight off infections, and to higher rates of maternal and child deaths. . . . These changes might contribute to the rise in obesity, as people eat increasingly starchy plant-based foods, and eat more to compensate for the lower mineral levels found in crops."

The sad reality is that our food is mineral deficient not just because the minerals are not in the soil to the extent that they were in the past but also because our modern CO_2-laden atmosphere is causing the plants themselves to take up less of those minerals. Can you see now how the food we are all eating today is very different than that of our ancestors? It's lower in the essential minerals and protein we all need to maintain health, and it is higher in sugar and other carbohydrates.

MORE REASONS YOUR FOOD IS NOT THAT OF YOUR ANCESTORS

Do you remember that list of foods we mentioned earlier that our ancestors might have eaten—the fresh, unadulterated local vegetables, fruits, eggs, meats, fish, dairy products, and naturally pressed oils? Notice that this list does not include any of the following:

- Highly processed packaged foods or anything from a different country or continent
- Genetically modified, pesticide-laden vegetables and fruits
- Hormone- and antibiotic-laden meat and dairy from animals confined to a cage and fed genetically modified food
- Genetically modified fish confined to a cage and fed genetically modified food pellets
- Eggs from poultry confined to a cage and fed genetically modified food
- Genetically modified oils that have been heated, bleached, and hydrogenated to the point of creating poisonous trans fats

Today our food is fighting a losing battle not only against depleted mineral levels in the soil and ever-increasing CO_2 levels, but also against GMOs, global distribution, factory farming, and food processing and cooking methods, which all further deplete the few micronutrients that are left.

Genetically Modified Organisms (GMOs)

The genetic modification of organisms (creating GMOs) takes place in a laboratory and involves artificially inserting genes from bacteria, viruses, insects, animals, or even humans into the DNA of food crops or animals in order to improve their resistance to pests, make them heartier to survive changes in weather, increase yield, and reduce maturation time. GMOs are a controversial topic for many reasons, but what is not often talked about is the danger of consuming these foods as it relates to micronutrient deficiency. Current statistics show that GMOs are found in more than 80 percent of packaged foods in the United States.[21] While it may be hard to imagine how that is possible, when you think about the fact that 94 percent of all soy, 90 percent of canola, 88 percent of corn, 100 percent of sugar beets, 80 percent of Hawaiian papaya, and 25,000 acres of zucchini and crookneck squash are grown using GMO seeds, it's actually surprising that there is still 20 percent of foods that don't contain GMOs.[22]

So, how do GMOs contribute to the micronutrient deficiency pandemic?

Some GMO crops have been genetically engineered not to die when sprayed with an herbicide called glyphosate, better known as Roundup. You may have heard of it. That is why these GMO crops are often referred to as "Roundup Ready." The way glyphosate works is it actually kills weeds by latching onto, or chelating to, the essential minerals they need to live, thus starving them of micronutrients. The problem is that it does the same thing to the Roundup Ready crops themselves. Then these micronutrient-depleted crops, in turn, do the same thing to both the animals and humans who eat them.

Here is what Don Huber, PhD, a GMO expert and emeritus professor of plant pathology at Purdue University, had to say on the subject: "I have been doing research on glyphosate for 20 years. . . . Glyphosate kills weeds by tying up essential nutrients needed to keep plant defenses active. . . . Micronutrients such as manganese, copper, potassium, iron, magnesium, calcium, and zinc are essential to human health. All of them can be reduced in availability by glyphosate; mineral nutrients are less in glyphosate treated plants. We are seeing a reduction in nutrient quality (in food crops). . . . The [Roundup Ready] gene will reduce micronutrient efficiency up to 50 percent for zinc and manganese. . . . If we continue to abuse the use of glyphosate, it's just a matter of time before we see more serious negative ramifications."[23]

Disturbingly, according to the US Department of the Interior, "Glyphosate is currently the world's best selling herbicide, used in more than 90 countries and on more than 150 crops." Can you see how this rarely discussed aspect of GMOs can have a very negative effect on your ability to become sufficient in essential micronutrients? There is no need to worry, though; the Micronutrient Miracle plan shows you how to avoid GMOs as well as the GMO-derived ingredients hiding in every aisle of the grocery store.

Our New Global Food System and Factory Farming

Let's move on now to global distribution and factory farming, two other modern realities that rob our food of micronutrients. According to Joel Salatin, author of *Folks, This Ain't Normal*, "In 1945, 40 percent of all vegetables consumed in the United States were grown in backyards."[24] Today, backyard gardens are, for the most part, a thing of the past. Instead, most of our food (fruits, vegetables, meats, and poultry) are produced on factory farms many states away or even in other countries, often traveling the distance between New York City and Dallas (1,400 miles) before reaching your table. For example, a report from the Leopold Center for Sustainable Agriculture at Iowa State University notes that the average potato has traveled 1,155 miles to reach your grocery store. Similarly, a tomato travels

1,569 miles, and a carrot travels an exhausting, micronutrient-depleting 1,838 miles prior to being served.[25] Additionally, the USDA Economic Research Service database reveals that the typical American meal contains, on average, ingredients from at least five countries *outside* US borders. The USDA estimates that 39 percent of fruits, 12 percent of vegetables, 40 percent of lamb, and 78 percent of fish and shellfish are imported each year from other countries.[26] And this micronutrient-depleting factor is not limited to the United States. Over the last 40 years, the world population has doubled while the amount of food shipped between countries has quadrupled. In the United Kingdom, for example, food travels 50 percent farther than it did 20 years ago.[27]

This wouldn't be a problem if it weren't for the fact that our food's micronutrient levels are greatly affected by heat, air, and light. This means that during every minute of every mile that your food is exposed to the hot temperatures of a shipping truck or a cargo ship or the fluorescent lights in a storage warehouse, it is losing the very micronutrients we need for good health. Additionally, in order to make sure that the food being transported looks "fresh" when it hits store shelves and can better withstand the bumps and bruising that can occur with mechanical harvesting and long-distance travel, farmers often pick their crops prematurely, before they have fully ripened. This also impacts the food's overall micronutrient levels. According to Harvard School of Public Health's Center for Health and the Global Environment, "While full color may be achieved after harvest, nutritional quality may not."[28] Tomatoes, for example, will have some increase in vitamin C after being prematurely harvested; however, they will never reach the micronutrient levels of those that ripen on the vine. When you take into consideration that tomatoes make up one-quarter of Americans' total vegetable consumption, that is a lot of vitamin C we are all missing out on. And then there is the taste of these micronutrient-depleted foods. Have you ever bitten into a red, seemingly juicy, delicious-looking tomato or strawberry only to be shocked that it tasted like nothing? That's because micronutrients are at least in part also responsible for flavor! When we lose micronutrients, we lose the essence of the food itself—we lose the soul. That is why we want you to choose naturally ripened, locally grown produce while on the 28-day program. It will greatly increase your total micronutrient intake as well as ensure your food is flavorful and delicious.

Farm Animals or Farmed Animals

As you have seen so far, factory farming has changed how our food is grown and what our food is exposed to, but it has also changed what farm animals are being fed and the environments in which they live. And as you may have guessed, these unnatural feeds and environments can also have devastating effects on the micronutrients that are in the burgers, fish fillets, and "farm fresh" eggs eaten by millions of people.

Here is a fact we hope you know: Cows are supposed to eat grass. Everyone knows this, right? Well, evidently someone forgot to tell that to the huge factory farms that are responsible for raising the majority of cattle here in America. That's because these cows are no longer roaming free, allowed to eat a natural diet of green grass. Instead, they are caged together in pens with floors of mud and manure and forced to eat a diet of genetically modified corn and soy. And that's not all: According to Randy Shaver, PhD, a professor in the department of dairy science at the University of Wisconsin, factory-farmed cattle are often fed up to 5 pounds of stale chocolate and 2 pounds of candy per cow per day due to their low cost and high fat content. While this practice reduces feed costs, it also produces beef that is artificially high in fat and low in vitamin E, beta-carotene, omega-3 fatty acids, and conjugated linoleic acid (CLA), a healthy fat with the potential to fight cancer and metabolize fat! [29] Holy cow!

Sadly, chickens and fish are not faring any better. Factory-farmed chickens that are housed indoors and deprived of natural sunlight and open pastures where they can peck in the dirt and eat insects produce micronutrient-deprived eggs. According to the USDA National Nutrient Database, pasture-raised eggs contain two times more omega-3 fatty acids, four to six times more vitamin D, two-thirds more vitamin A, three times more vitamin E, and seven times more beta-carotene. Another study in the *British Journal of Nutrition* found that pastured hen eggs had 170 percent more B_{12} and 150 percent more B_9 (folate) than their confined commercial counterparts.[30]

Did you know that nearly 90 percent of the salmon served in the United States is factory farmed?[31] When did this happen? These fish are raised in "aqua farms," and, sadly, the same mistakes that are happening in land-based factory farms are happening there, too. For example, sea lice are a big problem in these aqua farms, and even though salmon are carnivores, these fish are being fed food pellets packed with GMO corn and soy, and some farms have even stooped so low as to feed pig and goose feces often contaminated with salmonella. The results are sick, micronutrient-depleted fish that don't even produce the natural red color they are known for anymore and instead must be artificially colored to look more appetizing. Wild-caught fish can have up to 380 percent more omega-3 than factory-farmed fish according to the USDA National Nutrient Database. Additionally, the omega-3 to omega-6 ratio is far less health promoting in factory-farmed fish. For instance, while the ratio of omega-3s to omega-6s in wild coho salmon is 15.3 to 1 (optimal), farm-raised coho salmon has been shown to have a far less optimal ratio of only 3 to 1.[32]

Food Processing: Processing Out Your Micronutrients

Okay, now let's turn our gaze to the last modern food practice we are going to cover in this chapter, and this is a big one: food processing and cooking methods. Here is something you may never have thought of. Did you know that nearly everything you do to food depletes its micronutrients in some way? It's true. Every time you slice it, dice it, peel it, sauté it, microwave it, steam it, fry it, process it, refine it, boil it, bake it, or anything else you can think of, you are exposing the food to either heat, air, or light; and as you may remember from our earlier discussion, these three factors can really reduce the amount of micronutrients in our food. Think about even cutting an apple into six or eight pieces. When you do that, there is a lot more of the apple's surface area being exposed to those elements—and the longer the pieces are exposed, the more micronutrients are lost. None of those things, by the way, reduce the overall calorie content of the food. It's just the micronutrients that are reduced, and even though our ancestors processed and cooked their food to a certain extent, food manufacturers today take it to a whole new level.

It is usually pretty easy to identify heavily processed foods in the grocery store. If it comes in a box, bag, or bottle, there is a good chance food manufacturers have had their hands all over it. Cereals, chips, crackers, soda, juice, processed cheese (the name gives it away with this one), candy, dried potatoes, pasta, and even many deli meats are all heavily processed these days. But there are some other foods that are being robbed of their essential micronutrients in ways that may not be so obvious. Dairy products, for instance, almost always contain milk that has been pasteurized, or worse, ultra-pasteurized. Pasteurization is a heat process that "cleans" the milk and extends its shelf life. The problem is that it also kills the friendly bacteria in milk and reduces many of its important vitamins and minerals. For example, unpasteurized, natural, raw milk contains:

- Up to 60 percent more vitamin B_1 (thiamine) and B_6 than pasteurized milk
- Up to 100 percent more B_{12}
- Up to 30 percent more vitamin B_9 (folate)
- Increased amounts of calcium and phosphorus

And as if pasteurization wasn't bad enough, have you ever heard of something called irradiation? Irradiation is often referred to as "cold pasteurization" because, like pasteurization, it is used to "clean" the food—only instead of heat, it uses radiation! And because the Food Safety Modernization Act that President Obama signed into law in 2010 actively encourages irradiation of all fruits and vegetables, we are going to be seeing a lot more irradiation in the near future. So how bad is irradiation? Really bad! To start with, irradiation is the process of exposing food to radiation to destroy microorganisms, bacteria, viruses, or insects that might be present in the food, something our ancestors definitely did not worry about.

How much radiation? Oh, not much, just the equivalent of between 33 million and 150 million chest x-rays. This huge blast of radiation then disrupts the structure of everything it passes through, breaking up a food's DNA, vitamins, minerals, and proteins and creating something called free radicals (atoms, molecules, or ions that contain unpaired electrons and crash into each other, multiplying exponentially), which have been shown to contribute to many degenerative diseases, including heart disease, dementia, cancer, and cataracts. And as America is getting ready to significantly increase the number of foods that will be irradiated, back in February 2003, the European Parliament revoked its earlier approval of irradiation and voted to allow spices, dried herbs, and seasonings as the "only approved foods for irradiation until adequate scientific evidence proving its safety is conducted."[33]

The other side effect of irradiation is that it extends shelf life, making foods that are far past their natural "expiration dates" still appear fresh and vibrant. But like the Oscar Wilde character Dorian Gray—whose youthful, attractive outward appearance did not match his rotting, centuries-old interior—irradiated food on store shelves can also entice us for an extended period of time without sharing its true nature. All the while, this fresh-looking food continues to lose micronutrients long after nonirradiated food would have spoiled and been discarded. In fact, according to Joseph Mercola, MD, of the world's #1 natural health Web site, "Irradiation destroys vitamins, nutrients, and essential fatty acids, including up to 95 percent of vitamin A in chicken and 86 percent of vitamin B in oats."[34]

So what does this mean for those of us lucky enough to live here in America? Well the following quote from The Food Commission, Britain's leading independent watchdog on food issues, offers this warning: "Food irradiation can result in loss of nutrients. . . . This is compounded by the longer storage times of irradiated foods . . . which can result in the food finally eaten by the consumer to contain little more than 'empty calories.' This is potentially damaging to the long- and short-term health of consumers."[35]

Now, we understand that this can all be a bit overwhelming, but we cannot overemphasize the importance of knowing how truly micronutrient deficient the vast majority of our food really is. However, that does not mean all is lost. Recognizing that food is depleted puts you in the unique position of understanding the importance of finding the most micronutrient-rich foods (or as we will refer to them later on, Rich Foods) available. These foods increase micronutrient content by avoiding or eliminating GMOs, global distribution, and unnatural feed and environments, as well as food processing and cooking methods. *The Power Nutrient Solution* is filled with these vitamin- and mineral-rich foods, and later, in Chapter 5, we will give you all the tools you need to choose the foods with the most micronutrient bang in every bite.

Unveiling the First Law of Nutritional Science

Now that we have proven to you that micronutrient deficiency is the most *widespread* health condition of the 21st century, it's time to show you why we believe that micronutrient deficiency is also the most *dangerous* health condition of our time.

Here is a scientific fact to consider: **Micronutrients are so powerful that being deficient in even one can kill you.** It's the truth. Take scurvy (a deficiency in vitamin C), beriberi (a deficiency in vitamin B_1, or thiamine), and pellagra (a deficiency in vitamin B_3, or niacin): These diseases killed millions upon millions of people all around the world until medical science discovered that they were not caused from bacterial infection, as had been previously suspected, but were instead a direct result of a single micronutrient deficiency. A Centers for Disease Control and Prevention article titled "Achievements in Public Health, 1900-1999: Safer and Healthier Foods" sheds some light on the advancement of nutritional sciences and puts it this way:

> *Nutritional sciences also were in their infancy at the start of the century. Unknown was the concept that minerals and vitamins were necessary to prevent diseases caused by dietary deficiencies. Recurring nutritional deficiency diseases, including rickets, scurvy, beri-beri, and pellagra were thought to be infectious diseases. By 1900, biochemists and physiologists had identified protein, fat, and carbohydrates as the basic nutrients in food. By 1916, new data had led to the discovery that food contained vitamins, and the lack of 'vital amines' could cause disease.*[36]

In 1912, the relationship between micronutrient deficiencies and disease was hypothesized by two of the leading researchers of the time. After studying the effects of deficiency on disease, scientists Casimir Funk and Sir Frederick Hopkins published the *Vitamin Hypothesis of Disease*, which stated that certain diseases are caused by a dietary lack of specific vitamins.

What we want you to understand is that today, approximately 100 years later, nothing has changed regarding the causation of disease. While many people want to believe that our modern health conditions and diseases are somehow different from those of the past and that our current epidemics of cancer, osteoporosis, blindness, heart disease, diabetes, dementia, and obesity (to name but a few) are caused by something more than a micronutrient deficiency, this is not the case. Thousands of peer-reviewed studies over the last century show that, in the vast majority of cases, these diseases are not infectious or genetic but are instead caused by a deficiency in essential micronutrients.

Being passionate about the true power of micronutrients, we published a new hypothesis in 2012—exactly 100 years after Funk and Hopkins's *Vitamin Hypothesis of Disease*—that not only identifies the cause of today's most prevalent health conditions and diseases but also offers a realistic and sustainable method of preventing and reversing them. We call it the *Micronutrient Sufficiency Hypothesis of Health*. It states:

> **If a condition or disease can be directly linked to a micronutrient deficiency, then it can be prevented and/or reversed through sustained sufficiency of the deficient micronutrient(s).**

Our hypothesis is different from Funk and Hopkins's in that it includes all micronutrients (not just vitamins), and, perhaps most importantly, it points to the ability to prevent and reverse deficiency diseases through sustained micronutrient sufficiency. This is why the Micronutrient Miracle plan has but one objective—to achieve and sustain a state of micronutrient sufficiency. By identifying which micronutrients you are likely deficient in, as well as which current health conditions they may be causing or could potentially cause, and then by taking the necessary steps to fill in those micronutrient gaps and become micronutrient sufficient, the 28-day plan puts you on the path to preventing future disease or reversing any ill health you may be experiencing.

Within each scientific discipline, theorists strive to discover a universal truth. In physics, for example, there is the law of conservation of energy, which states that energy can be neither created nor destroyed, but can change form. In the field of nutritional science, it is very difficult to find a universal truth, but we believe there is one. We want to introduce you to what we call the Micronutrient Sufficiency Law of Optimal Health. It states:

Micronutrient sufficiency is a requirement of optimal health.

It's not fancy or particularly poetic, but we believe it is true. If essential micronutrients are, as their name implies, essential, then anything other than a sufficient state is insufficient at providing the body with what it needs to carry out whatever function the deficient micronutrient is essential to performing. In short, no micronutrient sufficiency, no optimal health—just like in our "all roads lead to Rome" story. But, the good news is that by understanding this Micronutrient Sufficiency Law of Optimal Health and working toward creating a state of micronutrient sufficiency within your body during your personalized 28-day program, you are taking control of your own health and setting the stage for a miracle in your life.

Micronutrient Deficiency Equals Disease

At this point you may be saying to yourself, "So if all this were true, then why wouldn't the American Medical Association (AMA) be yelling this from the highest mountaintop? Why wouldn't thousands of research papers point to micronutrient deficiency as a major causative factor of today's diseases? I've never seen one shred of evidence from any reputable source that says all I have to do to prevent disease is just get enough micronutrients." Well, hang on to your hats, because we're about to show you that evidence.

Let's start with a statement by Robert H. Fletcher, MD, MSc, and Kathleen M. Fairfield, MD, writers of the guidelines for the *Journal of the American Medical Association*: "Insufficient vitamin intake is apparently a cause of chronic diseases. Recent evidence has shown that suboptimal [below standard] levels of vitamins, even well above those causing deficiency syndromes, are risk factors for chronic diseases such as cardiovascular disease, cancer, and osteoporosis. A large proportion of the general population is apparently at increased risk for this reason."[37]

So, as you can see, the AMA is fully aware of the fact that micronutrient deficiency is a risk factor for modern diseases and that a large proportion of the general population is at risk, but the real question is—how much of a risk factor? Could micronutrient sufficiency be the missing piece of the puzzle we have all been searching for? Here are several studies from various esteemed institutions highlighting the connection between a variety of health conditions and diseases and micronutrient deficiencies.

In a study published in the *Proceedings of the National Academy of Sciences*, researchers concluded that congestive heart failure (from a wide variety of causes) is strongly correlated with significantly low blood and tissue levels of the accessory micronutrient coenzyme Q10 (CoQ10). The study determined that the severity of heart disease correlates with the severity of CoQ10 deficiency and concluded, "CoQ10 deficiency might be a major if not the *sole cause* of cardiomyopathy [heart disease]."[38]

Michael Holick, MD, of Boston University School of Medicine, notes in his study on vitamin D and sunlight that women who are vitamin D deficient have a 253 percent increased risk for developing colorectal cancer and a 222 percent increased risk for developing breast cancer. He suggests that blood levels of vitamin D at the time of diagnosis of breast cancer accurately predict a woman's survival.[39] Another study out of Mount Sinai Hospital in Toronto, Canada, showed that women with low levels of vitamin D at diagnosis of breast cancer are 94 percent more likely to have the cancer metastasize and 73 percent more likely to die within 10 years of diagnosis.[40]

In a study published in the *European Journal of Neurology*, researchers concluded that individuals with elevated homocysteine levels caused by a vitamin B_{12} deficiency had more than twice the risk of developing Alzheimer's disease.[41] And in the largest study yet to find an association between low levels of vitamin D and dementia, published in the journal *Neurology*, researchers determined that individuals with low vitamin D levels may have twice the risk of developing Alzheimer's as individuals with sufficient levels.[42]

Studies out of the Arizona Cancer Center and Cornell University determined that total cancer mortality was reduced by 50 percent in those taking 200 micrograms of selenium daily. The risk of developing prostate cancer was reduced by as much as 74 percent, colorectal cancer by 58 percent, and lung cancer by 48 percent.[43]

In a study published in the *Lancet*, vitamin E supplementation was shown to reduce the risk of myocardial infarction (heart attack) by 77 percent in patients with existing coronary artery disease.[44] Additionally, in a 2014 study published in the *American Journal of Clinical Nutrition*, researchers determined that a daily dose of just 800 international units (IU) of vitamin D_3 reduced the risk of heart failure by 25 percent.[45]

In 2011, New Zealand researchers from the obstetrics and gynecology department at the University of Auckland reviewed more than 30 studies on the correlation between subfertile men and antioxidant supplementation. They discovered that antioxidants—such as vitamins C and E and zinc—reduced infertility and increased the odds of conception more than fourfold.[46] And fertility studies focusing on female participants have fared even better. In a recent

British study, daily supplementation with 200 micrograms of selenium along with 400 milligrams of magnesium allowed 100 percent of the previously infertile women in the study to conceive and give birth.[47]

Vitamin K_2, which is only found in animal sources and is often deficient in the American diet, can reduce incidents of heart disease by directing calcium out of your arteries and into your bones. Researchers at Erasmus University Medical Center in Rotterdam, Netherlands, studied 4,807 men and women for over 7 years and determined that supplementation with vitamin K_2 improved cardiovascular health by reducing arterial calcium accumulation by 50 percent and slashed the risk of a cardiovascular event by 50 percent. Additionally, according to a 2012 study out of Harokopio University of Athens in Greece, vitamin K_2 serves up added bone benefits and induces positive changes in bone mass by allowing for proper use of calcium.[48, 49]

A 2013 scientific review of seven randomized controlled trials found that an average of 101,028 cardiovascular events could be avoided each year if all US adults over the age of 55 diagnosed with coronary heart disease were to supplement using B_6, B_9 (folate), and B_{12} at protective intake levels.[50]

That sure is a lot of evidence, and it all points to the fact that a lack of essential micronutrients increases the risk of a wide variety of health conditions and diseases, including heart disease, cancer, Alzheimer's, infertility, and osteoporosis. Now, when you think about being micronutrient deficient, does any word

Mark Hyman, MD,

Chairman of the Institute for Functional Medicine,

Tells It Like It Is

"[Today] vitamin deficiency does not cause acute diseases such as scurvy or rickets, but [it does] cause what have been called 'long-latency deficiency diseases.' These include conditions like blindness, osteoporosis, heart disease, cancer, diabetes, dementia, and more.

"What's remarkable is how most conventional doctors have it completely backward when it comes to vitamins and minerals. . . . Doctors tend to only use vitamins if medications don't work. They should be prescribing the vitamins in the first place. . . . Imagine a drug that could cure within days or weeks a fatal disease using a very small dose, without toxicity and with a 100 percent success rate. Such a drug does not exist and will never exist. But that is the power and potential of nutrients."[51, 52]

come to mind? How about *dangerous*? It certainly sounds *dangerous*, doesn't it? Micronutrient deficiency is the most dangerous health condition in the world because it has been shown to be a causative factor for nearly every health condition and disease we are all trying to avoid.

And there you have it. Because micronutrient deficiency impacts nearly every man, woman, and child on the planet and touches the lives of nearly double the number of people who are currently diagnosed with today's most prevalent and deadly health conditions and diseases—including heart disease, cancer, osteoporosis, and diabetes—combined, it is certainly the most *widespread* health condition of the 21st century. Additionally, because being deficient in essential micronutrients greatly increases the risk of developing today's most debilitating diseases, micronutrient deficiency is also the most *dangerous* health condition we face. And given the supporting research presented in this chapter, we feel that we have proven, beyond a shadow of a doubt, that the statement on which we founded our nutritional philosophy is indeed accurate: Micronutrient deficiency is the most widespread and dangerous health condition of the 21st century.

Discovering the Micronutrient Deficiencies Likely Affecting Your Health

We've shown you the big picture, but now it's time to set the stage for your very own Micronutrient Miracle to occur. It's time to create a list of the specific micronutrients that you, personally, should be paying special attention to as we move through this program. We will call this your Personal Micronutrient Deficiency List. Your list will be as unique as you are since the health conditions, illnesses, ailments, or diseases that you currently suffer from will determine the deficient micronutrients on it. Your goal throughout the Micronutrient Miracle plan will be to become micronutrient sufficient, paying extra attention to the specific micronutrients on your personalized list.

To begin, you must first assess your current state of health to determine which micronutrients you may be deficient in. In order to do this, we want you to look at Table 1.3 on page 24 and place a check (✓) next to the health conditions or diseases you are currently suffering from. For example, if you suffer from allergies, you would put a check in the box next to allergies. If you also suffer from anxiety, you would put an additional check in the box next to anxiety, and so on. The number of checks is determined by the number of conditions on the list you have or experience on a regular basis. For example, if you get a cold once every couple of years, you would leave the box next to "colds" unchecked, but if you get a cold every year or more than once a year, you would put a check in that box. Be as thorough as you can.

You will notice that next to each condition there is a second box containing the names of the micronutrients science has shown to be beneficial in the prevention and treatment of that condition. These are the specific micronutrients that you will want to focus on becoming sufficient in moving forward. Once you have checked off all the boxes that apply to you in Table 1.3, move on to Table 1.4 on page 27 and write in the number of times each micronutrient listed there was included in a grouping next to a condition or disease you put a check next to.

For example, if vitamin A was included in the group of micronutrients for only one of the conditions you placed a check next to, then you would write the number 1 next to vitamin A in Table 1.4. However, if vitamin A was included in the groups of micronutrients for three of the conditions you checked off, then you would write the number 3 next to vitamin A in Table 1.4. Take your time and be as accurate as you can. Once you complete this chart, you will be able to quickly identify which micronutrient deficiencies are likely at the root of many of your current health conditions and diseases.

TABLE 1.3
CONDITIONS AND KEY MICRONUTRIENTS USED IN PREVENTION AND TREATMENT

CONDITION	MICRONUTRIENTS USED IN PREVENTION AND TREATMENT	✓ IF CONDITION EXISTS
Acne	A, B_1, B_2, B_3, B_5, B_6, B_7, B_9, B_{12}, C, E, zinc	
ADHD	B_6, B_9, magnesium, zinc, omega-3, carnitine	
Allergies	A, B_5, B_6, C, E, calcium, magnesium, selenium, zinc, omega-6 (GLA)	
Alzheimer's disease/dementia	A, B_1, B_2, B_6, B_9, B_{12}, choline, C, D, E, chromium, copper, silicon, zinc, omega-3, alpha-lipoic acid, carnitine	
Anemia	B_9, B_{12}, copper, iron	
Anxiety	A, B_1, B_2, B_3, B_5, B_6, B_7, B_9, B_{12}, choline, C, D, E, calcium, chromium, copper, iodine, iron, magnesium, potassium, selenium, zinc, omega-3, carnitine	
Arthritis	B_1, B_2, B_3, B_5, B_6, B_7, B_9, B_{12}, C, D, boron, calcium, magnesium, silicon, omega-3, omega-6 (GLA)	

	TABLE 1.3 (cont.)	
CONDITION	**MICRONUTRIENTS USED IN PREVENTION AND TREATMENT**	**✓ IF CONDITION EXISTS**
Asthma	A, B_6, B_9, choline, C, D, E, magnesium, selenium, silicon, zinc, omega-3, carnitine, CoQ10	
Autism	A, B_1, B_6, B_9, B_{12}, C, D, magnesium, zinc, carnitine	
Blindness/night blindness	A	
Cancer	A, B_1, B_3, B_9, B_{12}, C, D, E, K, calcium, iodine, molybdenum, selenium, silicon, omega-3	
Cardiovascular disease/ heart condition	B_1, B_2, B_3, B_6, B_9, B_{12}, C, D, E, K, calcium, chromium, copper, magnesium, potassium, selenium, silicon, zinc, omega-3, omega-6 (GLA), CoQ10	
Carpal tunnel syndrome	B_6	
Cataracts	B_1, B_2, C, E, selenium, silicon	
Chronic fatigue	B_1, B_2, B_3, B_5, B_6, B_7, B_9, B_{12}, C, D, E, iodine, iron, magnesium, carnitine	
Cognitive function	A, B_1, B_2, B_6, B_9, B_{12}, choline, C, D, E, chromium, copper, silicon, zinc, omega-3, alpha-lipoic acid, carnitine	
Colds	C, D, zinc	
Constipation	B_1, C, E, magnesium	
Depression	A, B_2, B_6, B_7, B_9, B_{12}, C, D, E, calcium, chromium, iodine, iron, magnesium, selenium, silicon, zinc, omega-3, carnitine	
Dermatitis/eczema	A, B_3, B_7, C, E, zinc	
Diabetes type 1	B_3, B_7, D, K, zinc, carnitine	
Diabetes type 2	B_3, B_5, B_6, B_7, C, D, E, K, chromium, magnesium, manganese, zinc, alpha-lipoic acid	
Fibromyalgia	B_1, D, magnesium, selenium, silicon, zinc, CoQ10	
Frequent bruising	A, C, E, zinc	
Gout	B_6, zinc	
High cholesterol	B_3, B_5, E, chromium, copper	
HIV	B_3, selenium, silicon, zinc	
Hypertension (high blood pressure)	B_6, B_9, C, D, E, calcium, chromium, magnesium, potassium, selenium, silicon, omega-3, omega-6 (GLA), alpha-lipoic acid, carnitine, CoQ10	
Immunoglobulin A nephropathy	Omega-3	

TABLE 1.3 (cont.)		
CONDITION	**MICRONUTRIENTS USED IN PREVENTION AND TREATMENT**	**✓ IF CONDITION EXISTS**
Impaired immunity/ frequent illness	A, B_1, B_2, B_3, B_5, B_6, B_7, B_9, B_{12}, C, D, E, copper, iron, phosphorus, selenium, silicon, zinc	
Infertility (female)	B_6, B_9, B_{12}, C, D, E, copper, magnesium, selenium, silicon, zinc	
Infertility (male)	A, B_9, B_{12}, C, D, E, copper, manganese, selenium, silicon, zinc, carnitine, CoQ10	
Inflammation (conditions that end in -itis)	B_2, B_3, B_5, B_6, B_7, C, D, E, magnesium, manganese, zinc, omega-3, alpha-lipoic acid	
Insomnia	A, B_1, B_3, B_6, B_9, B_{12}, D, E, calcium, magnesium, zinc	
Kidney stones	A, B_6, D, calcium, magnesium, potassium	
Macular degeneration	A, lutein, E, zinc, omega-3	
Menopausal symptoms	B_6, C, E, magnesium, zinc, omega-3	
Migraines/headaches	B_2, B_3, B_9, B_{12}, iron, magnesium, CoQ10	
Muscle aches and cramps	B_1, B_2, B_3, B_5, B_6, B_7, B_9, B_{12}, E, calcium, magnesium, potassium	
Obesity	A, B_3, B_6, B_{12} C, D, E, K, calcium, chromium, iodine, iron, magnesium, potassium, zinc, omega-3, alpha-lipoic acid, CoQ10	
Osteoporosis/osteopenia	A, B_9, B_{12}, D, K, boron, calcium, copper, fluoride, magnesium, manganese, phosphorus, potassium, silicon, zinc, omega-3, omega-6 (GLA)	
PMS	B_6, E, magnesium, zinc, omega-3	
Psoriasis/skin disorders	A, E, selenium, silicon, omega-3, CoQ10	
Restless leg syndrome	Iron	
Schizophrenia	Omega-3	
Seizure disorders/epilepsy	B_6, B_7, magnesium	
Stroke	C, D, potassium	
Thyroid problems	A, B_1, B_2, B_3, B_5, B_6, B_7, B_9, B_{12}, C, D, E, iodine, iron, manganese, potassium, selenium, silicon, zinc, omega-3	
Ulcers	B_{12}, C	
Varicose veins	C, E, copper	

TABLE 1.4
YOUR PERSONAL MICRONUTRIENT DEFICIENCY LIST

MICRONUTRIENT	# OF TIMES LISTED AFTER A CHECKED HEALTH CONDITION	MICRONUTRIENT	# OF TIMES LISTED AFTER A CHECKED HEALTH CONDITION
Vitamin A		Chromium	
Lutein		Copper	
Vitamin B$_1$ (thiamine)		Iodine	
Vitamin B$_2$ (riboflavin)		Iron	
Vitamin B$_3$ (niacin)		Magnesium	
Vitamin B$_5$ (pantothenic acid)		Manganese	
Vitamin B$_6$ (pyridoxine)		Phosphorus	
Vitamin B$_7$ (biotin)		Potassium	
Vitamin B$_9$ (folate)		Selenium	
Vitamin B$_{12}$ (cobalamin)		Silicon	
Choline		Zinc	
Vitamin C		Omega-3	
Vitamin D		Omega-6	
Vitamin E		Alpha-lipoic acid	
Vitamin K		Amino acids (carnitine)	
Boron		CoQ10	
Calcium			

Have any patterns emerged? Are there any micronutrients in Table 1.4 that caused you to write a very high number? This is your Personal Micronutrient Deficiency List, and those micronutrients with the highest scores are the ones that you are likely the most deficient in and will want to pay special attention to throughout this plan. You will be referring back to this list while you work through the chapters in this book. As you examine your current dietary choices, lifestyle habits, and supplements to see if they may be contributing to your specific micronutrient depletions, we will show you how to make simple adjustments in each of these areas so that you can quickly and easily reduce or even eliminate those depletions. Additionally, you will use your Personal Micronutrient Deficiency List to identify the micronutrients you will be focusing on when you are making your Micronutrient Miracle menu choices. Bottom line: Your personal list will allow you to focus on the vitamins and minerals that will best benefit you, and this is great news, because the more focused you are, the better your aim, and the greater the likelihood you will hit your target—micronutrient sufficiency.

My Personal Micronutrient Miracle: Jeff R.

Sometimes people come into your life when you need them the most—what is it called, divine intervention? That is what happened when I met Mira and Jayson while on my honeymoon in Punta Cana. Through our casual conversation, I became very interested in the Micronutrient Miracle lifestyle (because it isn't just a diet—it's a lifestyle). What piqued my interest the most was that I was having ankle reconstruction surgery the following week and was going to be bedridden for 6 weeks after surgery. I was afraid I was going to put on 20 to 30 pounds while laid up because there was nothing I could do exercise-wise and I'd just be laying around snacking the entire time. Plus, I was already a bit bigger than I'd like to be.

After talking it over with my wife, I decided to give the Micronutrient Miracle Ketogenic protocol a shot. If I didn't lose any weight, or I just lost 5 pounds, I figured that was better than putting on 30. My wife changed her eating habits with me because we agreed it'd be easier to do together. It really was a miracle, because I didn't gain weight lying around for those 6 weeks. Instead, I dropped 20 pounds with no physical activity at all!

Now, I am down a total of 56 pounds. I have gone from a 44 to a 38 in the waist, and I lost 2 inches in the neck, as well. My wife says I don't snore anymore, and I notice I sleep much better every night. I feel much more focused at work and just feel great all around! The brain fog is gone, and I have a sense of mental clarity that I've never experienced before. We drink our Triple Threat Shakes every day with our nutreince multivitamin right in it; the chocolate is delicious! We also started shopping at farmers' markets for organically grown produce and meats. I am very aware of products and the chemicals in them and what to steer clear of. Generally, if it has more than three ingredients and I can't pronounce any of them, then forget it. We really enjoy this way of eating and living! I love to cook, and I've found very creative ways to make some of the most boring things exciting while keeping them ultra healthy. We love to entertain, and it's been fun to turn our friends and family on to delicious recipes that they may not have realized are also nutrient dense and natural!

My wife calls me an all-or-nothing person. I'm either "pot committed" or not interested at all, and this was one poker game I'm glad I went all in! And to think it all happened on our honeymoon!

2

How the 28-Day Micronutrient Miracle Can Work for You

LIKE SO MANY CLIENTS before them, married couple Stacy and Mark wanted to go through the Micronutrient Miracle plan together. And as so many others had in the past, they sat opposite us at our desk, full of questions. What they wanted to know most of all was how the 28-day Micronutrient Miracle could work for Stacy to eliminate the food cravings, mood swings, and poor sleeping habits that were driving her mad while addressing Mark's recently diagnosed prediabetes and the fact that his belt buckle had finally reached its last notch. And although they had faith in the program because we had previously helped Mark's mother lower her cholesterol levels and get off statins, they did not yet understand how following the same program would produce such personalized and seemingly different health benefits.

To help them understand this truly amazing phenomenon, we shared with Stacy and Mark our "orchestra analogy" (see page 30). We explained how each micronutrient is like a different instrument in the orchestra, and that in order to successfully play a specific piece of music (the equivalent to the body carrying out a specific essential function—like bone building or hormone production), all the instruments (or micronutrients) that are required for that specific piece of music must be present. When one or several instruments (micronutrients) are missing, the orchestra (body) will not be able to successfully play

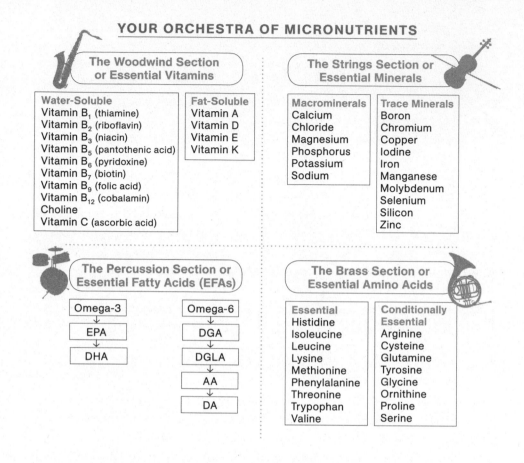

YOUR ORCHESTRA OF MICRONUTRIENTS

The Woodwind Section or Essential Vitamins

Water-Soluble	Fat-Soluble
Vitamin B_1 (thiamine)	Vitamin A
Vitamin B_2 (riboflavin)	Vitamin D
Vitamin B_3 (niacin)	Vitamin E
Vitamin B_5 (pantothenic acid)	Vitamin K
Vitamin B_6 (pyridoxine)	
Vitamin B_7 (biotin)	
Vitamin B_9 (folic acid)	
Vitamin B_{12} (cobalamin)	
Choline	
Vitamin C (ascorbic acid)	

The Strings Section or Essential Minerals

Macrominerals	Trace Minerals
Calcium	Boron
Chloride	Chromium
Magnesium	Copper
Phosphorus	Iodine
Potassium	Iron
Sodium	Manganese
	Molybdenum
	Selenium
	Silicon
	Zinc

The Percussion Section or Essential Fatty Acids (EFAs)

Omega-3	Omega-6
↓	↓
EPA	DGA
↓	↓
DHA	DGLA
	↓
	AA
	↓
	DA

The Brass Section or Essential Amino Acids

Essential	Conditionally Essential
Histidine	Arginine
Isoleucine	Cysteine
Leucine	Glutamine
Lysine	Tyrosine
Methionine	Glycine
Phenylalanine	Ornithine
Threonine	Proline
Trypophan	Serine
Valine	

the piece (carry out the specific essential function), and this will lead to a subpar performance (health condition or disease).

Just as a standard orchestra generally has four sections—woodwinds, brass, percussion, and strings—the human body plays its sweet music through processing and using four specific types of micronutrients: vitamins, minerals, essential fatty acids, and amino acids. And like the orchestra, each of the four sections is made up of similar, yet vastly different, instruments.

For example, the string instruments include violin, guitar, sitar, electric bass, viola, cello, harp, double bass, rebab, banjo, mandolin, ukulele, and something called a bouzouki, which we hear is the central string instrument in Greek music. They all create music through the vibration of strings. However, while they have that trait in common, the resulting sound that each produces is vastly different. When Beethoven composed his "Ode to Joy" for the violin, he didn't assume any string instrument could represent the ethereal nature of the melody—certainly not a banjo or an electric bass. Because each string instrument offers such a unique tone, they are not interchangeable.

The same is true of minerals. All minerals are found in the earth's soil and water. Plants don't create minerals; they must extract them from the soil as they grow. So all minerals have that in common. However, much like the instruments we mentioned earlier, they too are not interchangeable. For example, calcium, one of the essential minerals, is required for muscle contraction, while zinc, another essential mineral, supports smell and taste. If your body is deficient in calcium, zinc won't help your muscles contract. And, conversely, if your body is short on zinc, calcium cannot aid in flavor or smell perception.

Offering Stacy and Mark one more example, we explained that just as all instruments in the woodwind section make music by blowing air (wind) through a tube once made of, well, wood, of course, vitamins have something in common, as well. Vitamins are not found in soil or water. Instead, they are produced by the plants and animals we consume. Additionally, while some woodwind instruments, like the oboe or the clarinet, use reeds to cause their musical vibrations, others, like the flute or piccolo, are reedless. The vitamin family can also be subdivided by characteristics. Vitamins can be either fat-soluble or water-soluble. The fat-soluble vitamins—A, D, E, and K—are absorbed with the help of bile acids and can be stored in significant amounts in your body fat and liver until they are needed. All of the other vitamins are water-soluble, which means they cannot be stored in the body in significant amounts (B_{12} is an exception). Instead, water-soluble vitamins travel through the bloodstream, and if the body does not use them, they are eliminated through urination; they are not readily stored for a rainy day, like fat-soluble vitamins. Again, our point here was that one vitamin cannot take the place of another vitamin. Their functions are as unique as the pitch of an instrument. Vitamin A, for example, aids in night vision, while vitamin B_9, also called folate, helps prevent spina bifida in newborns.

We paused to examine their faces. Both Mark and Stacy seemed to be following along, so we continued. We explained how if, for example, a piece of sheet music requires a trombone, flute, cello, and violin, and the violin and flute are missing, it does not matter how many cellos or trombones are present at the time of the performance. The music will never sound as it should. Additionally, it would not matter if a tuba and a xylophone were present in their stead, because only the violin and the flute can produce the correct sound required for the musical piece.

Both Stacy and Mark nodded their heads in unison to indicate their understanding. Likewise, we told them, if an essential bodily function requires calcium, magnesium, vitamin K, and zinc, and the calcium and zinc are deficient, then regardless of how much magnesium, vitamin K, or any other micronutrients are present, the bodily function will never be carried out as it should be, and this will leave the door open to health conditions and diseases in the future.

Using this example, we explained that when all the essential instruments (micronutrients) are available, then the orchestra (body) can once again perform the piece of music (specific essential function) it was once unable to properly perform, and the subpar performance (health condition or disease) that was manifesting itself because of the deficiency will be greatly improved or reversed completely. We then explained our *Micronutrient Sufficiency Hypothesis of Health*, which we had stated many times, to many people, both in consultations such as this as well as in worldwide media. In short, a deficiency in an essential micronutrient will leave the body unable to perform necessary tasks, and, over time, this can lead to a serious health condition or disease. Conversely, achieving a state of micronutrient sufficiency ensures that the body has the essential micronutrients it needs to perform critical tasks and can prevent or reverse a health condition or disease being caused by a micronutrient deficiency.

The light in Stacy's eyes and the smile that had slowly appeared on Mark's face told us they were both starting to understand the potential health enhancing power of micronutrient sufficiency and how the 28-day Micronutrient Miracle plan could deliver such incredibly different benefits to each of them. They understood that regardless of which micronutrient gaps they each had, our program would create a full orchestra in their bodies from which any song, and every bodily function, could be perfectly performed.

Then came the inevitable question: "So, this program of yours…what kind of diet do we follow? Which one of us gets to eat the foods that we like?" Stacy informed us that she preferred a low-fat, high-protein diet. Her trainer at the gym mentioned that this was best for lean muscle. Mark, on the other hand, wanted to try a low-carb program. He had done Atkins with success in the past, and eating burgers and chicken wings really appealed to him. The couple asked us about fat, carbohydrate, and protein ratios and went on for a while about their past diet programs that forced them to measure everything, down to the last grain of rice. And we answered, like we had a thousand times before under similar circumstances, "You both can eat whatever style of diet you want."

The usual silence and blank stares came next, and then we explained that the 28-day Micronutrient Miracle plan is not based on one particular philosophy of eating (like low-fat or low-carb) but instead can be followed by everyone, regardless of what diet they follow. So Stacy can have her favorite low-fat, high-protein meals, and Mark can live on his low-carb burgers and chicken wings. As long as they followed the three simple guidelines we outline in the 28-day plan, their personal dietary habits were completely theirs to choose.

Welcome to the Nutrivore Lifestyle

Are you more aligned with Stacy, preferring to eat a low-fat, high-protein diet? Or does the idea of eating chicken wings and burgers while dieting excite you as much as it did Mark? Regardless of what type of diet you choose to follow, the 28-day Micronutrient Miracle plan will work for you. This is because being deficient in vitamins, minerals, essential fatty acids, and amino acids is detrimental for vegans, vegetarians, low-fat, Primal/Paleo, Mediterranean, and low-carb dieters alike. Therefore, becoming sufficient in the essential micronutrients should be the goal of each and every one of us.

In fact, because this shift in thinking is so unique, we coined a new term to describe the person who embraces this goal. The good news is that regardless of your dietary philosophy, we want to personally invite you to join this group of health-conscious visionaries. By reading this book now and embarking on the 28-day Micronutrient Miracle journey, you are officially welcome to call yourself a *nutrivore.*

So what is a nutrivore? Nutrivores are people, like you, who have decided to take control of their health and stop blaming it on genetics or searching for it at the bottom of a prescription bottle. Simply stated, a nutrivore is someone who recognizes that micronutrient deficiency equals poor health and disease and that micronutrient sufficiency is the foundation of optimal health, regardless of one's preferred dietary philosophy.

Additionally, nutrivores are environmentally conscious and tolerant of the nutritional preferences of others. Our vision is to empower everyone to come together behind one core nutritional belief that holds true for all people, regardless of dietary philosophy—the health-producing, disease-preventing power of micronutrient sufficiency. By doing so, we hope to create a workable environment where we can stop the arguing, fighting, and finger-pointing that has held us back from being able to slow down, stop, or reverse the ever-increasing deluge of chronic health conditions and diseases that are now plaguing all nations of the world. We hope that through respect, patience, and a true understanding of the role micronutrients play in the prevention and reversal of today's chronic health conditions and diseases, humanity may one day soon usher in an age of optimal health.

The reality is that the health-promoting power of micronutrients has the potential to prevent and reverse countless diseases within the next century, but only if we use it. So, we are going to teach you the exact steps to harness their power to potentially transform your health. We know you can do it. The best part is that the three steps we are going to teach you are really pretty simple. You don't have to change the things you love to eat or the way that you live your life. You simply have to change your focus. It is time to make the little things count. It's time to learn how to maximize your micronutrients!

Step 1:
Switch to Rich Food

Your goal is to get as many micronutrients as possible from your food. That is because food is your first line of defense against micronutrient deficiency. However, on the Micronutrient Miracle plan, the quality of food is not measured by whether it is plant or animal or low carb or low fat; instead, foods are graded on their ability to supply their inherit micronutrients. In Chapter 1, you learned that certain environmental factors have depleted the micronutrients in your food. Whether you're eating an apple or an egg, as a nutrivore, your goal is to attempt to obtain the freshest choice with the highest micronutrient content while striving to avoid nutritionally impaired foods, such as those that have traveled long distances or that are highly processed and have little to no nutritional value. As you begin to prep for your Micronutrient Miracle plan in Chapter 3, we will show you how to purge your pantry of micronutrient-robbing foods (we will call these *Poor Foods*) so that in Chapter 5 you can restock your kitchen with foods that give you the most micronutrient bang in every delicious bite (we will call these *Rich Foods*).

Remember, micronutrient-rich foods can be found in every dietary philosophy. This allows you to follow the program while eating the foods you enjoy and never feel like you're missing out. Your personalized Micronutrient Miracle plan will be as unique as you are.

Step 2:
Drive Down Micronutrient Depletion

Choosing to eat Rich Foods (which have the most micronutrients) is a fantastic first step, but it is really just that—a first step. Your health depends on your willingness to make small but strategic changes in your life. No one can do it for you. Part of being a nutrivore entails taking a good look at your life and identifying the habits that are acting as roadblocks on your highway to health.

In upcoming chapters, you will learn how even some "healthy" high-quality foods and lifestyle habits may also have leaching effects, and we will encourage you to limit obvious micronutrient-depleting habits, like smoking and excessive coffee and alcohol intake. Additionally, you will learn to evaluate the toxins in your life so that you can take an active approach to switching out common, everyday products that are adding to your overall toxic load. While this includes pesticides and chemical additives in your food, it also includes numerous toxins that can be found in things like toothpaste, shampoo, deodorant, cleaning supplies, and even your cookware and food storage containers.

Don't worry about all the details just yet, and don't get nervous thinking we are going to expect you to make too many changes. Some things may be too difficult for you to change right away. This second step is really about awareness. Ultimately, you are in total control of which lifestyle habits and products you want to alter during your first 28 days. But remember, the fewer of these micronutrient depleters you have in your life, the more likely you are to achieve a micronutrient sufficient state.

Step 3: Supplement Smart—Learn the ABCs

In Chapter 1, you were introduced to the global prevalence of micronutrient deficiency and learned how our soil and modern farming practices are literally starving us of our essential micronutrients. You also learned how the human body becomes susceptible to diseases and health conditions when hidden hunger takes hold. And while "switching to rich" (the first step) and "driving down micronutrient depletion" (the second) will certainly take you a long way toward your goal of micronutrient sufficiency, wouldn't you prefer to *ensure* micronutrient sufficiency is met? We sure do, and that makes this third step absolutely essential.

A quality multivitamin is only a supplement and not a substitute for a healthy diet and lifestyle. Its job is to help ensure minimum micronutrient sufficiency and protect you from micronutrient deficiencies when your diet or your daily actions don't always go as planned. Similar to choosing a quality car insurance or life insurance policy, choosing a quality multivitamin can be a confusing task. You want to find the policy (or multivitamin) with the best and most complete coverage. In Chapter 6, we will share with you our fail-safe guidelines to choosing smart supplementation, and we will make it as easy as learning the ABCs—the ABCs of Optimal Supplementation Guidelines, that is.

By using the ABCs when purchasing supplements, you will have the tools to sidestep the four major flaws we identified in most multivitamins on the market. Avoiding these pitfalls will guarantee that the product you choose can be absorbed and utilized by your body. No more multivitamins or other supplements that are literally flushing your money down the toilet. We will arm you with the knowledge you need to purchase the highest-quality multivitamin that can best set you on the road to personal micronutrient sufficiency.

Striving to become micronutrient sufficient is the cornerstone of the nutrivore lifestyle. By taking our simple three-step approach to maximizing your micronutrients throughout your 28-day plan, you are opening the door to amazing possibilities.

What Will Your Miracle Look Like?

How are you hoping to transform your own health? In the previous chapter, we asked you to identify some of the health conditions and diseases that you are currently suffering from. Additionally, we had you create your Personal Micronutrient Deficiency List to identify the specific micronutrients that are likely playing a role in these deficiency ailments. Whether they are serious diseases, like osteoporosis or heart disease, or aggravating health conditions, like poor sleep or brittle nails, by becoming sufficient in the micronutrients that may be at the root of your conditions, you are providing your body with the tools it needs to improve your health with every step of your journey. And more likely than not, you may even start to see health enhancements in areas of your life that you had not even marked down or taken notice of.

Clients ask us all the time what they can expect to happen in these 28 days. Our answer may surprise you: We tell them that we really don't know. Not because we aren't experts in micronutrient therapies, but because we can't be sure what their miracles will look like. You see, when we first meet with clients, we don't know which micronutrients they may be deficient in. Because of this, we can't always predict the amazing results that they will receive after their 28 days. The truth is that we are often just as amazed by the extraordinary results as they are, as was the case with our client Mabel.

Meet Mabel

Mabel was a woman in her fifties. She was engaged to be married, and her life of international globetrotting was the envy of many of her friends. However, Mabel was unhappy. She lacked energy, often sleeping in late and missing out on her fiancé's planned excursions, which were too early for her to get moving. Her 5-foot-4 body lacked the energy she desired, and her weight had slowly been escalating. She came to us with the desire to lose weight before their wedding, a request we get quite often from excited brides-to-be.

After our initial face-to-face consultation, we put Mabel on the Micronutrient Miracle plan, knowing that it would help her regain the thinner body of her youth. Because Mabel was often abroad, we regularly met with her on Skype to review her progress. Through our numerous conversations, we knew that she was succeeding, but when we finally met in person again, the results were truly miraculous.

First, the 30 pounds she had dropped on the plan appeared dramatically greater on her small frame. She was gorgeous. But there was something else. She seemed peppier, lighter, and full of energy. She explained that this plan had energized her once-sleepy self, turning her into a woman she was thrilled to become and her fiancé was looking forward to getting to know. She eagerly awoke every morning at 7 a.m.—a time unimaginable to her earlier self. She walked in the mornings and readily joined her fiancé on tours and expeditions during their travels. We were thrilled to see this unexpected bonus she had experienced. But there was something else different about Mabel. We just couldn't put our fingers on it. Then it hit us.

Mabel had incredible style. She was always accessorized head to toe, and her signature piece had always been her glasses. She must have owned dozens of pairs. Her edgy frames were always perfectly matched to her outfits, and today was the first time we had ever seen her without them on. When we mentioned this to her, this pint-size powerhouse nearly jumped out of her chair.

Over the past few months, Mabel had started getting headaches when reading. She hadn't wanted to worry us, so she made an appointment with her eye doctor with no mention to us. He tested her and then decided to retest her because he could not believe the results: Her glasses were giving her headaches because she no longer needed them. Mabel had completely reversed her poor vision, something she'd had her entire life. She had never before considered that her impaired vision was due to a lifelong deficiency in specific micronutrients. By following our three-step plan of eating Rich Foods, eliminating depleting lifestyle habits, and supplementing smart using our specific micronutrient therapy protocol, Mabel was now a thinner, happier, more energetic woman with twenty-twenty vision.

So what will your unexpected miracles be? For Mabel it was limitless energy and improved eyesight; perhaps for you it will be improved sleep patterns, a clearer complexion, or reduced arthritis. Extraordinary and unexpected benefits await you, as well. Only time will tell how becoming sufficient will improve your health—and your life. And, speaking of time, it is crucial to keep in mind that it might have taken years of deficiency to create some of the health conditions you are currently experiencing. While micronutrients are miraculous, we want you to have realistic expectations. Mabel didn't lose 30 pounds or regain perfect vision in her first 28 days. Remember, micronutrient deficiencies manifest themselves differently in each individual. What can Mabel teach you as we set out together on this 28-day plan? **Expect the unexpected!**

To Test or Not to Test: That Is the Question

In a later appointment, Mabel told us that she wished she'd known earlier that her eyesight was impaired due to her body being deficient in specific micronutrients. She felt it could have saved her bullying as a youth and thousands of dollars in eye appointments and glasses throughout her life. She asked us why more doctors don't test micronutrient levels. It seemed to her an obvious solution that could have spared her much agony. We explained that some doctors do test levels of a few micronutrients, and as pertinent research showing the health-producing power of vitamins and minerals is seen more frequently in the news, more and more doctors are starting to test for micronutrient deficiencies. However, the testing typically done through physicians' offices, called *serum testing*, is often limited to iron, vitamin D, vitamin B_{12}, calcium, and magnesium.

There are a few innate problems with this type of testing. First, analyzing blood levels of these five micronutrients leaves one in the dark about the more than 20 other essential vitamins and minerals that were not tested. Secondly, because serum testing only measures the amount of the micronutrient in the sample of blood taken, these tests don't always show the full picture. Here's how.

Darcie, a 47-year-old vegan, contacted us through Facebook. She wanted to share a story with us about how information she had learned through following us and reading our book *Naked Calories* had made her question her physician's lab results. Darcie, who had followed a vegan diet for 25 years and was an avid triathlete, went to her physician for her annual exam. After her blood tests were run, her physician told her that she was very low in vitamin D but that her calcium levels were perfect. Having learned from us about foods and lifestyle habits that deplete calcium (information we will share with you in upcoming chapters) and realizing that her diet was very high in these depleters, as well as recognizing that her vegan diet was not supplying a great amount of calcium in the first place, Darcie began questioning how her blood calcium levels could have possibly come back in the sufficient range.

She also remembered us teaching how some foods can cause calcium to leach from the bone into the blood. Curious now about her bone strength and her doctor's lab results, Darcie decided she wanted a DEXA scan, a test that measures bone mineral density and thus the test for osteoporosis. The results were devastating. This seemingly healthy, athletic woman was now diagnosed with osteoporosis and degenerative scoliosis! She also learned that she was no longer 5 feet 8 inches but rather 5 feet 6.5 inches. Had Darcie not questioned the calcium levels reported in her blood work, this deficiency would have gone unchecked for a longer period and likely left her in far worse shape.

So, as you can see, serum testing—the common blood testing done by most physicians—can produce false calcium readings. It is problematic for other reasons, as well. A 2009 study from the University of Oxford proved that even though some patients' serum blood levels of B_{12} may appear normal, they might still have a B_{12} deficiency if their bodies do not produce enough transcobalamin-2 (proteins in the salivary glands that are meant to protect vitamin B_{12} from acid degradation in the stomach).[1] So, here again, an individual might have a blood test that shows sufficient levels of B_{12} and still be suffering from a B_{12} deficiency, which can lead to fatigue, memory problems, and cardiovascular disease.

A third problem with serum blood tests is that the results can vary depending on how much inflammation the body is experiencing. According to a 2012 study in the *American Journal of Clinical Nutrition*, a reliable clinical analysis of plasma (in blood) micronutrients can be made *only* when the degree of inflammation in the body is known. This is because the levels of several vitamins and minerals decrease by up to 40 percent when inflammation is present. Thus, low values do not necessarily indicate deficiency.[2] So, if your body is fighting an infection, for example, this causes an inflammatory response, which will make your blood levels of certain micronutrients appear lower. While this can be temporary, it may lead you to think you are more deficient than you really are, causing you to perhaps contemplate megadosing the deficient micronutrients (not good) or other more serious interventions. The bottom line is, at least in these circumstances, serum blood testing can fall short.

So, as you can see, serum blood work isn't perfect for identifying micronutrient status. However, in many cases, it is a decent starting point as long as you don't take it as gospel and rely on it alone. So, is there a better test? We would want one that looks at a greater spectrum of micronutrients so that it could offer a more complete analysis. Additionally, we would desire a test that measures the micronutrients in a whole new way, one that would have indicated that Darcie's calcium levels were deficient. Well, guess what? That technology is available, and it can really shed some light on whether your body has enough of the specific micronutrients it needs and if it is using them properly. This high-tech testing that we often suggest to clients is called a nutritional analysis, and a company called SpectraCell Laboratories performs it using patented technology.

Similar to serum testing, it all begins with a prick of the needle and blood being drawn. However, traditional serum testing only checks the amount of a specific micronutrient in the sample, whereas SpectraCell uses a method called essential metabolic analysis, which doesn't simply test the amount present in the sample but also measures how well a micronutrient works. It is a very complicated patented process, but through this, SpectraCell can determine the functionality of a specific micronutrient within a cell. And that information is far more important than the measurements given with a serum test, and it more closely estimates the status of a micronutrient, because the reason our cells use that micronutrient is to perform one of the functions necessary for life.

The Perfect Choice for Our Calculating Clients

We all know someone, or maybe you are that someone, who likes to see the data on things and measures progress by analyzing the numbers. We call these clients, who, by the way, are often some of the most successful, our "calculating clients." These individuals feel best when things are precise, so they thrive by turning in meticulous food journals, weight charts, and blood pressure measurements. For this group, a chart that shows quantified health improvements or precise amounts of weight loss is a great motivator for continued success on the plan. Are you one of these people? Would being able to chart precise improvements made in your sufficiency levels of specific micronutrients be motivating to you? If you can see yourself in this category, then a nutritional analysis prior to starting the Micronutrient Miracle plan may be right for you. If you do the blood work before starting and then retest a few months later, you will be able to see the progress you have made toward becoming sufficient in all of the micronutrients.

Several micronutrient analysis options can be purchased in the Micronutrient Miracle Motivation and Resource Center by visiting our Web site at mymiracleplan.com.

While many of our clients do choose to partake in some form of micronutrient testing and use it to measure their progress, we don't mandate this before starting the plan. Some people are squeamish about having their blood drawn. Others would rather invest the cost of the testing into upping their food quality or purchasing quality supplements. Either way, the testing is a bonus rather than a requirement. However, that doesn't mean that you don't have to take a test before starting your 28-day Micronutrient Miracle plan—it's just not a blood test.

The Personal Micronutrient Sufficiency Analysis

You already learned in the previous chapter that, statistically speaking, there is a high likelihood that you are deficient in micronutrients due to soil depletion from overfarming; GMOs; global food distribution; factory farming; and our modern food processing system, which further depletes the few micronutrients our food has left. But the story doesn't stop there. Each and every one of us is in some way either contributing to these deficiencies or reversing them through the choices we make in our diet, lifestyle, and supplementation habits each and every day. To help you identify (and then disarm) the micronutrient-depleting habits in your life, we created our Personal Micronutrient Sufficiency Analysis.

The first thing that we do when a client is interested in starting our plan is give them the very same micronutrient sufficiency analysis that we have provided here for you. It doesn't matter if that client already had a blood test of any

You can also take this exact analysis for free in the Micronutrient Miracle Motivation and Resource Center when visiting our Web site (mymiracleplan.com) and let us do the math, or you may choose to take our advanced diagnostic test called the Micronutrient Matrix, also on our site, for an additional fee. The Micronutrient Matrix is a much more detailed diagnostic tool, which examines your prescription medication and over-the-counter drug use, dietary habits, skin tone, and current multivitamin or supplement choices to help identify specific micronutrients you may be depleting. It also identifies the health conditions these deficiencies may be putting you at risk for. Many clients prefer the Micronutrient Matrix to blood testing for analyzing current micronutrient status as it considers both ingested micronutrients as well as risk factors for micronutrient depletion.

kind. Our analysis is different. We look at your dietary, lifestyle, and supplementation habits along with information on your current health status to identify the areas where you most need to improve. All you have to do is answer the questions honestly. Don't worry about how you score. Even if you don't score as high as you would like this time around, when you take the analysis again at the end of your 28-day plan, after implementing everything we are teaching you, your score is sure to impress. It may not be as scientific as blood work, but it does offer great insight into the likelihood of your being sufficient or deficient, and the more you learn about yourself and your micronutrient levels, the better equipped you will be to lose weight, improve your sleep, kill those food cravings, prevent disease, and finally have the knowledge to improve all aspects of your health.

Time to Test!

YOUR DIET	OFTEN	SOMETIMES	NEVER
1. I eat locally grown food.			
2. I eat organically grown food.			
3. I eat my food raw.			
4. I buy the majority of my food from a chain grocery store.			
5. I peel my fruits and vegetables.			
6. Fruits, vegetables, cheese, and meats may sit in my refrigerator or the grocery store refrigerator for a few days before being used.			
7. I eat out at restaurants more than two times a week.			
8. I eat grain-fed beef and store-bought cheese, eggs, and butter.			
9. I use canned or frozen vegetables.			
10. I eat potato chips, french fries, tortilla chips, nuts, or other salty snacks.			
11. I eat candy (gummy, hard, or anything else made of sugar).			
12. I take home and eat leftovers.			
13. I eat white bread, rolls, or traditional pasta.			
14. I drink carbonated sodas.			
15. I use products containing high fructose corn syrup (including salad dressing and ketchup).			
16. I eat dessertlike baked goods (muffins, croissants, cakes, biscuits, crepes, quiche).			
17. I eat spinach, collard greens, sweet potatoes, rhubarb, or beans.			

YOUR DIET	OFTEN	SOMETIMES	NEVER
18. I eat whole grain breads, corn, beans, grains (including cereal), or soy isolates.			
19. I eat nuts, apples, carrots, seeds (including flaxseeds), or oats.			
20. I drink pasteurized (grocery store–bought) milk.			
21. I drink alcohol (beer, wine, or spirits).			
22. I drink coffee, tea, or coffee drinks.			
23. I drink caffeinated sodas or energy drinks.			
24. I drink fruit juices or sports drinks sweetened with sugar or enhanced with high fructose corn syrup.			
YOUR LIFESTYLE	OFTEN	SOMETIMES	NEVER
25. I have stress in my life.			
26. I take any prescription medication (including birth control and medication for erectile dysfunction).			
27. I take aspirin or other over-the-counter pain and fever reducers (including acetaminophen and ibuprofen).			
28. I take antacids or laxatives.			
29. I smoke cigarettes, cigars, or a pipe or live with (or spend a large amount of time with) someone who does.			
30. I purchase conventional moisturizer, toothpaste, shampoo, or household cleaning products at the local grocery store.			
31. I live in a large or highly polluted city.			
32. I am physically active in a gym, at home, or outdoors (walking, bike riding, swimming).			
33. I skip meals.			
34. I follow a low-carbohydrate, low-fat, Paleo, Primal, Mediterranean, medically founded, or calorie-restricting diet.			
35. I eat at least 23,566 calories a day. (Twenty-three thousand five hundred and sixty-six calories. That's no typo! We'll explain this in Chapter 4.)			
36. I eat 5 servings of fruit and 5 servings of vegetables every day.			
37. I take fat burners, diuretics, or appetite suppressants.			
38. I have had surgery to help me lose weight. (Check "never" for no, "often" for yes.)			
39. I eat vegetarian, vegan, or gluten-free.			
40. I prepare meals ahead of time and refrigerate or freeze them to be eaten at a later date.			

(continued)

YOUR CURRENT HEALTH STATUS	OFTEN	SOMETIMES	NEVER
41. I feel lethargic.			
42. I have type 2 diabetes or have been diagnosed with prediabetes. (Check "never" for no, "often" for yes.)			
43. My physician has warned me about my elevated cholesterol levels. (Check "never" for no, "often" for yes.)			
44. My blood pressure is too high. (Check "never" for no, "often" for yes.)			
45. I feel depressed or anxious.			
46. I have been diagnosed with low bone density or have been told I am at risk for it. (Check "never" for no, "often" for yes.)			
47. I am currently overweight or obese. (Check "never" for no, "often" for yes.)			
48. I am currently underweight. (Check "never" for no, "often" for yes.)			
YOUR SUPPLEMENTATION ROUTINE	OFTEN	SOMETIMES	NEVER
49. I take a daily multivitamin/mineral supplement in a pill or capsule form.			
50. I take a liquid multivitamin supplement that is labeled to include Anti-Competition Technology.			

Time to Tally!

Step 1: Look at statements 1, 2, and 3. If you answered "often," give yourself a round of applause and **add 10 points** for each time you answered "often." **Add 5 points** for each time you answered "sometimes." Don't add any points if you answered "never." **TOTAL** _____

Step 2: For statements 4 through 34, **deduct 5 points** for every time you answered "often." **Deduct 3 points** for every time you answered "sometimes." Don't deduct any points if you answered "never." **TOTAL** _____

Step 3: Look at statement 35. If you answered "often," **add 100 points**. If you answered "sometimes," **add 50 points**. Don't do anything if you answered "never." **TOTAL** _____

Step 4: Look at statement 36. If you answered "often," **add 10 points**. If you answered "sometimes," **add 5 points**. Don't do anything if you answered "never." **TOTAL** _____

Step 5: For statements 37 through 46, **deduct 5 points** for every time you answered "often." **Deduct 3 points** for every time you answered "sometimes." Don't deduct any points if you answered "never." **TOTAL** _____

Step 6: Look at statements 47 and 48. If you answered "never," do nothing. If you answered "often" to either question, **deduct 20 points**. TOTAL _____
Step 7: Look at statement 49. If you answered "often," **add 10 points. Add 5 points** if you "sometimes" remember to take a multivitamin in pill or capsule form. **Deduct 10 points** if you answered "never." TOTAL _____
Step 8: If you answered "often" to statement 50, then bravo! **Add 100 points** to your score. You must be one very informed supplement consumer. And we'll tell you why that's important in Chapter 6. If you answered "sometimes," **add 50 points** and try to remember to take it more often. Do nothing if you answered "never." TOTAL _____
Step 9: Add up all the totals from Step 1 through Step 8.
GRAND TOTAL _____

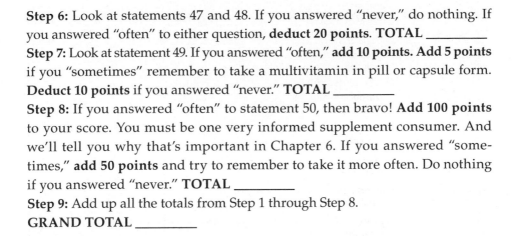

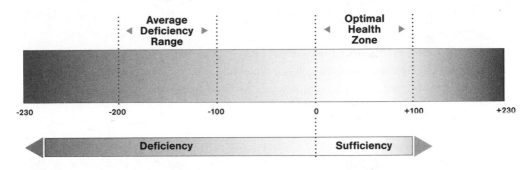

A Snapshot of Your Sufficiency Level

IF YOUR SCORE WAS NEGATIVE:

Your score indicates that you are not reaching micronutrient sufficiency. But don't worry if you have a low score, or even a *really* low score. If this is the case, get excited because the lower your score, the more you can improve. By reading this book, you'll learn our secrets to increase your micronutrient sufficiency level and dramatically improve your health.

Each chapter of this book will continue to offer you insight concerning the details of the analysis you just took, while building on one another to offer you the big picture on how your dietary, lifestyle, and supplementation habits impact your personal micronutrient sufficiency and, ultimately, your health. Our goal for you is to get your score into the Optimal Health Zone, where you'll be primed to see fast, dramatic results that can last a lifetime. Don't forget to take the analysis again at the end of your 28 days. When you follow the plan exactly as we outline it, your score and sufficiency level will both greatly improve. We believe in you!

IF YOUR SCORE WAS BETWEEN 0 AND 100:

Bravo! You are in the Optimal Health Zone, and for that, we salute you. Your score indicates that you are making great decisions to consume high-quality micronutrient-dense foods (maybe you read *Rich Food, Poor Food* already). It is likely that you have also eliminated a few micronutrient–robbing lifestyle habits, and perhaps you supplement using a properly formulated multivitamin. (You may even be taking our patented multivitamin nutreince already.)

Now, our goal for you is to keep your score in the Optimal Health Zone. You may not even know which things you have done right or how you scored so high. Following our Micronutrient Miracle plan will reveal to you the "healthy habits" that got you here, so you can make sure to continue them. It will also give you some great information on how to improve your score even further. This is a great starting point. Your sufficiency level means that you are primed to see fast, dramatic results that can last a lifetime.

IF YOUR SCORE WAS GREATER THAN 100:

Well, you actually scored over 100, above our Optimal Health Zone. And while it appears you are avoiding many everyday micronutrient depleters, you may also be missing some of these depleters' *positive* health benefits. For example, you may remember that in statement 32 we asked you about your physical activity level. Points would have been deducted for being physically active; however, the benefits of exercise far outweigh the micronutrient depletion from such exertion.

Pretty sneaky of us, huh? Although some of the healthier habits actually contribute to a lower level of micronutrient sufficiency, the truth is that we don't want you to give up all of these habits. As you continue reading this book, you will learn that while many of these lifestyle choices, or "healthy habits," deplete micronutrients, they also offer health benefits that should not be overlooked, and you may decide to add them back into your everyday life. Our goal for you is to get your score into the Optimal Health Zone (between 0 and 100), where your body can transform in exciting, unexpected, and, yes, miraculous ways.

Ready, Set, Go!

Up until this point we have been sharing with you the reasons why micronutrient sufficiency is so important. Now you understand that by becoming a nutrivore, you are taking personal responsibility for your health as well as taking a stand against the most widespread and dangerous health condition of the 21st century—micronutrient deficiency. You've personally examined which health issues in your life you might be able to reverse by becoming micronutrient sufficient, and you've analyzed, using our Personal Micronutrient Sufficiency Analysis, your own dietary, lifestyle, and supplementation habits to get a snapshot of where you currently fall on our micronutrient deficiency/sufficiency scale. You are now *ready* to start making some important changes in you life.

We know you will succeed, because we are going to be with you the whole time. In fact, this is a great time to come and explore our Micronutrient Miracle Motivation and Resource Center and sign up for our free, personally guided 28-day plan, which comes with money-saving coupons, bonus material, and daily tips and motivation. It's like having us as your personal concierge nutritionists, and it will put you on the fast track for success, so don't forget to sign up at mymiracleplan.com! But before you can start your plan, we need to arm you with the necessary tools and knowledge. In other words, we need to make sure that you are *set* up for success. Preparation is important for any great journey, and your 28-day Micronutrient Miracle plan is no different. It's now time for you to begin the prep work, such as purging micronutrient-poor foods from your pantry and restocking the shelves with micronutrient-rich choices. You will also need to pick which micronutrient-depleting lifestyle habits you can't live without and which ones you can say goodbye to. Lastly, you will want to get any supplements you are going to be using to help you reach micronutrient sufficiency during your 28-day plan so you can make sure you have them before you begin. Don't worry; on the next two pages, we supplied you with everything you need to successfully prepare for the 28-day Micronutrient Miracle plan. Just follow the timeline and you will be set up for success.

Once the prep work is complete, it's *go* time! Armed with fabulous recipes specifically designed to target your health concerns, your 28-day journey will begin to transform your health in ways you may never have imagined. Remember to expect the unexpected! Now, let's get that pantry purged. Who knows what we might find in there; this is going to be fun!

Your Micronutrient Miracle Program Planner

READY, SET, GO

We created the schedule below as a checklist that you can use to make sure you are ready to start your Micronutrient Miracle plan. It reviews all the things that you should do before starting and gives you a timeline that you can use to set yourself up for success. You may have already completed some of these tasks as you have been reading this book. However, in case you haven't, here are the tasks we want you to consider for your final week before "go day."

7 DAYS BEFORE "GO DAY"

TASK LIST

1. Make sure that you have read this book from the intro to the conclusion. After all, you can't eliminate the EMDs if you don't know where they are hiding or practice ZMT if you don't know what it stands for.

2. Go to the Micronutrient Miracle Motivation and Resource Center online at mymiracleplan.com and sign up for your free personally guided 28-day plan. This will allow us to send you daily tips that we couldn't fit into this book, as well as valuable Rich Food coupons, discounts on Calton Nutrition products, and a plethora of videos and downloads to help you succeed.

3. Purchase any supplements and products that you will need to start the plan. Make sure to include:
    a. Multivitamin (see page 178)
    b. Protein powder (see page 142)
    c. Fat source (see page 146)
    d. Omega-3 (see page 202)
    e. Any additional supplements noted under the special health conditions section you are going to follow (see Chapter 8)

4. Review the Top 10 Terrific Tips to Reduce Household Toxins on page 103. Choose which products you want to replace with nontoxic, healthy alternatives, and purchase any of the nontoxic specialty brands listed. Once you have them, purge your home of the toxic substances you are replacing.

5. **Optional:** Purchase a scale designed to measure body fat (see page 197).

6. **Optional:** Are you a "calculating client"? Purchase the nutritional analysis (see the box on page 41) from our Micronutrient Miracle Motivation and Resource Center and schedule your blood work. Alternatively, you may choose instead to take the Micronutrient Matrix online. This advanced micronutrient sufficiency analysis will give you a greater understanding of your current levels of deficiency for each micronutrient as well as the

health conditions and diseases that these deficiencies may currently be causing or can cause in the future.

5 TO 7 DAYS BEFORE "GO DAY"

TASK LIST

1. Purge the pantry following the guidelines in Chapter 3.
2. Look in the Micronutrient Miracle Motivation and Resource Center at mymiracleplan.com for online shopping suggestions and discounts to make the plan easier and more enjoyable. Ordering early guarantees that any speciality products ordered over the Internet will arrive to your home in plenty of time.

2 TO 5 DAYS BEFORE "GO DAY"

TASK LIST

1. Make sure your exercise plan is in place. Which days will you do your Zero Movement Training cardio workout? What are the One Set To Failure weight-training exercises you plan on starting with for each of the 4 days?
2. Review the first week's menu plan. Decide whether you will be following the Signature 28-day Micronutrient Miracle plan or one of the health condition–specific protocols. Swap out any foods or recipes you don't love and make a Rich Food shopping list.
3. Identify which de-stressing activities you are planning on using. Watch related videos in the Micronutrient Miracle Motivation and Resource Center to learn these beneficial techniques.
4. Print out the Fab 14 and Terrible 20 wallet guide at mymiracleplan.com to take on your grocery shopping expeditions.

1 TO 2 DAYS BEFORE "GO DAY"

TASK LIST

1. It's time to go shopping. Stock your fridge with all of the Rich Foods you will need to create meals that will build micronutrient sufficiency. Don't forget anything that you wrote down on your shopping list.
2. Soak or sprout any nuts, seeds, or grains you plan on using in the first week unless you purchased them already soaked or sprouted.
3. Premake any SKINNYFat Oil Infusions, Miracle Butters, Miracle Pestos, mayonnaise, and SKINNYFat salad dressings that you may want to enjoy during the plan (see pages 282 to 289). You can freeze your butters and pesto in ice cube trays to reduce your meal prep time.

3

The Pantry Purge

SO, ARE YOU READY to get started? Our first step is to set you up for success. Right now, there are likely a lot of products in your kitchen that could hurt your chances of reaching micronutrient sufficiency over the next 28 days. While some are easy to spot because the micronutrient-robbing ingredients are listed right on the label, other mischievous miracle blockers may be hiding in less obvious places. Get ready to take your first giant step toward sufficiency. It is time to Switch to Rich. So off we go to pass on the Poor Foods, oust the obesogens, and eliminate your Everyday Micronutrient Depleters. (Don't worry—we'll explain all of these terms as we go.)

It's Hard to Say Goodbye

Just as it's normal to get attached to the coworkers we see regularly at the office, it's also normal to get attached to familiar products that you purchase week after week for your home. That bag of your favorite chips or box of irresistible cookies that always seems to find its way into your shopping cart may be like a friend you can't wait to see after a hard day or a trusted shoulder to cry on after a fight with a loved one. However, some friends don't always have your back the way you'd want them to, and you have to reconsider the friendship. Is it a healthy relationship? Is this old friend even good for you?

Saying goodbye to an old friend can be hard, but we are going to ask you to be honest when you evaluate the products that you have befriended and invited into your home. As you will learn in this chapter, many of these products may have been taking more from you than they were giving back. Unlike other books that judge whether a food is "healthy" or not based on its calories, sodium, or fat content, our definition of healthy is based on how the food affects your micronutrient levels—in other words, whether a food contributes to or interferes with your ability to achieve micronutrient sufficiency.

Start this purging process early if you can, perhaps a week before your "go date." This will allow you time to decide which foods you want to gobble up before beginning the plan and which ones you want to bag up and give to coworkers or a local food bank. We suggest grabbing those large black lawn sacks and literally filling them with all of the unwanted Poor Foods you uncover. But it is your choice how you handle it. We have some clients who simply push things to the back of the fridge. We suggest you don't do that, though, since many people just don't have the willpower to pass by old friends as they call out to say hello. We prefer you take the Poor Foods out of the house. Out of sight, out of mind, as the saying goes.

Now, this might not be possible for those of you who have family members or roommates who are not starting the plan with you. To that we say, "Why aren't they?" We love when whole families take this extraordinary journey together. Parents are often amazed at the changes they see in their children, as their once hyperactive child, used to a diet filled with artificial colors and micronutrient-depleted food, calms almost overnight and exhibits a mental focus never before seen. And couples who have chosen to experience the Micronutrient Miracle together have reported extraordinary results, often with beneficial side effects they never counted on, as was the case with Winona and Rock (page 52).

If your family and friends still aren't convinced to join you for this transformation, then we suggest clearing out a shelf in the fridge *and* an area of the pantry to claim as your own for the next 28 days. Make sure to be firm with those sharing your home. Tell them that you would appreciate their support during this plan and that the best way for them to help is to make sure your designated space is a "no-touch zone" so that your foods are not disturbed in any way. Then, just wait—we bet your food is going to look so good to them and your results will be so impressive that they may just decide to join you after all!

Our Personal Micronutrient Miracle: Winona and Rock Keim

My name is Winona Keim. I am a 62-year-young wife, mother of three, and grandmother of eight. My husband, Rock, is the second youngest of six siblings, and I'm the second youngest of five. And we are the *only* ones in our families who are not on any medication. We cannot thank the Caltons enough for what their knowledge has done to help us stay healthy and lose weight, too!

I wish I could remember the exact day, but I don't. What I do remember is my exact reaction. I woke up one morning, kissed my sweet hubby, and sat down to a cup of coffee and the morning news, when Rock said he had something for me to see. He had recorded a segment from *Fox News* with Jayson and Mira Calton on their book *Rich Food, Poor Food*. I could not believe what I was hearing about the ingredients in our foods! I didn't even finish watching the news. I went straight to my cupboards and started reading every label. I threw out a ton of food that day and actually wondered what we were going to eat.

That day changed our lives forever. We started working with Jayson and Mira and began learning about reading labels and eating Rich Foods. I always thought we ate healthy, but now I know we do! Everything gets cooked or baked from scratch from healthy Rich Food ingredients. At first I wondered about the transition, but it was actually quite easy for us. Since starting the Micronutrient Miracle plan, we haven't eaten conventional store-bought beef; we eat wild game. And I do as much home canning as possible.

But what I didn't expect to happen actually started happening quickly—so quickly, at first, that I wondered if I was sick! I started losing weight. We hadn't thought of this as a weight-loss plan at all—simply a plan to get healthy. I struggled with 20-plus pounds for years, and Rock was overweight from inactivity due to some injuries. But we both started losing quite a bit of weight. And the thrill of realizing we could actually get our arms around each other again brought us further excitement, because I began to feel just a little bit sexy again! To date, Rock has lost 25 pounds and I've lost 20. I went from wearing a size large to a size small and have lost five pants sizes. And the fun part is that I didn't gain my normal "winter fat" storage of about 15 pounds.

People are surprised when they see me and wonder how I did it. And I don't hesitate to blast it all over the Internet! Thank you, Jayson and Mira, for all that you are doing. Thank you for sharing your knowledge and for opening my eyes. I pray that God will open people's eyes and ears to seeing and hearing your words of wisdom!

The Rich Food, Poor Food Philosophy

During the pantry purge, your goal is to identify the foods that could block your path to micronutrient sufficiency over the next 28 days. To help you with this evaluation, we created the Rich Food, Poor Food philosophy. We define Rich Foods as foods that help increase your micronutrient sufficiency levels and that are natural, unprocessed or minimally processed, high in micronutrients, and low in or devoid of problematic ingredients that can put your health at risk. Poor Foods, on the other hand, are highly processed and low in or devoid of micronutrients, and they often contain problematic ingredients such as everyday micronutrient depleters (EMDs), stealth thieves that rob you of vitamins, minerals, and essential fatty acids. (We will discuss EMDs in depth later in this chapter.) During your Micronutrient Miracle 28-day plan, your goal will be to eat as many Rich Foods as possible and to steer clear of Poor Foods.

Pass on the Worst Poor Food Perpetrators

Some foods are worse for you than others, so we'll tackle the very worst of the bunch first—the three Poor Food Perpetrators that we want you to completely eliminate for the next 28 days: sugar, wheat, and soy.

SACK THE SUGAR

Sugar is one of our absolute least favorite ingredients in the grocery store—and there are so many reasons why. A recent study conducted by the Wall Street bank Credit Suisse revealed the bitter truth about global sugar consumption. The study found that sugar makes up 17 percent of the global diet. The daily average consumption for the world is 17 teaspoons (68 grams), which is 45 percent higher than 30 years ago. In the United States, which tops the list for consumption, the amount is far greater; Americans average 40 teaspoons (160 grams) a day, or 3 pounds of sugar per week.[1, 2, 3] In 2014, the World Health Organization (WHO) recognized the not-so-sweet dangers of sugar and drafted guidelines recommending that people around the world limit consumption to 5 percent of their diets. This means that one of the most highly respected global health organizations thinks that 5 percent, or 25 grams, is the maximum amount of sugar you should take in daily. Did you know that a 16-ounce can of soda usually contains 40 grams? That is nearly double the amount deemed safe for an adult, and you don't even want to think about how damaging the amount of sugar in a single can of soda would be for a child.

So what makes sugar top of our list of Poor Food Perpetrators? Remember, on this plan, the micronutrients come first. And this perp is one of the biggest roadblocks on your path to micronutrient sufficiency because it can deplete your body's micronutrients as well as block micronutrients from being absorbed. Additionally, unlike other micronutrient-leaching ingredients you will meet later on, there is absolutely no evidence of any health or nutritional benefit to eating refined white sugar.

The Crave Cycle

While sugar's sweet flavor may be appetizing, its depletion of calcium, magnesium, chromium, and copper is not, especially when you consider the negative side effects of becoming deficient in these essential minerals. And vitamin C is also affected by sugar; because of similar chemical structures, vitamin C and glucose (a type of sugar) compete for entry into your cells. Even slightly elevated blood sugar levels can block vitamin C from getting in and can cause a weakened immune system. Take a look at the table below to get a better idea of just how many health conditions and diseases your sugar consumption could be putting you at risk for.

TABLE 3.1
MICRONUTRIENTS DEPLETED BY SUGAR[4]

MICRONUTRIENT	WHAT IT DOES	SYMPTOMS AND PROBLEMS
Vitamin C	Protects from cardiovascular diseases, cancers, joint diseases, cataracts, and the common cold; aids in collagen and elastin synthesis, both necessary elements in bone matrix, skin, tooth dentin, blood vessels, and tendons; protects against oxygen-based damage to cells (free radicals); required for fat synthesis; has antiviral and detoxifying properties; helps to heal wounds	Inability to heal wounds; frequent infections, colds, or flu; lung-related problems; easy bruising; tender, swollen joints; lack of energy; bleeding gums; nosebleeds; anxiety; tooth decay; visceral (belly) fat
Calcium	Required for bone and tooth formation, muscle contraction, blood clotting, and nerve transmission; reduces the risk of colon cancer; prevents hypertension	Osteoporosis, osteomalacia, osteoarthritis, rickets, muscle pain or cramps, tooth decay, colon cancer risk, high blood pressure, PMS, sugar and salt cravings, bone pain, numbness or tingling in extremities, insomnia

TABLE 3.1 (CONT.)		
MICRONUTRIENT	**WHAT IT DOES**	**SYMPTOMS AND PROBLEMS**
Chromium	Assists insulin function, increases fertility, required for carbohydrate/fat metabolism, essential for fetal growth/ development, helps lower elevated serum cholesterol and triglycerides	Metabolic syndrome, insulin resistance, decreased fertility, diabetes, obesity, hypoglycemia, cold hands, cardiovascular disease, high cholesterol, cold sweats, need for frequent meals
Copper	Required for bone formation, energy production, hair and skin coloring, and taste sensitivity; involved in healing process; aids in iron transport; helps metabolize several fatty acids	Osteoporosis, anemia, baldness, diarrhea, general weakness, impaired respiratory function, myelopathy, decreased skin and hair pigment, reduced resistance to infection, elevated LDL cholesterol, binge eating, fatigue, low body temperature
Magnesium	Involved in 300 essential metabolic reactions; necessary for muscle activity and nerve impulses; regulates temperature and blood pressure; essential for detoxification; aids in creating strong bones and teeth	Sugar cravings, nausea, vomiting, fatigue, cramps, numbness, tingling, seizures, heart spasms, personality changes, increased heart rhythm, hypertension, coronary heart disease, osteoporosis, asthma, constipation, insomnia, depression

Do you crave sweet foods and then find that one bite leads to two and then three? If you answered yes, then you are not alone. In fact, according to research from Philadelphia's Monell Chemical Senses Center, "food cravings are extremely common. . . . Close to 100 percent of young adult females and about 70 percent of young men report having experienced one or more food cravings at some time in the past year."[5] This is an important fact because uncontrollable cravings are one of the major reasons people fall off their diets. Researchers found that "food cravings are clearly a separate phenomenon from hunger." So if those unyielding cravings that wake you up in the middle of the night insisting on a bowl of ice cream are not from hunger, then what is causing them? Would you believe it is a deficiency in specific micronutrients?

As you can see from the table above, when your body ingests sugar, your calcium and magnesium levels can become diminished. And guess what scientists discovered happens when those levels fall short? You crave sugar! That is why one bite leads to another and then another. And with every bite, your levels of calcium and magnesium are further reduced, increasing your desire for more sugar. Your internal "cravings monster" calls out louder and louder, and there are only two ways to quiet him. First, you can continue on the path to deficiency and obesity by eating more and more sugar (with every bite making it more likely you will get osteoporosis and other deficiency diseases),

My Personal Micronutrient Miracle: Evelyn Mann

I've been working with the Caltons for over a year now. It all began when I read their second book, *Rich Food, Poor Food*, after my mother-in-law passed away from colon cancer. I'd always found reading food labels to be confusing, and to be honest, I didn't read them at all. Reading that book gave me the key to understanding food labels and taught me the importance of the micronutrients in the foods I eat. I took the first step on my own and began eating Rich Foods as well as eliminating sugar and wheat from my diet. It was a miracle. I was amazed at how my sugar cravings were wiped out within just weeks. My need for a nightly bowl of ice cream simply vanished. No more late-night runs to the store for my must-have ice cream.

However, I knew I had to do more. I suffered from intense headaches and was diagnosed with an ovarian cyst. I contacted Mira and Jayson and began my own Micronutrient Miracle plan. I added in supplementation with nutreince, their multivitamin drink, and within 10 days the headaches were gone. Could it have been that I was getting headaches due to a lack of adequate vitamins and minerals? It sure seemed so. The biggest miracle of all, though, was that my cyst went away, as well. My prayers, and those of my friends and family, had been answered.

On top of having lost my cravings, my headaches, and my cyst, I realized I had lost something else. I had lost 10 pounds of weight without any additional effort. My husband was so impressed that he joined in, and immediately I noticed he had a lot more energy. (Who wouldn't want a husband with more energy?) I thought that was just great! Now my brother and his wife are on the program and loving it. They are experiencing huge increases in energy, as well as noticeable improvements in eyesight. I knew I had to share my knowledge, so I started teaching what I had learned from the Caltons in church, and I have personally witnessed the joy in others as they report losing weight and experiencing decreased pain and inflammation by adopting this micronutrient sufficient way of life.

or you can stop the cycle altogether by simply becoming sufficient in calcium and magnesium. It really is that easy.

But wait, there's more good news. Not only will you kill the cravings for sugar with this one easy step, but if you are a person who craves salty snacks, like pretzels or chips, research shows these cravings will be eliminated as well. Monell researchers determined that salt cravings are also caused by a deficiency in calcium.[6] They found that when you snack on something salty, the sodium temporarily increases calcium in the blood, which tricks your body into thinking the calcium deficiency is over. However, while your salt craving may be temporarily satisfied, the secreted bone calcium leads to an exacerbated calcium deficiency, further salt cravings, and possibly more cravings for sugar, as well!

The Micronutrient Miracle plan is about to take you out of "The Crave Cycle" and put you and your willpower back in control. First, through eating Rich Foods and supplementing smart, any calcium or magnesium deficiencies you may have will be eliminated. And no deficiencies mean no cravings. Additionally, by avoiding sugar, you will be avoiding any further micronutrient depletions, which will help to break the vicious Crave Cycle and quiet that crave monster for good.

High Fructose Corn Syrup: A Syr-*up* You Should Put *Down*

Sugar has a sweet little sidekick that we also want you to sack. It's high fructose corn syrup (HFCS)—also known as glucose/fructose in Canada or glucose/fructose syrup in the United Kingdom—which is made by refining cornstarch. HFCS's popularity has skyrocketed by 472 percent since the 1970s, when, due to manufacturing advances, it became cheaper to produce than sugar.[7]

While it's bad enough that the excessive production of this monoculture crop (corn) robs the soil of its micronutrient content, that is nothing compared to the micronutrient-depleting effects this ingredient has on your body. Fructose has been shown to have a negative effect on calcium, chromium, magnesium, zinc, and copper levels in the body. The more fructose you take in, the more your body becomes depleted of these micronutrients. So how much fructose is hiding in your HFCS? A 2010 study published in the *International Journal of Obesity* shed light on the true levels of fructose found in the HFCS in 23 common sweetened beverages. While federal law specifically defines HFCS as a "mixture containing either approximately 42 or 55 percent fructose" (the ingredient depleting our micronutrients), the researchers found that many soft drinks contain HFCS with fructose levels as high as 65 percent. [8,9] Remember, the greater the amount of fructose, the greater the risk for micronutrient depletion. And to make matters worse, in 2014 food manufacturers figured out that seeing HFCS on labels was a real turnoff. So what did they do? They created a new product to get around this stigma. HFCS-90 is the name of this new villain, which you will simply see as "fructose" on labels, and it is 90 percent fructose syrup. This new sweetener, found now in numerous products touting no HFCS,

Six More Reasons to Sack the Sugar and Syrup

As if micronutrient depletion and overeating aren't enough, here are six more reasons to eliminate sugar and HFCS from your diet.

1. **It is most likely genetically modified (GMO).** When you think of sugar, what comes to mind? Do you imagine a sugarcane plantation? Well, if you do, we need to introduce you to the sad reality of 21st century sugar. The truth is that 55 percent of the time you see sugar on the ingredients list it's coming from the juice of a sugar beet, and, unfortunately, 100 percent of US sugar beets are genetically modified.[10, 11] And with 88 percent of all US corn being genetically modified, your odds aren't much better when HFCS is on the label.[12] (See more on the dangers of GMOs on page 122.)

2. **Sugar is an addictive drug.** Researchers in Bordeaux, France, demonstrated that "intense sweetness can surpass cocaine reward."[13] Yes, your gummy bears are more addictive than cocaine. No wonder so many people just can't stop with one. Scientists from Princeton University explain that, like many drugs, sugar causes a dopamine (or pleasure) surge in the brain and that removing sugar causes an opiate-like withdrawal symptoms "indicated by signs of anxiety and behavioral depression."[14]

3. **Sugar can cause insulin resistance.** When you eat sugar, your blood sugar levels increase and your body secretes the hormone insulin to help regulate the levels. A diet filled with sugar causes the cells to become deaf, or resistant, to insulin, and insulin resistance, as it is termed, can lead to metabolic syndrome, obesity, cardiovascular disease, and type 2 diabetes.[15] And surprisingly, it doesn't take very much sugar to see these negative effects. In a Harvard University study, researchers reported that drinking just one sugar-sweetened beverage a day increased the risk of type 2 diabetes by 83 percent.[16]

4. **Sugar can cause cancer.** Cancer, one of the leading causes of death worldwide, is characterized by uncontrolled growth and multiplication of cells. According to Lewis Cantley, PhD, director of the Cancer Center at Beth Israel Deaconess Medical Center in Boston, as much as 80 percent

such as cereals by General Mills, adds an even higher level of micronutrient-depleting fructose to every bite.

Additionally, HFCS is an obesogen (pronounced obese-o-gen)—a natural or man-made chemical that affects the regulatory system that controls your weight (endocrine system), increasing the fat cells you have, decreasing the calories you burn, and even altering the way your body manages hunger. A 2013 study of all cancers are "driven by either mutations or environmental factors that work to enhance or mimic the effect of insulin on the incipient tumor cells."[17] As we just revealed, increases in sugar result in increases of insulin. For this reason, many scientists believe that having constantly elevated insulin levels (a consequence of sugar consumption) can greatly increase the risk of cancer.[18, 19] Additionally, research has shown that cancer only has one fuel source. Can you guess what it is? Sugar! Not only is sugar compromising your immune system and creating a favorable environment for cancer to start, but it's also providing the fuel that cancer needs to grow.[20]

5. **Sugar intake correlates to heart disease.** Thank goodness science is finally calling it like it is. For many years, saturated fat had been vilified as the cause of heart disease, the number-one killer in the world. But recently, the truth has come out that sugar, in all of its forms, is really to blame. According to a 2014 study in the journal *JAMA Internal Medicine*, individuals who received between 17 and 21 percent of their calories from added sugar had a 38 percent higher risk of dying from cardiovascular disease compared to those who consumed just 8 percent of their calories from added sugars.[21]

6. **Sugar shortens your lifespan.** If you are looking to live a long life, then stop with the sodas and sugary beverages. A 2014 study published in the *American Journal of Public Health* found that telomeres—protective DNA caps on the ends of chromosomes—were shorter in people who reported habitually drinking more sugary beverages. Shorter telomeres are linked to accelerated DNA aging, and individuals who drank only 12 ounces of soda a day (a typical bottle) were found to have DNA changes typical of cells 4.6 years older. Kick the sugar habit before this soda-induced telomere shortening strikes years off your life.[22]

Whoa! Both sugar and HFCS really do deserve to be ditched. Due to sugar's micronutrient-depleting effects, as well as all of the other health conditions and diseases it can increase your risk for, we are going to sack the sugar for the next 28 days.

out of Yale University revealed that volunteers who ingested fructose did not have activity in the part of the brain that recognized satiety and therefore felt hungrier. This is because, unlike sugar, fructose does not trigger the secretion of leptin, a hormone that tells your brain when you are full.[23] To add insult to injury, a 2013 study in the *Journal of Clinical Endocrinology & Metabolism* determined that this is compounded due to the fact that fructose-laden beverages increase circulation of the hormone ghrelin, whose primary job is to signal hunger to the brain,[24] meaning that eating foods high in fructose, including HFCS, not only will cause your body to *not* feel full but will actually make you hungrier, setting the stage for overeating.

The Sinister Sugar Substitutes

Companies know how attracted we are to sweet foods. That is why food chemical companies have spent millions of dollars creating sugar substitutes that satisfy your sweet tooth without increasing your muffin top. While these sinister sugar substitutes don't rob you of your micronutrients, like sugar and HFCS do, scientific data suggests that they too can be detrimental to your health. In fact, a 2014 study warns that the artificial sweeteners saccharin, sucralose, and aspartame—more commonly known by the popular brand names Sweet'N Low, Splenda, and Equal, respectively—are likely disrupting the microbiome, a vast and enigmatic ecosystem of bacteria in our guts. This is extremely dangerous, as this microbial world plays a fundamental role in one's ability to fight disease, and 57 percent of volunteers who ingested these sweeteners for only one single week saw significant glucose intolerance, a condition that can lead to diabetes. These offenders will also be off-limits.

TABLE 3.2	
SINISTER SUGAR SUBSTITUTES TO SACK	
SINISTER SUGAR SUBSTITUTE	**AKA—KNOWN ALIASES**
Sucralose	Splenda, Sukrana, SucraPlus, CandyS, Cukren, Nevella, and E955 (European Union)
Acesulfame potassium	Acesulfame K, Sunett, Sweet One, and E950 (European Union)
Aspartame	NutraSweet, Equal, AminoSweet, Canderel, Spoonful, Equal-Measure, and E951 (European Union)
Neotame	Newtame and E961 (European Union)
Saccharin	Sweet'N Low, Sugar Twin, and E954 (European Union)
Advantame	The newest (2014) and sweetest addition to the aspartame/neotame family

Send All the Sugars Packing

Don't think that it's just your sweet treats—such as sodas, sugar-laden cereals, cookies, and cakes—that contain sugar. Did you know that condiments, like ketchup and mayonnaise, are likely filled with sugar, too? In fact, even many brands of table salts, including the popular brand Morton with the cute little girl with the umbrella logo, contain sugar. Almost everything from frozen pizzas, canned soups, and "healthy" juices and yogurts are sneaking in sugar these days. It's true! So in order to eliminate this Poor Food Perpetrator from your home, you are going to have to get in the habit of reading all your ingredients lists carefully for the next 4 weeks.

But watch out: Food manufacturers can be really sneaky, using numerous aliases on their packaging. However, you are going to outsmart them using the list below. If you find any of these sneaky aliases on the ingredients list, the food needs to be exiled—out of the fridge and pantry and into the giveaway or throwaway sack. Your pantry purge starts now. Remove all of the products in your refrigerator, freezer, and pantry that contain the ingredients listed below, as well as those sinister sugar substitutes in Table 3.2. If you see stevia, stevia rebaudiana, xylitol, monk fruit, loa han (guo or kuo), erythritol, sorbitol, mannitol, or coconut sugar in the ingredients list without any of the names listed in Tables 3.2 and 3.3, you can keep that food in your pantry for now. We will talk more about stevia and other Rich Food sugar substitutes in Chapter 5.

TABLE 3.3
THE MANY NAMES FOR SUGAR

Don't let manufacturers fool you. All of these aliases need to be avoided.

Barley malt	Demerara sugar	Invert sugar
Beet sugar	Dextrin	Lactose
Blackstrap molasses	Dextrose	Maltodextrin
Brown sugar	Diastase	Maltose
Cane juice crystals	Diastatic malt	Malt syrup
Cane sugar	D-mannose	Maple syrup
Caramel	Evaporated cane juice	Molasses
Carob syrup	Fructose	Raw sugar
Castor sugar	Fruit juice concentrate	Rice syrup
Confectioner's sugar	Galactose	Sucrose
Corn sweeteners	Glucose	Syrup
Corn syrup	High fructose corn syrup (HFCS)	Treacle
Crystalline fructose	Honey	Turbinado sugar
Date sugar		

WHACK THE WHEAT

Imagine you are sitting at an Italian restaurant waiting for your entrée to arrive. The conversation with family or friends is flowing as the waitress brings over a basket filled with warm, fresh bread. The yeasty aroma entices you, and you quickly reach in and grab a small piece. When your entrée arrives, you glance down at your bread plate, shocked to realize that you have already eaten two slices. Sound familiar? The addictive nature of food is quite amazing, when you start to think about it.

Wheat's addictive nature is due to a protein called gliadin that, when digested by stomach acids and enzymes, becomes an exorphin, a morphinelike compound that binds to opiate receptors in your brain. Unlike other opiates that relieve pain, these exorphins cause addictive behavior and appetite stimulation that can result in the consumption of more than 400 additional calories every day![25] So that waitress is unknowingly acting as a drug dealer—serving up warm breadbaskets filled with obesity-inducing exorphins.

While gliadin makes wheat addictive, like sugar, it is really the other micronutrient-depleting parts of wheat that we want you to focus on. First, wheat naturally contains phytic acid, which binds to and blocks the absorption of calcium, magnesium, copper, manganese, chromium, iron, zinc, and niacin and accelerates the metabolism of vitamin D, causing the body to use up this important antiobesity vitamin at a faster rate. Secondly, wheat contains oxalic acid, which binds to calcium, magnesium, and iron and blocks their absorption. Thirdly, wheat contains lectins, which are a plant's natural self-defense mechanism. While lectins are good for plants, they are not good for humans to eat. Their stickiness causes them to bind to your intestinal tract, and because we require a clear intestinal tract to properly absorb vitamins and minerals, lectins have been shown to reduce micronutrient absorption and should be avoided.

Lectins also work alongside gluten, another bothersome protein in wheat. You may have already heard of gluten or be among the 30 to 50 percent of the population that has a gluten sensitivity. You may even be the 1 out of every 133 Americans that is diagnosed with celiac disease, a genetic condition resulting in intestinal damage whenever gluten is ingested. However, you may also be one of the people needlessly suffering from digestive problems, headaches, eczema-like skin symptoms, brain fog, and fatigue who have not yet realized that the gluten in your food is causing these conditions.

Lectins and gluten work together to give you a real one-two punch to the stomach, causing a condition known as leaky gut. *Leaky gut* is the term for a breach in the intestinal lining. You see, your gut should be a tightly sealed area so that the undigested food you eat stays inside, where it belongs. When you ingest wheat, lectins throw the first punch by causing intestinal permeability. Then, gluten throws the second punch by triggering the release of zonulin (no, we aren't making up these intergalactic-sounding names). The evil zonulin destroys the seals in the walls of the intestines, making it possible for an intestinal breach to occur.[26]

Once the intestinal breach exists, lectins, along with other particles, like partially digested food and toxins, can "leak" into the bloodstream. Your body views these escapees as unwelcome foreign invaders and begins a direct attack on these particles, leading to autoimmune mayhem and opening up the door to disorders like irritable bowel syndrome, Crohn's, colitis, thyroiditis, fibromyalgia, chronic fatigue syndrome, and arthritis.

The final downfall of wheat is something called amylopectin A, which is responsible for the expansion of visceral fat (unhealthy fat that surrounds the organs) in the abdomen, often referred to as the "wheat belly." It is also responsible for the high blood sugar spike caused by eating wheat. Yes, wheat! Did you know that eating a slice of whole wheat bread can spike your insulin more than a candy bar?[27] It's true. And what did we just learn about spiking insulin in our discussion on sugar? This very high wheat-induced insulin spike can lead to insulin resistance, obesity, diabetes, heart disease, and even cancer.

Say Goodbye to All the Glutenous Goons

We hope you can now understand how all the various components of wheat work together to deplete your micronutrients and increase your risk for serious illness and disease. So, what are you waiting for? For the next 28 days, we want you to whack the wheat as well as all of the other products in which wheat and its most notable sidekick, gluten, are hiding. Table 3.4 on page 64 lists products where wheat and gluten most commonly hide. Read the ingredients lists carefully. Luckily, label reading for wheat has become much easier since the Food Allergen Labeling and Consumer Protection Act was passed in 2004. This regulation requires that the top eight allergens be clearly identified, wheat being one of them. So, if a food product contains a derivative of wheat, such as modified food starch, it must clearly indicate that wheat is the source. *Wheat* can appear either in parentheses in the ingredient list or in a separate "contains" statement. Regardless, it must always be labeled, so you can rest assured that you will get the facts if you check the label. Now get to it. Pack away those products. These glutenous goons have to go!

TABLE 3.4
WHERE GLUTEN IS HIDING

Bread crumbs

Baked beans

Biscuits or cookies

Bread and rolls

Brown rice syrup

Bulgur wheat

Cakes

Cheap brands of
chocolate

Chutneys and pickles
(made with malt
vinegar)

Couscous

Crispbreads

Crumble toppings

Farina

Gravy powders and
stock cubes

Hydrolyzed vegetable
protein (HVP)

Imitation crab meat

Instant coffee

Kamut (ancient grain)

Licorice

Lunch meat (may
contain fillers)

Malted drinks

Malt vinegar

Many salad dressings

Matzo flour/meal

Meat and fish pastes

Most breakfast cereals

Muesli

Muffins

Pancakes

Pasta

Pastry or pie crust

Pâtés

Pizza

Potato chips

Pretzels

Pumpernickel

Rye bread

Sauces (often
thickened with flour)

Sausages

Scones

Seitan (doesn't
contain gluten;
it *is* gluten!)

Self-basting turkeys

Some blue cheeses

Soups (often
thickened with flour)

Soy sauce

Spelt (ancient grain)

Spice mixes

Stuffing

Waffles

White pepper

Yorkshire pudding

SAY IT AIN'T SOY

Looking for a nice set of "man boobs"? Trying to slow down your metabolism? If you answered yes to either of those questions, then make sure to keep soy *in* your diet. Did you know that eating soy products—including soy milk, soy sauce, and even that soy lecithin that somehow snuck into your protein shake or chocolate bar—can disrupt your sex hormones?[28, 29] Now, that should make both the men and women reading this perk up and pay attention. It's true. Soy contains isoflavones, a class of compounds known as phytoestrogens, meaning an estrogen that comes from plants. And phytoestrogens have been shown to mimic the effects of the female hormone estrogen in the body.

For the ladies out there, a study in the *American Journal of Clinical Nutrition* looked at the effects of soy on menstruation and determined that eating soy products significantly delayed menstruation and shortened cycles. While that may sound appealing, in reality, science shows that this results in a higher risk for breast cancer.[30] And for you gents out there, or wives that care about the masculinity of your man, a recent study found that men who took 56 grams of soy protein powder over 28 days experienced a 19 percent drop in testosterone. It makes sense, doesn't it? Give a man isoflavones mimicking estrogen, a female hormone, and what would you expect to happen? This hormone imbalance (excessive estrogen in relation to testosterone) can also lead to sexual dysfunction, reduced body hair, and even gynecomastia—the abnormal enlargement of breast tissue in males (aka man boobs). A 2004 National Cancer Institute study even revealed that men eating high levels of soy (megadosing) experienced "nipple discharge, breast enlargement, and hot flashes."[31]

Now, if the threat of breast cancer and man boobs is not enough, how about weight gain? For both genders, testosterone is a vital hormone for growth, repair, red blood cell formation, healthy sleep cycles, and immune function, in addition to proper sexual function.[32] Low levels of testosterone have also been linked to low thyroid function, another unwanted and common side effect of soy consumption. And as if all this wasn't enough, soy contains goitrogens, substances that further suppress the function of the thyroid gland and interfere with the absorption of iodine. This can cause an enlarged thyroid gland and result in weight gain—especially for the two out of three women who have borderline hypothyroidism.

A 2013 study published in the *Journal of Clinical Endocrinology & Metabolism* found that a diet high in soy reduced levels of adiponectin—a hormone involved in regulating blood sugar and fat levels.[33] This increases the likelihood that your body will store fat rather than burn it for fuel. While storing fat is bad, making additional fat cells might be even worse, and that is exactly what eating soy can do for you. Soy also contains two naturally occurring chemicals, genistein and daidzein, both of which are estrogenics that can spur the formation of fat cells. This means that your soy latte for breakfast is a real loser for your muffin top. Due to all of these changes to your endocrine system and metabolism from eating soy, it is considered one of those nasty obesogens for sure.

Oh, there's one more thing we didn't want to leave out: Low levels of testosterone in both men and women lead to a low libido. So, say sayonara to soy to increase your sex drive.

Soy's Abundance of Antinutrients

Above and beyond the numerous drawbacks we just outlined, this Asian import also contains an abundance of antinutrients just waiting to deplete your micronutrient levels. First off, soy contains Everyday Micronutrient

Depleters—phytic acid, oxalic acid, and lectins, which you learned about earlier in the section on wheat. So, that edamame starter (yes, edamame is soybeans) at the Japanese restaurant is lowering your levels of calcium, magnesium, copper, manganese, chromium, iron, zinc, niacin, and vitamin D. The depletion of the bone-builders (calcium, magnesium, copper, manganese, zinc, and vitamin D) alone makes soy a poor choice for anyone looking to improve or maintain bone health.

Soy also contains trypsin inhibitors, a fourth type of antinutrient. Trypsin is an enzyme produced in the pancreas that is needed to digest protein and break it down into its constituent parts, known as amino acids. Trypsin inhibitors have been shown to prevent the pancreas from producing the amount of trypsin necessary for the normal breakdown of protein into amino acids. Remember, amino acids are one of the four types of essential micronutrients. They are the building blocks of life—chemical units that enable the cells to maintain their structure. They are responsible for a variety of functions in the body, from building muscle to protecting your heart to transporting, metabolizing, and storing macronutrients (fat, carbohydrates, and proteins). As you can see, amino acids really are *essential* for your good health. Because of this, we recommend eliminating soy (as well as other foods that contain a high amount of trypsin inhibitors) from your diet.

Miso (Me So) Sorry—GMO Soy Is Everywhere!

Since the 1950s, global production of this "king bean" has skyrocketed, increasing 15 times over. Together, the United States, Brazil, and Argentina produce about 80 percent of the world's soy.[34] Unfortunately, according to 2014 USDA statistics, 94 percent of the US soy produced is genetically modified.[35] (Make sure to see Chapter 5 to read up on all the reasons to avoid GMOs.) This new supercheap soy is pervasive in our foods. You can find it in obvious spots, like soy sauce and tofu burgers, but because many farmers use GMO soymeal as an inexpensive feed to fatten up cattle, we are consuming a great deal of it through the animal sources and dairy that we eat and drink. Additionally, soybean oil, often listed as vegetable oil on labels, makes up 27 percent of the worldwide oil production, making it one of the most common forms of oil at the dinner table. In order to avoid soy for the next 28 days, you are going to have to read labels carefully. Because it is an allergen, just like wheat, it must always be clearly labeled on packaging. So grab your throwaway sacks and send the soy packing now.

TABLE 3.5
WHERE SOY IS HIDING

Animal feed of nonorganic meats	Protein bars and shakes	Tea bags
Asian foods	Salad dressings	Tempeh and miso
Chocolate bars	Soy lecithin (Watch out for this!)	Teriyaki sauce
Mayonnaise		Tofu
Prepared foods	Soy protein powders	Vegetable oil
	Soy sauce	Veggie burgers

OUST THESE OBESOGENS

You have now removed the worst Poor Food Perpetrators from your home. And as we mentioned, two of these perpetrators (HFCS and soy) are also considered obesogens because they contain chemicals that disrupt the endocrine system and promote weight gain. They make you pack on the pounds by increasing the number of fat cells in the body, promoting fat storage, altering metabolism in favor of storing calories as opposed to burning them, and directly affecting the hormones responsible for appetite and satiety. Both HFCS and soy have obesogenic and micronutrient-depleting effects, but they aren't alone. We will now turn our gaze to additional obesogens to oust from your home—all of which can not only increase your weight but also decrease the likelihood of you reaching micronutrient sufficiency.

Menacing Monosodium Glutamate (MSG)

Food manufacturers just love it when you can't stop with a single serving. For them, it is the sound of cash registers ringing in sales. But what does this mean to us? It means that somehow the food is now in control. Somehow it has been manipulated to cause you to overeat. Monosodium glutamate is the go-to add-in to create this desired effect. So much so that this menacing flavor enhancer is found in almost all processed and packaged foods in the United States. MSG-induced obesity is such an accepted concept in scientific circles that when studies require obese animals, the first thing they are given is MSG. Scientists in Spain found that giving laboratory rats MSG increased food intake by 40 percent.[36]

MSG works as an obesogen in three distinct obesity-inducing ways. The most obvious way is that it intensifies the tastiness of any treat, and this makes you desire it even more. Second, MSG has been shown to make us leptin resistant. Remember that leptin is the hormone that makes you feel full. Why would you ever put down a snack if your brain never gets the message to stop eating it? Finally, MSG causes the secretion of insulin, your fat-storage hormone, which drops your blood sugar and makes you hungrier faster.

However, this Poor Food ingredient also reduces our micronutrient levels because it is an *excitotoxin*. This means it can cross the blood–brain barrier and overexcite your cells to the point of damage or death, causing brain damage to varying degrees and potentially even triggering or worsening learning disabilities, Alzheimer's disease, Parkinson's disease, Lou Gehrig's disease, and more. It's true—and your micronutrient levels pay the price because your available antioxidants are used at an accelerated rate when trying to repair MSG brain toxicity. Rather than performing other important functions in your body, available antioxidants—such as vitamins C and E and selenium—are called on to repair the damage. Additionally, magnesium, chromium, and zinc are all very important protectors of neural cells, so their use is also accelerated in the presence of MSG.[37, 38] Can you imagine how many other essential bodily functions may not be able to be performed properly because food manufacturers snuck MSG into the recipe?

TABLE 3.6
THE MANY NAMES FOR MSG

Don't let manufacturers fool you. All of these aliases need to be avoided.

Autolyzed yeast	Magnesium glutamate	Soy sauce
Autolyzed yeast protein	Monoammonium glutamate	Textured protein
Calcium glutamate		Vegetable extract
Carrageenan	Monopotassium glutamate	Yeast extract
Glutamate		Yeast food
Glutamic acid	Natural flavors (ask manufacturers their sources, to be safe)	
Hydrolyzed corn		
Ingredients listed as hydrolyzed, protein fortified, ultra-pasteurized, fermented, or enzyme modified	Pectin	
	Sodium caseinate	
	Soy isolate	

Pitch the Plastics

The final obesogens we are going to discuss will not be listed on labels, but chances are you have recently ingested these plastics. What? You don't eat plastic? Fat chance! Odds have it that you're among the 93 percent of Americans with detectable levels of bisphenol A (BPA) in their bodies and also among the 75-plus percent of Americans with phthalates in their urine.[39, 40] Statistics seem to show us that we are not only what we eat but also what we touch *and* what touches what we eat.

Both BPA and phthalates are synthetic chemicals that mimic estrogen in the body. BPA can be found in reusable drink containers, toilet paper, DVDs, cell phones, eyeglass lenses, and automobile parts. In the grocery store, you are most likely to come in contact with it in its polycarbonate plastic form in water bottles and in its epoxy form in the linings of food cans. It is even in the thermal paper used for cash register receipts. Phthalates can be found in food packaging, plastic wraps, pesticides, many children's toys, PVC pipes, air fresheners, laundry products, personal care products, and even in medical supplies. Each year about 6 billion pounds of BPA and 18 billion pounds of phthalate esters are created worldwide—that's a lot of problematic pound-producing plastics![41]

In a 2012 study published in the journal *PLoS ONE*, research indicated that BPA triggers the release of almost double the insulin actually needed to break down food.[42] High insulin levels can desensitize the body to this hormone over time, which in some people may then lead to weight gain and type 2 diabetes. Research published in the *Journal of Clinical Endocrinology & Metabolism* in 2014 proved that men, women, and children exposed to high levels of endocrine-disrupting phthalates tended to have reduced levels of testosterone in their blood compared to those with lower chemical exposure. And in a recent study, several prevalent phthalate metabolites showed statistically significant correlations with abdominal obesity and insulin resistance in American men.[43] But, here again, the damage isn't only to your waistline. Research indicates that both BPA and phthalates affect calcium absorption at the cellular level.[44, 45]

You know the drill: It's time to oust those obesogens. Pack them up and ship them out!

TABLE 3.7
PLASTICS PREVENTION TIPS

Here are some quick tips to help you avoid both BPA and phthalates.

1. Don't microwave plastic food containers—ever!
2. Look for the recycle codes on the bottoms of plastic containers. Some, but not all, plastics that are marked with recycle codes 3 or 7 may be made with BPA.
3. Reduce your use of canned foods. Look for products in glass jars or, when necessary, cans labeled as BPA-free.
4. Opt for porcelain, glass, or stainless steel containers.
5. Go old school and tell your butcher to wrap your meat in paper to keep the PVC plastic wrap that most supermarkets use out of your cart.
6. Don't touch cash register receipts unless absolutely necessary.

INTRODUCING ALL OF THE ANTINUTRIENTS WE CALL EMDS

Once you put everything you just learned into practice, your house should be free of all sugar, wheat, soy, and MSG-laden products, as well as many plastics and canned foods. While we identified the many ways that Poor Food Perpetrators negatively affect your health, it's the Everyday Micronutrient Depleters (EMDs) hiding inside of them that can really derail your 28-day plan and ultimately block your ability to achieve micronutrient sufficiency. Remember, these EMDs are like stealth thieves that pop up in your foods and reduce the amount of micronutrients you will find inside; because of this, they are often referred to as antinutrients. Both sugar and high fructose corn syrup are EMDs in and of themselves. Their chemical structure reduces your micronutrient levels dramatically. Wheat, on the other hand, contains a trifecta of EMDs. Wheat is made of phytic acid, oxalic acid, and lectins, three micronutrient thieves you want to avoid, while soy takes the prize due to the "quad"-fecta: phytic acid, lectins, oxalic acid, and trypsin inhibitors.

How many other foods do you think these EMDs are hiding in? Are there other micronutrient depleters that work in similar ways? Should you be avoiding all of them, all of the time? First of all, it would be nearly impossible—or at least prohibitively difficult—to completely remove all of them from your diet, as they can be found in most foods. And we aren't sure we would want you to avoid all of these foods anyway. You see, there are naturally occurring EMDs in some of the "healthiest," most micronutrient-rich foods. Foods like kale, chia seeds, nuts, sweet potatoes, and berries all contain EMDs. Some EMDs can be reduced by proper preparation methods, making the foods safer to consume while allowing you to enjoy them and their micronutrient benefits, as well. Let's take a closer look at the EMDs found in our foods and drinks.

Phytates (Phytic Acid)

You've already seen how both wheat and soy contain our first EMD, phytic acid. Phytic acid works similarly to fiber, in that it binds to substances in our intestinal tracts. However, unlike fiber, which lowers cholesterol by binding to cholesterol-like compounds in the digestive tract, phytic acid reduces micronutrient absorption by binding to vitamin B_3 (niacin), calcium, chromium, copper, iron, magnesium, manganese, and zinc. Additionally, phytic acid accelerates the metabolism of vitamin D. Rickets, caused by a vitamin D deficiency, as well as osteoporosis are common in populations with high phytic acid intake.[46]

Where it is found: Wheat and soy are among the worst offenders, but we have already eliminated them from your diet. Other foods high in phytic acid include corn, beans, seeds (including flaxseed and chia seeds), nuts, cereal grains, brown rice, and oats.

Proper preparation: Sprouting and fermenting grains, beans, flaxseed, nuts, and chia will reduce phytic acid. According to a 2010 article that appeared in the Weston A. Price Foundation journal called *Wise Traditions in Food, Farming, and the Healing Arts,* "research suggests that we will absorb approximately 20 percent more zinc and 60 percent more magnesium from our food when phytate is absent."[47]

Oxalates (Oxalic Acid)

Did you know that your morning green smoothie may be contributing to your osteoporosis, high blood pressure, or kidney stones? It's true. All those raw greens may be to blame. As with phytic acid, oxalic acid also binds, or chelates, to specific micronutrients in the intestinal tract. Oxalates in your food bind to the calcium, magnesium, and iron in that same food (or in foods eaten with it), and they block their absorption. In the case of spinach, this results in leaving a mere 2 and 10 percent of the seemingly plentiful supply of iron and calcium, respectively, and it reduces the absorption of magnesium by 35 percent. However, it is the ability of oxalates to bind with calcium that brings 1 out of every 1,000 Americans annually to the hospital with kidney stones. Seventy-five percent of all kidney stones in patients in the United States are made of calcium oxalate, crystalized oxalate acid bonded to calcium.[48]

Where it is found: The foods highest in oxalates include spinach, wheat, buckwheat, peanut butter, beets, beet greens, Swiss chard, nuts, rhubarb, and beans (green, waxed, or dried). Oxalates can be found to a lesser extent in many other foods, including collard greens, sweet potatoes, quinoa, celery, green rutabagas, soy, white potatoes, okra, tomatoes, and carrots.

Proper preparation: Make sure to cook oxalate-rich foods. According to a study in the *Journal of Agricultural and Food Chemistry*, "boiling markedly reduced soluble oxalate content by 30 to 87 percent and was more effective than steaming (5 to 53 percent) and baking (used only for potatoes, no oxalate loss)."[49]

Lectins

Lectins are a plant's most powerful weapon. Believe it or not, plants don't really want us to eat them. A plant's goal is self-preservation, and lectins are its premier defense system. Lectins are sticky proteins that coat your intestinal tract, making it difficult to properly absorb micronutrients.

While micronutrient loss is our key concern, it is also important to understand the other ways that lectins can negatively affect our health. To begin with, lectins make us fat in two unique ways. First, they attach to insulin receptors on fat cells. Remember, insulin is the fat-storage hormone. And once attached, lectins never detach, indefinitely telling the fat cell to store more fat! To add insult to injury, lectins also attach themselves to the receptor sites for leptin, the hormone that tells your brain when you are full, and block its effect on satiety. The end result is that you are prone to overeating because you never get full and more of what you eat gets stored as body fat. That harmless bowl of lectin-containing nuts over cocktails hardly seems harmless anymore, does it?[50, 51, 52, 53, 54, 55, 56]

Lectins also aid in the creation of leaky gut by binding to your intestinal walls and acting like chisels, forcing apart the cells that protect the rest of you from the undigested foods inside. Many food allergies are actually immune system reactions to lectins.[57]

Still not convinced that these plants mean business? The type of lectin found in red kidney beans is so dangerous that only five raw beans can seriously hurt or even kill you! And speaking of deadly lectins, the lectin found in castor beans is one of the most deadly poisons known to man and has even been used in international espionage. It is called ricin, and a single dose of purified powder—the size of a few grains of table salt—can kill an adult human.

Where it is found: Lectins are present in about 30 percent of the American diet.[58] Foods with high levels include brown rice, wheat, spelt, rye, barley, tomatoes, beans, soybeans, seeds, nuts, corn, potatoes (skin), eggplant, and bell and hot peppers.

Proper preparation: Heat destroys some lectins, but not all. Pressure cooking is the only way to destroy lectins. Soaking, with frequent water changes, or sprouting can remove many lectins from beans, rice, and nuts.

Trypsin Inhibitors

While trypsin inhibitors are a plant's natural pest repellent, humans still consume them, not realizing the havoc they can have on digestion. Trypsin inhibitors put your amino acids as well as fat-soluble vitamins A, D, E, and K and vitamin B_{12} in jeopardy as they interfere with the pancreas's ability to create enzymes necessary for proper digestion.

They also put your pancreas in great danger. Your body responds to a lack of trypsin (which has been "inhibited") by increasing both the size and the number of pancreatic cells. Digesting too many of these trypsin inhibitors stresses the pancreas and can lead to pancreatitis and even pancreatic cancer, now the fourth-leading cause of cancer deaths in men and women.[59, 60, 61]

Where it is found: Most of the USDA studies performed over the years have looked at trypsin inhibitors in soybeans, but these antinutrients are also found in other beans, as well as grains, nuts, seeds, and vegetables of the nightshade family (potatoes, tomatoes, and eggplant).[62]

Proper preparation: Luckily, cooking deactivates most of the trypsin inhibitors. For example, when researchers heated sweet potatoes to 215°F (102°C), it led to rapid inactivation of their trypsin inhibitors.[63] However, while trypsin inhibitors are reduced by cooking, it is not completely removed. The cooked sweet potatoes still retained between 17 and 31 percent of their trypsin-inhibitor activity. Raw foodists and vegetarians who frequently consume large amounts of soy, beans, and nuts in their raw state are most at risk from these antinutrients.

Phosphoric Acid

This chemical additive that helps keep the carbonated bubbles in soda products from going flat is a real calcium depleter. Your body strives to maintain a 1 to 1 ratio of calcium to phosphorus. When phosphoric acid is ingested, your body leaches calcium from your bones or teeth in order to keep this balance. Then, when the phosphoric acid is passed in your urine, the calcium is also lost. However, the loss of calcium does not end there. Phosphoric acid also neutralizes hydrochloric acid in your stomach, and hydrochloric acid is needed to break down food and absorb micronutrients. Yes, you guessed it: Calcium needs an acidic environment to be properly absorbed, as do both vitamin B_9 (folate) and vitamin B_{12}. Finally, phosphoric acid binds with calcium and magnesium in our stomachs, creating insoluble salts and further micronutrient loss. So, if you are one of the 67 million Americans suffering from hypertension (high blood pressure) or one of the 40 million with osteoporosis, or, you are at risk for it due to low bone mass, steer clear of sodas because the leaching of both calcium and magnesium can have detrimental effects on both your blood pressure and your bone health.

Where it is found: Phosphoric acid is mostly found in bubbly beverages, like carbonated soft drinks, carbonated energy drinks, and some flavored waters.

Proper preparation: This EMD is simple to reduce and even eliminate. In fact, there is no need to drink these micronutrient-depleting beverages at all.

Alcohol

Remember earlier when we explained how trypsin inhibitors decrease the pancreas's secretion of digestive enzymes? Well, so does alcohol, which can cause the loss of both amino acids and fat-soluble vitamins. To make matters worse, excessive alcohol consumption can also damage the stomach lining and intestines. This may reduce the absorption of any vitamins and minerals that were made available for digestion by the digestive enzymes, such as vitamin B_1 (thiamine) and vitamin B_9 (folic acid).

However, don't let this information put a damper on your celebrations. Moderate alcohol consumption can be quite beneficial to your health. A recent study out of the University of Oregon showed that consumption of 19 grams of alcohol—about two small glasses of wine—helped preserve bone strength just as well as bisphosphonates, a type of drug used by hundreds of thousands of women to combat thinning bones.[64] Finnish researchers concur; in 2013 they determined that women drinking more than three alcoholic drinks a week had significantly higher bone density than abstainers.[65] Make no bones about it, moderate alcohol intake helps osteoporosis, but its benefits don't stop there. Two Harvard studies revealed that, compared to abstainers, the risk of death from all causes was reduced by up to 28 percent among men and women who drank alcohol moderately.[66, 67]

Where it is found: Beer, wine, hard cider, mead, and hard alcohol are the main culprits.

Proper preparation: Unlike other fermented foods, like kimchi and sauerkraut, which create "happy places" in your gut, the fermentation of alcohol makes your gut a poor host for proper micronutrient absorption. Alcohol is a micronutrient foe if you forget moderation! Reducing intake is the only way to enjoy it and benefit from its longevity-boosting perks.

Caffeine

While caffeine has been shown to deplete micronutrients, specifically calcium and iron, the levels of depletion are quite minor when consuming just two cups a day. A recent study determined that the calcium loss from a 6-ounce cup of coffee could be offset by supplementing with 40 milligrams of calcium—the equivalent of 2 tablespoons of milk in your cup of coffee.[68] Additionally, that same 6-ounce cup of joe can inhibit the absorption of nonheme iron (the main form of iron found in plants) by 24 to 73 percent.[69, 70] However, the micronutrient benefits of caffeine-laden beverages may far outweigh the minor depletion.

Coffee, for example, is the number-one source of antioxidants in the US diet, containing 300 percent more free radical–fighting antioxidants than even black tea. Coffee's antioxidant content has been shown to reduce the risk of heart disease, depression, Alzheimer's, Parkinson's, type 2 diabetes, stroke, cirrhosis of the liver, gout, dementia, and certain types of cancer. And there is good news for caffeine where frail bones are considered. A 2012 study presented at the Society for Experimental Biology reported that caffeine "boosts power in older muscles, suggesting the stimulant could aid elderly people to maintain their strength, reducing the incidence of falls and injuries."[71]

Where it is found: Caffeine can be found in caffeinated soft drinks, coffee drinks, tea, and chocolate, as well as in greater amounts in energy drinks.

Proper preparation: Opt for decaffeinated beverages or reduce your intake of caffeinated beverages while adding in milk or supplementing with other calcium sources, as well as iron sources, to offset the depletion.

Tannins

Do you enjoy a glass of red wine with your steak? Well, you may want to think about changing this habit, especially if you are anemic. The dry, mouth-puckering sensation you get from that cabernet or merlot tells you that tannins, our next antinutrient, are present. Like oxalates and phytates, tannins are naturally occurring molecules that bind with micronutrients—specifically vitamins B_1 and B_9 and the minerals calcium, magnesium, iron, and zinc—to inhibit their absorption. For this reason, UK researchers recommend that individuals wait at least 1 hour after eating before drinking tannin-laden tea, to lower the risk of anemia.[72]

Where it is found: In addition to coffee, tea, and red wine, these menacing molecules are also found in apples, grapes, and berries (including their juices), as well as rhubarb, beans, lentils, spices, barley (beer), nuts, and chocolate.

Proper preparation: Avoid at mealtimes if you are at risk for iron deficiency.

IT'S NOT ALL ABOUT ELIMINATION

Does it appear that EMDs are hiding in all of your foods, even some "healthy" ones? There sure are a lot of them, but when you take a really good look, you will see that many of them are hiding in the same foods. Some of those foods we have already eliminated, like wheat and soy. Sodas and energy drinks, which can contain phosphoric acid and caffeine, have been eliminated as well because of their sugar or sinister sugar-substitute content. You also saw that modest levels of some of the EMDs, like alcohol and coffee, can produce health benefits, as well.

Remember, we aren't telling you to simply cut out all of these foods all of the time. Just because a food is listed as containing an antinutrient doesn't mean you need to throw it in the trash sack immediately. You may be able to include it in moderation or replace it with a version that follows the proper preparation guidelines. For example, we don't want you to remove all nuts, even though they deplete you with oxalic acid, phytic acid, lectins, tannins, and trypsin inhibitors. There are some great micronutrients and healthy fats in a small handful of nuts. However, because those five EMDs are inherent to nuts, we want you to only purchase those that meet the proper preparation guidelines. So, we want you to either eliminate nuts and seeds or only purchase those that are properly soaked or sprouted for the next 28 days.

Additionally, because the EMDs are only reduced and not eliminated when properly prepared, we would still like you to minimize your consumption of the bolded foods in Table 3.8 (page 78), as these contain the highest levels of antinutrients. While on the Micronutrient Miracle plan, you will be eliminating sugar, soy, and wheat, and for the remaining bolded foods on this list, try to limit them and follow the preparation guidelines.

A Pattern Emerges—Your Personal EMD Intake Analysis

Take a look at Table 3.8 (page 78). Do you see any foods or beverages that you currently enjoy? Do you drink coffee, tea, or wine? Have you recently eaten spinach, nuts, sweet potatoes, or berries? Do you purchase water bottled in plastic? This part might take some calculating and perhaps 15 to 20 minutes of your time. But take the time to do it. It is very important to see how pervasive these EMDs are in your life.

Step 1: Place a check (✓) in the Tabulations column for each day of the week that you might consume or come into contact with BPA or an item listed containing that EMD. Be honest! If, for example, you browse the first EMD, phytates, and determine that you currently eat wheat, beans, flaxseed, and broccoli each once a week but snack on nuts daily, you should give yourself one check for each of the first four foods and seven checks for nuts. That would give you a total of 11 checks for phytates. You need to tabulate your usage of each EMD in the chart.

Step 2: Fill in Table 3.9 (page 80). This is your current Everyday Micronutrient Depleters Intake Chart. Using the checks you entered in Table 3.8, calculate how many times each micronutrient might be affected. For example, if you had 11 checks next to phytates, then you will need to put 11 points next to each vitamin and mineral phytates deplete. This means that you will write the number 11 next to B_3, D, calcium, chromium, copper, iron, magnesium, manganese, and zinc. Mark down your total for each EMD in every micronutrient it depletes. You will hit some micronutrients more than once. When you do this, simply mark the second number to the right of the first. For example, you could end up with something like this:

Calcium: 11 6 27 5 3

Step 3: Total the numbers listed for each micronutrient. For example:

Calcium: 11 + 6 + 27 + 5 + 3 = 52

Step 4: It is time to analyze your data. Are you surprised at how many EMDs you currently have in your life? Does the sheer amount of micronutrients being depleted by your current habits shock you? Are there some patterns emerging in the clusters of micronutrients most often lost through EMDs? Take note as to which micronutrients are being heavily depleted due to your current habits.

TABLE 3.8
EVERYDAY MICRONUTRIENT DEPLETERS FOUND IN FOODS AND DRINKS

EVERYDAY MICRO-NUTRIENT DEPLETER (aka antinutrient)	MICRO-NUTRIENTS DEPLETED	FOUND IN THESE FOODS/DRINKS	PROPER PREPARATION AND MICRONUTRIENT MIRACLE PLAN GUIDELINES	TABULATIONS (Place one ✓ for every day of the week you consume a food.)
Phytates (phytic acid)	B_3, D, calcium, chromium, copper, iron, magnesium, manganese, zinc	Breads (any wheat product), corn, beans, seeds (including flaxseed and chia seeds), nuts, grains (cereals), brown rice, soy products, oats, figs, artichokes, carrots, potatoes, broccoli, strawberries, rice, apples	Reduce phytates by sprouting, soaking, or fermenting grains, beans, seeds, and nuts.	
Oxalates (oxalic acid)	Calcium, iron, magnesium	Spinach, wheat, buckwheat, peanut butter, beets, beet greens, Swiss chard, nuts, rhubarb, beans (green, waxed, or dried), collard greens, sweet potatoes, quinoa, celery, green rutabagas, soy products, white potatoes, okra, tomatoes, sesame seeds (tahini), carrots	Cook oxalate-rich vegetables.	
Lectins	All vitamins and minerals (Check all.)	Rice, wheat, spelt, rye, barley, soy products, other beans, seeds, nuts, corn, potatoes, tomatoes, eggplant, hot and bell peppers	Reduce lectin levels by soaking, sprouting, and fermenting; cooking also reduces levels, but none of these will totally eliminate lectins. (Pressure cooking is the best.)	
Trypsin inhibitors	Fat-soluble vitamins A, D, E, and K, amino acids (carnitine)	Soy products, other beans, grains, nuts, seeds, vegetables of the nightshade family (potatoes, tomatoes, and eggplant)	Cooking deactivates most of them.	

TABLE 3.8 (cont.)				
EVERYDAY MICRO-NUTRIENT DEPLETER (aka antinutrient)	**MICRO-NUTRIENTS DEPLETED**	**FOUND IN THESE FOODS/DRINKS**	**PROPER PREPARATION AND MICRONUTRIENT MIRACLE PLAN GUIDELINES**	**TABULATIONS** (Place one ✓ for every day of the week you consume a food.)
Phosphoric acid	Calcium, iron, magnesium, manganese	**Carbonated sodas, carbonated energy drinks, some flavored waters**	Omit completely.	
Alcohol	A, B_1, B_2, B_3, B_5, B_6, B_7, B_9, B_{12}, C, calcium, chromium, magnesium, phosphorus, potassium, selenium, zinc, omega-3, omega-6	**Beer, wine, hard alcohol**	Limit to two drinks a day to reduce depletion while gaining health benefits; some condition-specific protocols may reduce the amount further.	
Caffeine	A, B_9, D, calcium	**Coffee, tea, soda, energy drinks, and chocolate**	Limit to 2 cups a day and replenish calcium; some condition-specific protocols may reduce the amount further.	
Tannins	B_1, B_9, calcium, iron, magnesium, zinc	**Coffee, tea, red wine, fruit juice, rhubarb, beans (red), lentils, barley (beer), nuts,** spices, chocolate, pomegranates, berries, apples, and grapes	If at risk for iron deficiency, avoid consuming tannin-containing beverages at mealtimes.	
Sugar and HFCS	C, calcium, chromium, copper, magnesium, zinc	**Almost all prepackaged goods in the grocery store under all the names listed on pages 60 and 61**	Do not consume.	
MSG	C, E, chromium, magnesium, selenium, zinc	**Almost all prepackaged goods in the grocery store under all the names listed on page 68**	Do not consume.	
BPA and phthalates	Calcium	**Plastic and Styrofoam food containers, water bottles, canned foods, receipts, many children's toys, PVC pipes**	Avoid whenever possible.	

TABLE 3.9
EVERYDAY MICRONUTRIENT DEPLETERS INTAKE CHART

MICRONUTRIENT	TABULATION TOTALS
Vitamin A	
Vitamin B₁ (thiamine)	
Vitamin B₂ (riboflavin)	
Vitamin B₃ (niacin)	
Vitamin B₅ (pantothenic acid)	
Vitamin B₆ (pyridoxine)	
Vitamin B₇	
Vitamin B₉ (folate)	
Vitamin B₁₂ (cobalamin)	
Choline	
Vitamin C	
Vitamin D	
Vitamin E	
Vitamin K	
Calcium	
Chromium	
Copper	
Iodine	
Iron	
Magnesium	
Manganese	
Phosphorus	
Potassium	
Selenium	
Zinc	
Omega-3	
Omega-6	
Amino acids (carnitine)	

Now revisit your Personal Micronutrient Deficiency List (page 27). Do the micronutrients you are depleting through your foods and drinks correlate with those on your list? If the answer is yes, then just think how removing some of these antinutrients could improve your health. Use this information as motivation as you move through your pantry and fridge identifying the Poor Food Perpetrators just waiting to trip you up on your path to extraordinary health.

4

Get Out of Your Own Way!

ARE YOUR CUPBOARDS LOOKING a little bare after that pantry purge? Did you expose some sneaky micronutrient-depleting foods and drinks that might have been putting your sufficiency at risk? Well now it's time to turn the spotlight back on you. That's right! You have seen how specific foods in your kitchen can negatively affect your micronutrient sufficiency levels, but now we are going to evaluate how your sufficiency levels are being influenced by your lifestyle habits. In the previous chapter, you took the first step to becoming a nutrivore by Switching to Rich and completing your pantry purge. While there is still a second part to that step, the Rich Food restock (which we will cover in Chapter 5), you took a big bite out of it already by getting rid of the Poor Food Perpetrators in your kitchen.

Now it is time to take the second step to becoming a nutrivore and focus on *driving down depletion*. It is time for you to take a good look at your life and take accountability for your actions. *Accountability!* Now that is a scary word. But unless we hold ourselves accountable for our actions, we never push ourselves to do better. It will always be someone or something that stopped us from achieving our goals. Accountability forces us to take responsibility for where our health is today and make the changes that will result in success tomorrow. As we continue this journey together, we want you to become aware of how your personal lifestyle habits may unknowingly be foiling your best intentions for optimal health. It's time to take a good look at how your dietary philosophy, daily habits, medication regimen, and toxic load may be packing on the pounds and holding your health hostage.

The Great Diet Debate

One of the many problems with nutrition today is that there is so much infighting between dietary philosophies. It makes sense, when you think about it. People are very attached to their belief systems, and when you make up your mind to follow a specific dietary philosophy, it becomes a large part of who you are. You go out of your way to find restaurants that cater to your particular preferences and often bond easily with others following the same dietary protocol. You may even join a designated Facebook or Meetup group to befriend others with the same dietary beliefs as you. So, when your dietary philosophy is challenged, you are bound to become a bit defensive.

We often find ourselves listening to arguments or intense discussions among our colleagues—writers and scientists in the nutritional arena—over which dietary philosophy is the best to follow. Eventually, someone in the group, trying to see if we are allies, asks us our opinion. And our response is always the same. We tell them that an individual has the right to choose whichever dietary philosophy they like, but based on our research, they all fall short in what really matters. No dietary philosophy provides the minimum amount of the vitamins, minerals, essential fatty acids, or amino acids we need every day to achieve micronutrient sufficiency.

Does it surprise you now that no diet meets micronutrient sufficiency? Perhaps after hearing how deficient the soil is, how far your food traveled, and how many antinutrients bind to and deplete vitamins and minerals, you may not be all that surprised. However, you have most likely heard people, be it on TV or in conversation, tell you that all you have to do to get all the vitamins and minerals you need is to just eat a balanced diet. How can they say that? Do they have scientific evidence or research studies to back that statement up? No, they don't. But we have studies that prove exactly the opposite.

In a study published in the *Journal of the American Dietetic Association* titled "Problems Encountered in Meeting the Recommended Dietary Allowances for Menus Designed According to the Dietary Guidelines for Americans," a group of dietitians were asked to create menus that met the RDAs (Recommended Dietary Allowances) for the essential micronutrients while providing 2,200 to 2,400 *palatable* calories. Remember, the USDA statistics we shared earlier showed that Americans were not reaching sufficiency in all of their micronutrients.

However, those statistics were based on average Americans eating random diets, not diets specifically designed by specially trained dietitians with the aim of reaching the goal of micronutrient sufficiency. So, when these professionals were given that task, surely they could create the perfect menu. Well, the sad truth is that they couldn't. Not one single person was able to reach the study's objective, not even when they used software designed specifically for creating a healthy diet. According to the researchers, "only 11 percent of the menus met the RDA for zinc. Half of the menus did not meet the RDA for vitamin B_6, and one-third did not meet the RDA for iron."[1] If these dietitians couldn't create a sufficient diet with that as their primary goal, then what is the likelihood that you will randomly be serving up sufficiency for supper?

If a random diet doesn't provide micronutrient sufficiency and trained dietitians couldn't create menus that meet sufficiency either, how do you think the world's best-selling diet books did at this same task? That is exactly what we wanted to know and exactly what we researched for Jayson's 2010 article published in the *Journal of the International Society of Sports Nutrition* titled "Prevalence of Micronutrient Deficiency in Popular Diet Plans."[2]

In this study, we examined the sufficiency levels of 27 essential micronutrients as recommended by the RDI (Reference Daily Intake) in four popular diet plans to see if the very act of dieting itself could be creating a micronutrient-deficient state in the average American. In order to be fair to all the dietary philosophies, we included Atkins (low carbohydrate), the South Beach Diet (Mediterranean), and the Best Life Diet (low fat). The fourth diet we chose was the DASH diet—a medically founded diet plan written by an amazing group of researchers from some of the country's top institutions, including Brigham and Women's Hospital; Harvard Medical School; Duke University Medical Center; Johns Hopkins University; Kaiser Permanente Center for Health Research; the National Heart, Lung, and Blood Institute; and the Pennington Biomedical Research Center at Louisiana State University. The best part about the DASH diet is that it was created to reverse disease, not merely lose weight. The entire concept of the DASH diet (DASH stands for Dietary Approaches to Stop Hypertension) was that one could lower blood pressure through gaining sufficiency in potassium, magnesium, and calcium. Surely a diet aimed at micronutrient sufficiency would perform well in our study. Later, we decided to add both the Primal and Paleo diets into the mix in order to include two of the hottest diet crazes in the bookstores.

In order to evaluate each diet plan's ability to reach micronutrient sufficiency, we measured the amount of every micronutrient in the respective menu plans, right down to the very last gram of salt. After all the computations were completed, it was revealed that not one of the popular diet plans reached micro-nutrient sufficiency for the 27 essential micronutrients we evaluated—vitamin A, vitamin B_1 (thiamine), vitamin B_2 (riboflavin), vitamin B_3 (niacin), vitamin B_5 (pantothenic acid), vitamin B_6, vitamin B_7 (biotin), vitamin B_9 (folate), vitamin B_{12}, vitamin C, vitamin D, vitamin E, vitamin K, choline, calcium, chromium, copper, iron, iodine, potassium, magnesium, manganese, molybdenum, sodium, phosphorus, selenium, and zinc. See Table 4.1, below, for our findings.

TABLE 4.1 INDEPENDENT RESEARCH ON SIX POPULAR DIET PROGRAMS			
NAME OF DIET	**% RDI SUFFICIENT**	**# OF MICRONUTRIENTS OUT OF 27 THAT MET RDI**	**# OF AVERAGE DAILY CALORIES**
Atkins for Life	44%	12	1,786
Best Life	56%	15	1,793
DASH	52%	14	2,217
Practical Paleo	56%	15	2,160
Primal Blueprint	56%	15	1,911
South Beach	22%	6	1,197
Average	**48%**	**13**	**1,844**

The study determined that a typical dieter using one of these six popular diet plans would be, on average, 48 percent sufficient at reaching RDI require-ments and would meet sufficiency in only 13 out of the 27 essential micronutri-ents required every day to prevent diseases from micronutrient deficiency. These diet plans were literally starving their followers of more than half of the micronutrients they needed to prevent disease, even when supplying them with up to six meals a day. We did notice, however, that there were big discrepancies in the number of calories that each program provided. The DASH diet, for example, supplied nearly twice the amount of calories as the South Beach Diet, so it made sense that it met RDI sufficiency in around twice the number of micronutrients. In order to compensate for the caloric differences, we decided to determine which diet would reach micronutrient sufficiency first. To accom-plish this, we increased the amount of each ingredient in each meal proportion-ally until RDI sufficiency for all 27 essential micronutrients were met. We never changed the macronutrient ratios or menu selections; we simply created the exact same meals as those suggested by each diet's daily menu plan, just larger. The results are in Table 4.2, below.

TABLE 4.2 NUMBER OF CALORIES NEEDED TO ACHIEVE 100% RDI SUFFICIENCY IN SIX POPULAR DIETS	
NAME OF DIET	CALORIES REQUIRED TO REACH 100% RDI SUFFICIENCY FOR ALL 27 MICRONUTRIENTS
Atkins for Life	37,500
Best Life	20,500
DASH	33,500
Practical Paleo	17,000
Primal Blueprint	14,100
South Beach	18,800
Average	**23,566**

Are you shocked? Did you think the number of calories needed to reach micronutrient sufficiency would be much lower? The truth is that the world's leading diet books, if followed perfectly to plan, would require you to eat—on average—23,566 calories a day in order to reach micronutrient sufficiency. You most certainly would not get any benefits out of any diet requiring that many calories, nor would we ever suggest this. Our point in sharing these studies with you is to show you that no matter how much we may all want to simply believe that a balanced diet can provide all the essential micronutrients we need to maintain our health day in and day out, it is not true. In fact, to our knowledge (and, believe us, we have searched), no study has ever been published proving that this is possible. The reality is that the balanced diet is a myth. The American Dietetic Association could not create a sufficient meal plan, even when using computer software designed to do so. And America's most trusted diet books written by doctors and nutritionists haven't been able to do it, either—regardless of which dietary philosophy they were following. This does not mean, however, that micronutrient sufficiency is impossible to achieve; it just means we have to work a little harder to get there, and understanding the shortcomings of your particular dietary philosophy is a good place to start.

Dietary Doctrine

What exactly is a dietary philosophy? What makes a vegan a vegan or the Paleo diet the Paleo diet? When you start to look at how a dietary philosophy is designed, you realize it basically comes down to one thing—elimination. A vegan diets eliminates food sourced from animals, while the Paleo diet eliminates dairy and legumes. Each dietary philosophy is designed to eliminate specific food groups that don't fit into their protocols. What do you think happens when foods get eliminated? Well, the vitamins and minerals that are abundant in those eliminated foods are also eliminated, and this can lead to certain dietary philosophies falling short in specific groups of micronutrients.

We aren't trying to suggest that simply because gluten-free diets are often low in vitamin A, the B vitamins, vitamin D, calcium, iron, magnesium, phosphorus, and zinc that one shouldn't follow this diet. In fact, we are gluten-free (*and after reading this book, you will be as well, if you aren't already*). The benefits of removing wheat from your diet greatly outweigh the fact that the foods eliminated are often high in specific micronutrients. It is the awareness that this diet may fall short at supplying enough of these essential vitamins and minerals that is important. Awareness is the key, so that you can focus on either eating foods that contain these missing micronutrients or supplementing them instead. So, because you will be gluten-free for at least the next 28 days, you will need to focus on your intake of vitamin A, the B vitamins, vitamin D, calcium, iron, magnesium, phosphorus, and zinc. We want you to specifically focus on vitamin B_6 and vitamin B_9 (folate) because in studies more than half of the individuals following a gluten-fee diet were found to be deficient in both.[3]

Remember, as a nutrivore, you can follow whatever dietary philosophy you believe in as long as you make micronutrient sufficiency your main goal. Do you follow a vegetarian or vegan diet? If you do, then you need to know that while you are taking in a lot of great micronutrient-rich produce, your diet has been shown to fall short in supplying adequate amounts of vitamins B_{12} and D, iron, calcium, zinc, and omega-3 fatty acids.[4] Diets that do not include fish, eggs, or sea vegetables (seaweeds) generally lack the essential fatty acids, which are important for cardiovascular health as well as eye and brain functions. Vegans as well as vegetarians who exclude dairy products should consider supplementation of vitamin D, because milk is the primary source of vitamin D in the United States. In the EPIC-Oxford study, which compared the nutrient intake of 33,883 meat-eaters (omnivores) to 31,546 nonmeat-eaters (vegans) in the UK, researchers found that the vegan diet only provided one-quarter the amount of vitamin D that the omnivore diet provided.[5] Additionally, in a study published in the *American Journal of Clinical Nutrition*, 73 percent of lacto-ovo vegetarians (vegetarians who do not consume animal flesh but do consume eggs and dairy) and vegans were found to be deficient in vitamin B_{12}, an essential vitamin that cannot be found naturally in any plant-based sources and is only found naturally in animal products.[6] And a B_{12} deficiency puts the vegetarian and vegan populations at risk for elevated homocysteine levels—a risk factor for cardiovascular disease, osteoporotic bone fractures, disorientation, dementia, and mood and motor disturbances. Furthermore, individuals following a vegetarian or vegan diet often increase their intake of foods like legumes, soy, spinach, and grains, which contain phytic acid, oxalic acid, and other antinutrients that can cause further micronutrient depletion.

And what about the Paleo and Primal diet crazes that are sweeping the nation? These ancestral-style diets encourage their followers to achieve better health by focusing on eating foods that would have been available to our Paleolithic ancestors. You would expect that a diet like this, which focuses on eating fresh, high-quality meat, fish, eggs, nuts, seeds, and vegetables, would be successful at providing a wide range of essential micronutrients—right? Well, here again, both the Paleo and Primal diets fall short. While these ancestral-style diets are among the most micronutrient-rich dietary philosophies we have found, because of key food group eliminations—including wheat (gluten), legumes, and dairy (for Paleo)—both diets were shown to be deficient in key micronutrients, including calcium, chromium, and B_7 (biotin).

Following a low-carbohydrate diet means nearly cutting out one of the three macronutrient groups (carbohydrates, fats, and proteins) altogether. When the Atkins diet was studied by researchers at the Children's Nutrition Research Centre of the Royal Children's Hospital in Australia, they found it to be significantly deficient in vitamin B_2 (riboflavin), vitamin B_9 (folate), calcium, magnesium, and iron.[7] Conversely, low-fat diets, which greatly reduce overall fat content, greatly decrease their followers' chances of reaching sufficiency in the essential fat-soluble vitamins A, D, E, and K, as well as calcium and omega-3 fatty acids.

WEIGHT REDUCTION AS A DIETARY PHILOSOPHY

Perhaps the most detrimental dietary philosophy, when it comes to micronutrient deficiency, is dieting strictly with weight loss as your goal. Many of these popular diet programs now recommend eating prepackaged diet-approved meals. As we mentioned in our conversation earlier about global food distribution and food processing and preparation, the modern convenience of frozen, processed, premade food in microwavable containers can often lead to diminished micronutrient intake. For example, a study published in *Nutrition Journal* evaluated dieters following the Weight Watchers protocol and found "significant declines" in vitamin B_2 (riboflavin), vitamin B_3 (niacin), potassium, calcium, magnesium, iron, and zinc. Other weight-loss-focused dietary philosophies simply try to reduce caloric intake by encouraging dieters to eat less food. Of course less food equals both fewer calories and fewer micronutrients. Research published by the National Institute of Hygiene in Poland evaluated the effects of a 1,000-calorie-a-day diet on a group of 96 overweight patients. This style of diet, which is typically prescribed for obesity, supplied participants with insufficient intakes of vitamins A, B_1, B_2, B_3, C, and E.[8] Additionally, skipping meals and the new, popular trend called intermittent fasting are not wise solutions either if micronutrient sufficiency is your goal. While they can reduce overall daily caloric intake, and likely reduce weight (mostly muscle, not fat), what are the chances that a dieter following these starvation-style weight-loss strategies can achieve micronutrient sufficiency in only two meals a day—especially if studies show no chance of becoming sufficient even when eating as many as six meals a day? However, if you are a fan of intermittent fasting, don't worry; later on we will show you how to incorporate a micronutrient-infused fast into your personalized plan.

Finally, when all else fails and weight loss is seemingly out of reach, many frustrated dieters turn to surgical procedures such as laparoscopic banding (lap band) and gastric bypass surgery. These procedures cut out or "band off" a portion of patients' stomachs so they cannot eat large portions, which in turn ensures they will not be able to fully absorb their micronutrients. While this can result in significant weight loss of 50 to 75 percent of excess body weight, due to the malabsorption created by virtue of the bypassed surface area, more than calories are lost. Deficiencies in vitamins B_1, B_9, B_{12}, and D, along with copper and calcium, are common postsurgery.[9] The resulting deficiency in B vitamins can leave the patient depressed and exhausted after surgery, while the lack of calcium causes sugar and salt cravings to take hold, often resulting in future weight gain.

As you can see, regardless of what dietary philosophy you may be following—be it the standard American diet (SAD), which the USDA sufficiency chart reflected back in Chapter 1; one of today's popular diet programs we outlined above; or a gluten-free, vegetarian, vegan, Paleo, Primal, low-carb, low-fat, low-calorie, or surgically induced diet, such as lap band or gastric bypass—there are inherent micronutrient deficiencies associated with each. However, your dietary philosophy is just one lifestyle habit that has been shown to affect your ability to achieve micronutrient sufficiency. Let's continue our journey and discover other areas in your life where you can drive down depletion.

Daily Habits

You can eat the most micronutrient-rich diet possible to greatly increase your chances of micronutrient sufficiency. However, that is the addition part of the equation. You are adding in all the micronutrients to see how close you are to reaching a micronutrient-sufficient state. Unfortunately, the equation doesn't end there. You see, throughout the day there is a sneaky little thing called "real life" that happens to each and every one of us. And life takes its toll—and the currency demanded is your micronutrients. Your daily habits act as Everyday Micronutrient Depleters (EMDs), subtracting the vitamins and minerals you thought you could count on, often unexpectedly leaving you further away from meeting your goal of micronutrient sufficiency.

Stress

Stress and anxiety plague 80 percent of Americans.[10] And the problem is a global one: According to the World Health Organization, more than 15 percent of the world population is suffering from a stress-related disorder.[11] In fact, it is hard to imagine that anyone today isn't affected by stress in some way. From traffic jams to business meetings, stress is hiding everywhere. While yoga, meditation, and exercise can do a lot to reduce your anxiety, the psychological conditions caused by stress can have profound physical implications. In fact, it is no exaggeration to say that stress can shorten your life. Studies show that the cumulative impact of stress has been linked to a host of age-accelerating conditions and degenerative diseases, including cardiovascular disease, diabetes, and various cancers.[12, 13, 14, 15, 16]

In times of stress, certain metabolic reactions occur, and this causes certain micronutrients to be used up at a faster rate by the body. The water-soluble micronutrients—such as the B vitamins, vitamin C, and all of the minerals—are generally excreted at a faster rate during stress, and because these micronutrients are not stored to any great extent in the body, deficiencies can develop rather quickly. In fact, the B vitamins have come to be known as antistress nutrients because they are often the first deficiencies to develop during times of stress.

While vitamins B_1 and B_5 help fight off stress by maintaining proper function of the adrenal glands (the most important glands in the fight against stress), vitamins B_6 and B_9 help equip you to better deal with the stress that you do experience by aiding in the formation of chemicals called neurotransmitters, which are necessary for balancing emotions. According to a study conducted by the Mayo Clinic and published in the *Archives of Internal Medicine* (now *JAMA Internal Medicine*), you don't need a great deficiency in the B vitamins to set in before you really start to feel it. The study revealed that subjects who were given just half the daily requirement of vitamin B_1 (thiamine) became "irritable, depressed, quarrelsome, uncooperative, and fearful that some misfortune awaited them."[17]

Similarly, the demand for vitamin C increases tenfold during stressful periods, which can cause this water-soluble vitamin to become depleted relatively quickly. And much like with the B vitamins, when you deplete vitamin C, you are depleting the very same micronutrient that can help to eliminate the stress in the first place. Research shows that people with high levels of vitamin C do not show the expected mental and physical signs of stress when subjected to acute psychological challenges. What's more, they bounce back from stressful situations faster than people with low levels of vitamin C in their blood. It all comes down to the relationship between vitamin C and cortisol.

Cortisol, often called the "stress hormone," is produced by your adrenal glands during stressful episodes. It is responsible for the fight-or-flight response

Making Sense of Stress Eating

Are you a stress eater? Have you been known to grab a bowl of ice cream or bag of chips when stress comes knocking at your door? While you might think you are eating to stifle your emotions or anxiety, we want you to know that stress and anxiety themselves may be physically responsible for your snacking. Remember in our earlier discussion of the Crave Cycle when we identified how magnesium and calcium deficiencies can cause food cravings for both sweet and salty foods? Well, stress causes both of these water-soluble minerals to be used quickly, resulting in rapid depletion. It is because of these mineral deficiencies that you begin stress eating. So know that you're not mentally weak, just mineral deficient. Make sure to supplement smart, and both the stress and cravings will be a thing of the past.

to stress that allows us to spring into action when we sense danger. As the body experiences stress, it secretes cortisol into the bloodstream, which spikes appetite and increases fat deposits in the belly region. *That's right, this stress-induced steroid may likely be the culprit behind your belly fat.* According to *Psychology Today* magazine, vitamin C can "abolish the secretion of cortisol."[18] Conversely, according to researchers at the University of Maryland, even slight deficiencies of vitamin C can increase cortisol output.[19] So while stressful situations cause the adrenal glands to release cortisol, which relays the news of stress to all parts of the body and mind, they also release vitamin C, which fervently attempts to squash the physiological and psychological stress you're experiencing. Humphry Osmond, MD, a former psychology professor at the University of Alabama, and Abram Hoffer, MD, a former psychiatrist from British Columbia, believe that weight for weight, vitamin C is "as active as Haldol," a drug prescribed to help people deal with stress.[20]

However, if you don't have enough vitamin C in your body, then cortisol sends the message of stress throughout your body. This is another way that stress can further reduce micronutrients, because when too much cortisol is present in the body for an extended period of time, your immune system is weakened. This causes your body to use your immune-boosting micronutrients, including your antioxidants, at a more feverish pace.

The final way that stress reduces micronutrients is by harming your friendly gut bacteria. A reduction in the beneficial organisms in your digestive tract can lead to both digestive upset and malabsorption of the micronutrients taken in through your food.

Does this remind you of the Crave Cycle we introduced earlier? When your body feels stress, it uses specific micronutrients faster—the same micronutrients that can help to alleviate stress in the first place. But you don't have to *stress out* over this fact. A 2013 study published in *Psychosomatic Medicine* concluded that individuals taking a multivitamin supplement for at least 28 days enjoyed a 65 percent and a 68 percent reduction in stress and anxiety, respectively.[21] (Hmm—28 days, eh?) So, the next time you are put on hold and the computerized operator tells you that you are caller number 73 or you get a flat tire while taking your screaming kids to school in the morning, take a deep breath and repeat this statement: "My 28-day Micronutrient Miracle plan has me covered."

OH YEAH—DON'T FORGET ABOUT YOUR OMEGA-3S

Recent research shows that omega-3 fatty acids can play a key role in keeping stress at bay. Unfortunately, our Western diet doesn't supply us with enough of these essential fats, primarily found in fish, eggs, and meat, so supplementation is a smart choice for anyone who doesn't eat fish daily. One study from Toyama, Japan, focused on how DHA, part of the omega-3 chain, affected aggressive behavior in young adults. Researchers proved that DHA prevented the study's 41 participants from becoming more frustrated, even when put under mental stress.[22] Scientists believe that omega-3 supplementation "inhibits the adrenal activation elicited by a mental stress," leaving cortisol levels "significantly blunted" when omega-3 levels are high.[23] In fact, omega-3 supplementation can reduce the body's stress-induced production of cortisol by 22 percent.

One study at Gettysburg College in Pennsylvania proved just how powerful omega-3 fatty acids can be. Study participants who supplemented with omega-3s had significantly lower cortisol levels compared to those taking a placebo. This resulted in them shedding three and a half times more body fat while increasing lean muscle mass.[24] This is great news—now by adding the omega-3 fatty acids DHA and EPA into either your diet or your supplementation regimen, you can quiet cortisol, reduce stress, and eliminate much of the micronutrient depletion that stress may have cost you (and perhaps lose a few pounds of fat and add a few pounds of metabolism-boosting muscle while you are at it!).

Exercise

When you think about hard workouts and professional athletes, what images come to mind? Is it those images in magazine advertisements and TV commercials that you often see trying to sell you those brightly colored sports drinks? You know, the ones where the pro athletes are literally sweating neon orange or bright blue liquid through the pores of their skin. Man, do they sweat. Now, when you exert yourself, you likely sweat as well. Maybe not in Technicolor, but your perspiration is a testament to the level of strenuous labor you are putting into your time either at the gym, in a cardio class, or hiking and biking on a warm summer day. And what do you think you are using faster the harder you work out? What does that Technicolor liquid represent? Yep, you guessed it. It's your micronutrients (yes, electrolytes are micronutrients too!), and the amount of micronutrients you lose directly correlates with the intensity and the duration of the activity you perform. Studies show that because they play key roles in energy metabolism, the utilization rate of these micronutrients may be increased by up to 20 to 100 times the resting rate during intense physical activity.[25]

Iron is a great example of this "intensity equals loss" principle. Strenuous exercise stimulates an increase in red blood cell and blood vessel production, which creates an increased demand for iron. Those individuals who work out

---

The Calcium Clock Is Ticking!

If "Your Personal Micronutrient Deficiency List," on page 27, indicated that calcium is of critical concern, then here is a tip for you. Always take your calcium supplements prior to your workout. (For those taking nutreince, our patented multivitamin, calcium is in the AM dose, so you are all set as long as you drink it down first.) Research has shown that those taking calcium supplements 30 minutes prior to a workout can offset some of the bone leaching caused by exercise.

---

fewer than 4 hours a week don't need to be concerned with this depletion; however, those exerting themselves over 6 hours a week need to be cautious of iron-deficiency anemia.[26] Calcium, another essential mineral/electrolyte, is also at risk for exercise-induced depletion. This should be of particular interest to the cardio kings and queens out there, who, like Mira back when she lived in New York City, love to spend hours sweating in the gym or dance studio. As an individual perspires, calcium is released, but where do you think the body finds more calcium to replenish it? That's right, it must leach the calcium from the bone to replace it. This means that as you increase intensity, you could be causing your own bones to weaken due to the large amounts of calcium that escape via your sweat. The great news is that findings presented at the 2013 meeting of the Endocrine Society found that athletes might be able to offset some of this bone loss by simply supplementing smart with calcium.[27]

However, iron and calcium aren't the only minerals affected by exercise. Both male and female athletes also have lower serum zinc levels compared to sedentary individuals, and studies show that those who train without days off lose zinc even more quickly.[28] Additionally, strenuous exercise increases urinary and sweat losses that may increase magnesium requirements by 10 to 20 percent. USDA research shows that marginal magnesium deficiency can both impair exercise performance as well as amplify the oxidative stress that exercise can cause.[29] Yep, not only is exercise hard to do, but it is also hard on your body. This is because when you perform aerobic activities, like cardio, your body undergoes oxidative cell damage, and this causes the formation of free radicals, and the more free radicals there are, the more cellular damage is done. So antioxidants—like vitamins A, C, and E; alpha-lipoic acid; and selenium—are extremely important for athletes because they are fabulous free-radical scavengers and can help to reduce this cellular damage. Reduced oxidative stress not only results in a lower likelihood of degenerative diseases—including heart disease, dementia, cancer, and cataracts—but also shortens recovery time and improves athletic performance.

Exercise activates a finely orchestrated interplay of the body's physiological systems to produce the desired skeletal muscle contractions at the right time. Yes, there it is again—that orchestra of essential micronutrients, all needed at just the right time to support you both during and after physical activities. But don't be mislead. Although exercise is an EMD, draining you of a wide variety of essential vitamins and minerals, we are in no way saying that it should be avoided. In fact, the exact opposite is true—we are huge advocates of exercise. We are not giving you permission to be a couch potato in the name of micronutrient sufficiency. In Chapter 7, we will tell you exactly how to exercise to get the greatest health benefits with the least amount of depletion. As we said earlier, there are some EMDs—like coffee and alcohol, for example—that have been shown to have some really healthy side effects. So it is the awareness of how exercise may be depleting you that we want you to understand and account for through diet and proper supplementation.

Smoking and Pollution

Hey, there are some habits that are simply bad for you. No sugarcoating this one. Smoking cigarettes has no benefits to your health. And while you have probably heard that smoking causes cancer, ages you, and wrecks your teeth and skin, you might never have considered the micronutrient-depleting aspects of cigarette smoke. Cigarette smoke causes a rapid depletion of vitamins A, C, and E. Smoke itself is an oxidant that creates free radicals, and the antioxidants play a protective role, trying to repair the damage that this oxidant (smoke) is causing. Again, and we hope you see a pattern here: The micronutrients that might be able to repair the damage from smoking are the very same ones you are using and depleting with every puff. If you are living with a smoker or work in a smoke-filled environment, you need to know that the secondhand smoke you are being forced to inhale is having a similar effect on your health. Research out of Johns Hopkins revealed that exposure to passive smoking (secondhand smoke) may also result in decreased concentrations of selected micronutrients, primarily antioxidants.[30]

Poor air quality is another daily habit that can negatively affect those living in large cities. According to the Environmental Protection Agency (EPA), at least

20,000 premature deaths occur every year in the United States due to air pollution. Globally, this number may exceed 500,000 per year.[31]

The polluted air you inhale—which can be caused by high ozone levels, smog, and car exhaust—is also acting as an oxidant. Luckily, the surface of the lungs is covered with a thin layer of fluid containing a range of antioxidants that appear to provide the first line of defense against oxidant pollutants. Studies show that supplementation of antioxidants can also help prevent damage from air pollution, and the EPA suggests antioxidant supplementation for those living in large, polluted cities.

Obviously we aren't going to suggest you leave your family, change jobs, and move to a new city for the next 28 days simply because you are an urban dweller. However, because your environment is not going to change, you need to recognize the inevitable micronutrient depletion your habitat invokes and that this greatly increases your need for antioxidants.

Prescription Medications

Have you noticed that prescription drug use is on the rise? We sure have. In fact, the odds are that most people you know are on at least one medication. According to a 2013 report by the Mayo Clinic and the Olmsted Medical Center, nearly 7 in 10 Americans are on at least one prescription drug, and more than half take two. A whopping 20 percent take five or more. According to the Centers for Disease Control and Prevention, 1 out of every 5 children and 9 out of 10 older Americans reported using at least one prescription drug in the past month.[32] While many of these prescriptions can be lifesaving, there is no denying that their use in this country has increased steadily over the past decade, and what's more, overdoses involving prescription drugs are at new epidemic levels, now killing more Americans than heroin and cocaine combined.[33] And America is not alone in this pill-popping party. According to a 2013 study, the average person in the UK takes 18 prescriptions a year, and approximately two-thirds of Australian seniors over the age of 60 are reported to take four or more drugs.[34, 35]

While many of these prescription drugs may make you "feel better," like a Band-Aid covering and protecting a wound, they likely will not fix the underlying problem. In fact, at a micronutrient level, they may be making matters quite a bit worse. The fact is that prescription medications can reduce micronutrient sufficiency in three unique ways.

First, some prescribed medications reduce appetite. This is the case for both Ritalin and Adderall, which are prescribed for attention deficit disorder. And as we stated with low-calorie starvation diets, reducing food intake reduces the likelihood that you will receive all the essential micronutrients you need throughout the day. Second, other drugs—such as antipsychotics, antidepressants, and steroids—have quite the opposite effect. They cause blood sugar swings, which can then cause cravings for simple carbohydrates—like white bread, pasta, and sugary snacks—and these are often filled with sugar and wheat, two EMDs we don't want in our diets. The third way prescription meds sabotage our sufficiency levels is by directly depleting the micronutrients from our bodies. In other words, the simple act of taking a prescription medication robs you of specific micronutrients, and these depletions are thought to cause up to 30 percent of all pharmaceutical side effects. Yes, your prescription medication may be an "antimicronutrient pill," depleting your essential micronutrients without you even knowing it. Over time, these depletions can cause new health conditions to arise, which may possibly require yet more medications to treat.[36] Let's look at two of the most commonly prescribed medications in the United States, Abilify and Crestor, to discover how they affect your micronutrient levels and hinder your chances of recovery.

First let's examine the most commonly prescribed medication in the United States. You may not have guessed this one, but it's the antidepressant sold under the name Abilify, and 1 out of every 4 women ages 50 to 64 is on an antidepressant. If you live in the United States, you have probably seen the commercials for this pill. It is the one with a woman who walks around depressed with her best friend, a small cartoon prescription drug pill, but he just can't cheer her up. Luckily, her doctor offers her a script for this exciting new pharmaceutical "add-on" called Abilify. In the ad, a giant cartoon letter *A* joins her and her prescription, and together the three live happily ever after. So, first of all, you need to know that this isn't a primary medication. This means that the most commonly prescribed drug in the United States, for which annual sales exceed 6 billion dollars, is only given to those already on depression medications that aren't working. Yes, that's billion with a *B*!

While studies have shown that Abilify reduces depression, it also has a slew of other unwanted side effects, including dizziness, nausea, vomiting, drooling, weight gain, seizures, and increased suicidal tendencies. Another side effect that is not often discussed is its depletion of the essential mineral selenium. And guess what? Selenium has important functions in brain metabolism. Selenium is so important to the brain that the body tries to maintain the concentration of selenium in the brain even when there is a deficiency in the peripheral organs. A low selenium status has a negative effect on the psyche and can be accompanied by an increased incidence of depression and other psychiatric conditions. So this medication actually eliminates the very micronutrient you need to fight depression naturally.

One UK study showed that "the lower the level of selenium in the diet, the more reports of anxiety, depression, and tiredness," and the researchers found that supplementation with this one micronutrient for a 5-week period significantly reduced these ailments.[37] Selenium has also been shown to reduce postpartum depression, as well as lift the spirits of and reduce clinical depression in elderly patients and those with cancer and HIV.[38] So, as you can see, adding this selenium-robbing thief into your prescription drug mix isn't smart if your goal is alleviating depression. Rather than depleting "feel-good" micronutrients, wouldn't it be better to add some in naturally through diet and supplementation? For example, studies show that eating selenium and omega-3–rich seafood two or more times a week may be linked with a 50 percent lower rate of depression. Eating super-delicious salmon certainly sounds better than taking a drug that depletes selenium and increases suicidal tendencies—don't you think?[39] In fact, just one 4-ounce serving of wild caught salmon contains more than 50 percent of the RDI for selenium and between 1,000 to 1,500 milligrams of omega-3.

The second drug we will discuss is Crestor, which is currently the fifth most commonly prescribed medication in the United States with just over $5.25 billion in annual sales. Crestor is classified as a statin and is often given to treat high cholesterol. You may also be aware of some other well-known statins, such as Lipitor, Levacor, Zocor, and Pravachol. And Lipitor is actually the

More Sad News For Those Trying To Get Happy

Currently, upwards of 50 percent of older people use benzodiazepines—a class of antidepressant medications that includes Xanax, Valium, and Klonopin—for some kind of mental health problem. However, a 2014 French study published in the journal *BMJ* found that use of benzodiazepines for 3 months or more increased one's risk of developing Alzheimer's disease by as much as 51 percent![40, 41] This shouldn't be surprising, as this class of drugs depletes vitamins B_6, B_9, B_{12}, and C and CoQ10. The B vitamins work in unison to lower homocysteine, which can cause atrophy in the part of the brain most affected by Alzheimer's. Both CoQ10 and vitamin C have been shown to fight the free radicals caused by oxidative stress, and evidence suggests that increased oxidative stress is common in Alzheimer's patients. Taking this class of micronutrient-depleting drugs will likely only supply a short-term smile and possibly much greater sadness later on.

world's all-time biggest-selling prescription medicine, with cumulative sales topping $130 billion.[42] According to a report from the National Center for Health Statistics, nearly 45 percent of people over the age of 60 now take cholesterol-lowering prescription medicines—a figure that has more than doubled since 1999. So the side effects of this type of medicine currently affect nearly half of America's aging population. To make matters worse, experts from the American Heart Association and the American College of Cardiology recently crafted new guidelines for prescribing statins, and these new guidelines are forecasted to widen the use of statins. In fact, under the new guidelines, nearly half of all Americans ages 40 to 75 and nearly all men over 60 now qualify to take statins.[43] Adding to the sales, and the prevalence of this class of drugs among the American population, the American Academy of Pediatrics now recommends statins for children over 8 years of age who are suffering from high cholesterol. And just because you may not call the United States home, don't think that you are off the hook. Australians take more cholesterol medication than any other developed country, with prescription rates 40 percent above the global average.[44]

Well, if so many people are taking statins, what could possibly be the problem? As it turns out, a lot! First, according to a 2015 study published in *Diabetologia*, researchers that studied the effects of statins for 6 years on more than 8,000 nondiabetic participants ages 45 to 73 found that "statin treatment increased the risk of type 2 diabetes by 46 percent."[45] Second, a 2015 study published in the journal *Movement Disorders* found that those taking cholesterol-lowering drugs (such as statins) are more than *twice* as likely to develop Parkinson's disease as those who do not.[46] Finally, Another side effect that is just starting to gain attention is muscle damage, which scientists believe is potentially "very serious." The industry insists that only 2 to 3 percent of patients get muscle aches and cramps, but according to one study, 98 percent of patients taking Lipitor and one-third of patients taking Mevacor (a lower-dose statin) suffered from muscle problems![47]

But while we want you to be aware of these major side effects, what we really want to focus on is this script's ability to deplete your micronutrients. Again, here in the United States, these depletions are commonly overlooked, but our northern neighbor, Canada, warns of this on prescription bottles: Use of this statin *"could lead to impaired cardiac function in patients with borderline congestive heart failure."* Why? This side effect is due to the depletion of CoQ10. It is well documented that the heart requires a sufficient amount of CoQ10 for energy production. However, when treating a patient with a bad heart thought to be due to high cholesterol, doctors give statins that deplete CoQ10, a micronutrient known to be essential to proper heart function—so essential, in fact, that some studies even suggest that congestive heart failure is primarily a CoQ10 deficiency disease. Here again, the one micronutrient absolutely critical for heart health is the one depleted in the treatment of heart disease.

We aren't trying to say that physicians are out to hurt you by offering you prescription medications. This is what they are taught in medical school and by the numerous pharmaceutical reps that visit them weekly. However, what if some of your health complaints are actually being caused by these doctor-prescribed medications? The micronutrient depletion caused by prescription drugs is well-documented, and for the next 28 days, while we don't want you to jump off of your medications, we want you to become aware of their depleting side effects. Pharmacists can be a big help in this area, as they are experts in drug-to-drug and drug-to-micronutrient antagonisms/competitions. Our goal is to help you fill in the nutritional gaps that your prescription medications may be causing. And as an added benefit, creating sufficiency will likely, over time, reduce your body's requirements for these medications, and slowly but surely, you may be able to get off of them altogether. Think of the micronutrient depletion you will avoid and the money you will save!

Don't forget to fill out the worksheet at the end of this chapter (Table 4.5, starting on page 108) to identify how your medications, both prescription and over-the-counter, are depleting your body of vital micronutrients.

Over-the-Counter (OTC) Medications

Just because the pills you pop are purchased over the counter at a drugstore doesn't mean you are out of the woods. Chances are you never thought medications that are so convenient, and so readily available, could be dangerous to your health. Wrong! In fact, while most Americans take prescription meds, the number popping over-the-counter drugs is much, much higher. These nonprescription medications—such as aspirin, acetaminophen, nonsteroidal anti-inflammatory drugs (NSAIDs), antacids, laxatives, and H_2 blockers (found in heartburn medications)—may seem harmless, but they also work to deplete your vital micronutrients in ways you likely have not imagined.

Let's examine how a simple case of heartburn may cause depletions leading to far more serious conditions. One class of medications commonly purchased at the local drugstore to treat heartburn is H_2 blockers. These include brand names such as Axid, Pepcid, Tagamet, Zantac, and others. Research indicates that these medications can deplete vitamins B_1, B_9, B_{12}, and D, as well as all of the following minerals: calcium, copper, iron, magnesium, phosphorus, potassium, and zinc.[48, 49] See Table 4.3, below, to discover how the "innocent" act of taking this type of OTC drug may be affecting your health.

TABLE 4.3	
MICRONUTRIENTS DEPLETED BY H_2 BLOCKERS	
MICRONUTRIENT DEPLETED	**SOME RELATED SIDE EFFECTS OF DEPLETION**
Vitamin B_1 (thiamine)	Depression, heart palpitations, eye pain, constipation, thyroid problems, muscle aches
Vitamin B_9 (folate)	Depression, hair loss, fatigue, periodontal disease, cardiovascular disease, insomnia, osteoporosis, arthritis
Vitamin B_{12}	Depression, fatigue, cardiovascular disease, Alzheimer's, osteoporosis, ulcers, insomnia, cancer
Vitamin D	Alzheimer's, anxiety, autoimmune disorders, depression, obesity, cancer, asthma, tooth decay, osteoporosis
Calcium	Bone loss leading to possible osteoporosis, bone pain, muscle cramps, irregular heartbeat, hypertension, sugar and salt cravings, insomnia
Copper	Anemia, changes in hair structure, heart damage, growth retardation, impaired bones, lung disease
Iron	Anemia, weakened immunity, dizziness, fatigue, irregular heartbeat
Magnesium	Muscle cramps, heart irregularities, insomnia, hypertension, diabetes, osteoporosis, sugar cravings, depression
Phosphorus	Bone pain, mental confusion, anorexia, anemia, low immunity, respiratory difficulties, seizures
Potassium	Loss of appetite, nausea, drowsiness, excessive thirst, irrational behavior, fatigue, muscle pain, weakness (especially in the lower legs), irregular heartbeat
Zinc	Loss of appetite or taste, impaired immunity, growth retardation, skin changes, increased susceptibility to infection

Did you happen to notice that many of the conditions on the list are in fact much worse than the heartburn itself? Again, OTC medications act similarly to prescription drugs: They deplete essential micronutrients and open the door for future illnesses and diseases that are often much worse than the condition you took the OTC medication to get rid of. While OTC medications may be easier to acquire, they are in no way any less dangerous where micronutrient depletion is concerned.

Heartburn Got You All Hot and Bothered?

Stop the burn! Simply take digestive enzymes before meals until the situation is under control. Truth be told, heartburn is almost always a case of too little acid for proper digestion, not too much. Antacids not only deplete you of your essential micronutrients, but they also don't address the real problem at all. If the condition persists, add in acid by taking betaine HCL with pepsin (available at health food stores). Caution: *Do not* take with aspirin, ibuprofen, or other nonsteroidal anti-inflammatory drugs, as this could damage the lining of your gastrointestinal tract.

Toxic Load

Look around. This is not the world of our ancestors. In fact, it isn't even the same world that our grandparents or great-grandparents enjoyed. Not only is our soil and our food supply becoming more and more micronutrient-depleted by the day, but the world around us, including the foods we eat and the items we surround ourselves with, are also filled with potentially dangerous toxins. How did this happen? To put it plainly—industrialization. In an attempt to make our human lives easier, we have destroyed the natural environment of our ancestors and replaced it with an unhealthy man-made environment filled with industrialized chemical runoff, animals forced to live in unnatural environments and given unnatural feed, and products sold globally with little to no testing and regulation for safety. On the following page, Table 4.4 outlines a few examples of toxins hiding in plain sight in your refrigerator and pantry. How many of these products do you buy at the grocery store and possibly feed to your family that contain these three toxins?

TOXINS IN HOUSEHOLD ITEMS

Just because you don't put something in your mouth doesn't mean that you aren't ingesting it! It's true. Your skin is constantly absorbing the things it comes into contact with, and the average person sure is giving it a lot to drink in. In fact, the average woman uses 12 beauty and skin products containing 168 different ingredients daily. Men aren't far behind, using six products daily with 85 unique ingredients. But who uses the most products? It might surprise you, but teen girls (whose smaller bodies are still developing hormonally) actually use an

TABLE 4.4

TOXINS FOUND IN FOODS AND THEIR DANGERS[50]

TOXIN	WHERE IT IS FOUND; HOW TO AVOID	CONCERNS	MICRONUTRIENTS TO PREVENT TOXICITY
Lead	**Found in:** Rice, protein powder, juice and foods containing synthetic nitrates (like bacon) **Avoid by:** Choosing meat products without synthetic nitrates and reducing rice and juice consumption; make sure the manufacturer of your protein powder can show you a heavy metal third-party lab analysis.	Fatigue, headaches, irritability, uneasy stomach, reduced IQ and attention span, impaired growth, reading and learning disabilities, hearing loss, mental retardation, coma, convulsion, death	Vitamins B_1, B_6, C, and E; calcium; iron; phosphorus; selenium; zinc; alpha-lipoic acid; and quercetin have the ability to scavenge free radicals and chelate lead ions. While vitamin D usually increases the absorption of calcium, magnesium, and zinc, if those minerals are deficient, it may work to increase intestinal absorption of lead instead. As lead and iron share a common absorptive mechanism, lead uptake is enhanced in iron deficiency.[51]
Mercury	**Found in:** Fish, usually the largest predatory fish, like swordfish and shark, that have eaten the greatest majority of toxin-containing smaller fish for the longest period of time **Avoid by:** Choosing smaller fish.	Sensory impairment (vision, hearing, speech), disturbed sensation, lack of coordination, profuse sweating, faster-than-normal heartbeat, increased salivation, high blood pressure	Selenium and vitamins C and E
Arsenic	**Found in:** Rice, juice, protein powder, foods containing synthetic nitrates, poultry from conventional farms **Avoid by:** Choosing meats without nitrates and organic poultry; make sure the manufacturer of your protein powder can show you a heavy metal third-party lab analysis.	Nerve damage; scaling skin; skin pigment changes; circulatory problems; increased risk of lung, bladder, kidney, skin, and liver cancer	Phosphorus, selenium, vitamins A and E

average of 17 personal care products each day—40 percent more than an adult woman.[52] And these numbers are only the beginning in terms of what your body is absorbing. Think about the dish detergent, stain-resistant chemically coated carpeting, cleaning products, Teflon-coated pans, laundry cleaners, dryer sheets, and air fresheners you come into contact with daily. It really adds up. According to the United Nations Environment Programme, approximately 70,000 chemicals are commonly used across the world, with 1,000 new chemicals being introduced every year. While many of these new industrialized chemicals act as obesogens, disrupting your endocrine system and causing weight gain and hormonal issues, all of them increase your toxic load.

And your body only has two ways of handling this toxic load: Either the toxins wreak havoc in your body—causing thyroid issues, neurological damage, or even cancer—or, preferably, you have enough essential micronutrients around for natural detoxification to occur. As it turns out, micronutrients work as the body's natural detoxifiers, affecting both the absorption and excretion of these toxic contaminants. So you may not be able to tell your boss that the air freshener has to go, but you can reduce its obesogenic effect by making sure you are sufficient in the essential micronutrients, specifically the antioxidants (vitamins A, C, E, and alpha-lipoic acid) as well as magnesium, selenium, and zinc. Zinc is actually an important immune strengthener and tissue healer and is necessary for the functioning of many detoxifying enzymes, thus helping to protect the cells from pollutant toxins.

The Top 10 Terrific Tricks to Reduce Household Toxins

Remember, the Micronutrient Miracle plan is all about driving down your micronutrient depletion by making changes in your diet and lifestyle. This is not meant to stress you out. If this is your first 28-day plan, we want you to make the changes that you can. Food and supplementation first, and changes to your lifestyle and environment second. However, if you already shop using our *Rich Food, Poor Food* philosophy and are ready for the next step, then jump right in and change out your household and beauty products for safer nontoxic ones. Make changes at your own pace; remember, you can always add in another great habit tomorrow! Here are our top 10 terrific tricks to get you started no matter where you begin your journey to micronutrient sufficiency. Note: Whenever you see an asterisk (*) next to a product, you can find a coupon for that product in our Micronutrient Miracle Resource Center at mymiracleplan.com.

1. **Find a new fragrance.** This goes for your house, your car, and your body. We want you to ditch any product that says "perfume" or "fragrance" on the label. Don't worry, this doesn't mean that you have to smell bad. Natural essential oils can be used to recreate perfume,

and burning them over an oil burner quickly fills a room with scents ranging from sweet vanilla to spicy cinnamon or woodsy eucalyptus. *Safe alternatives include* Aura Cacia aromatherapy mists* or Mrs. Meyer's Clean Day air fresheners. You can also try a lotion like Face Naturals Organic Creamy Coconut and Key Lime Body Butter* to keep your skin smelling delicious all day.

2. **Launder your detergent.** You want your clothes to come out clean, not coated with a film of irritants and potential carcinogens, right? Remember, you will likely be wearing these clothes for hours, so anything on them will surely end up in you. Always avoid products with labels that say "warning," "danger," or "poison." Forego fabric softener and instead add 2 cups of organic vinegar to the wash. *Safe alternatives include* detergent by GreenShield Organic,* Dr. Bronner's, Seventh Generation, and Mrs. Meyer's Clean Day.

3. **Ditch the dryer sheets.** You just don't need them, and you'll never know what is in them anyway. This is because manufacturers aren't required to tell you. While the box may just list the ingredients as "biodegradable cationic softeners," you may be coating your clothes with camphor, chloroform, or ethyl acetate, all of which are on the Environmental Protection Agency's hazardous waste list, or with alpha-terpineol, benzyl alcohol, or linalool, all of which are known to cause nervous system disorders. *Safe alternatives include* adding essential oils to a wet cloth before starting the dryer, purchasing wool balls, or using Mrs. Meyer's Clean Day dryer sheets.

4. **Toss the traditional toothpaste.** Your mouth and the rest of your body will thank you for choosing a product that does not contain fluoride, artificial flavors and colors, polysorbate-80, ethanol, titanium dioxide, benzoate or benzoic acid, or sodium lauryl sulfate. There are a plethora of options for your pearly whites. *Safe alternatives include* toothpaste by Redmond Clay,* JÂSÖN, Jack n' Jill (for the little ones), Just the Goods, and Tom's of Maine.

5. **Shun the traditional shampoos and body washes.** Here again, products are misleading you with promises. Herbal Essences commercials, for example, suggest a climactic shower experience, and with herbal in the name, what could possibly be wrong? However, the list of ingredients will really make you shake and shudder. Watch out for parabens, fragrances, sodium lauryl sulfate, and polyethylene glycol (often listed as PEG) in your shampoos and conditioners. The good

news is that the alternative "healthy" products are so gentle you can save cash by using them on both your hair and body. *Safe alternatives include* products by Beauty Without Cruelty (BWC), Maia's, Annemarie Gianni Skin Care,* Face Naturals,* and The Honest Company.

6. **Manage your makeup.** No, we aren't suggesting that you have to leave your face bare. There are plenty of responsible brands these days that realize that lead in lipstick is lousy and mercury in mascara is maddening. Take some time off, and allow your skin to breathe and detox naturally when at home or out with loved ones. And when you want to doll up, choose from brands that make you beautiful on the outside and keep you beautifully healthy on the inside. *Safe alternatives include* products by Maia's, Beauty Without Cruelty (BWC),* Au Naturale,* W3LL People,* and jane iredale. Some drugstore products like Revlon Colorburst lipstick and Almay Intense I-Color Volumizing Mascara also hit the mark.

7. **Drop the deodorant.** It is time to save those sweat glands from the estrogenic, and likely cancer causing, aluminum found in most antiperspirants. Many also add in unwanted parabens, triclosan, steareth, propylene glycol, and talc, which are all possible allergens—not to mention that unwanted mystery "fragrance" again. If natural crystals are your choice, opt for a Himalayan salt spray, like the one made by Face Naturals; they leave out the potassium alum found in most crystal sprays. *Safe alternatives include* Face Naturals Pink Salt Deodorant Spray or Grapefruit Natural Deodorant Stick,* Pure & Natural Crystal Mist Body Spray, Poofy Organics,* and Arm & Hammer.

8. **Set aside the dish soaps.** First things first: Clean your house of any product that says antibacterial, as the common ingredient triclosan has been shown to interrupt the endocrine system, even in very low doses. Whew! Now we can get to the nitty-gritty of getting clean. As always, skip artificially "fragranced" products and search out ones with the fewest and least unpronounceable chemicals listed on the back. *Safe alternatives include* Mrs. Meyer's Clean Day, GreenShield Organic,* Seventh Generation, and The Honest Company.

9. **Pass on plastic storage.** Toss the Tupperware and purge the plastic wrap. It's time to rethink how you can safely stow your leftovers. Purchase glass storage containers in a variety of sizes with covers to match. Make sure the lids are BPA-free, lead-free, PVC-free, and phthalate-free. Not only will you drive down your toxic exposure but

---

Don't Be Fooled by Misleading Marketing!

Products labeled "nontoxic," "biodegradable," and "earth friendly" aren't always safer choices. Even "organic" can leave you with a false sense of safety. There are no federal regulations to require that household products advertised as "natural" or "organic" actually live up to these claims. For safer nontoxic options in each category, visit the Micronutrient Miracle Motivation and Resource Center online at mymiracleplan.com. We have some great resources that will help you grade the products you are currently using and find safer ones.

---

you will also find that your food stays fresher longer, and that can save you money. *Safe alternatives include* glass storage containers with BPA-free lids (we use Pyrex, MightyNest, and Martha Stewart).

10. **Nix the nonstick pots and pans.** While Teflon nonstick coating can make cleanup a cinch, there is no easy way to get the toxins from it out of your system. The repelling action comes from a class of toxins called perfluorinated compounds (PFCs), and they are found not only on your favorite frying pan but also on your raincoats, your boots (think Gore-Tex), and popcorn bags and buckets to keep the grease from seeping through onto your lap in the movie theater. The harmful PFCs in Gore-Tex or Teflon, which can be found in the blood of 98 percent of the population, can remain in your body for 5 to 8 years! They have been shown to increase the risk of cancer, ADHD, heart disease, infertility, and obesity.[53] *Safe alternatives include* cookware made of glass, enamel, stainless steel, or "Made in the USA" cast iron. We love Xtrema Ceramic cookware. Look for clothes treated with Nikwax.

Accounting for Your Actions

It is now time to review your lifestyle habits to discover how they may be contributing to your current state of micronutrient deficiency. To reiterate, we don't want you to just up and quit all of your micronutrient-depleting habits; some habits, like living gluten-free and exercising, are encouraged. Other lifestyle EMDs, like living in a big city, you will not likely be able to change. This exercise is simply to help you realize which micronutrients you are unknowingly putting at risk so you can fully understand the need for more quality, micronutrient-dense foods, along with proper supplementation to fill in these gaps. Take your time and be as accurate as you can. Once you complete this chart, you will be able to quickly identify which micronutrients your current lifestyle is putting at serious risk of deficiency.

Step 1: To see just how many lifestyle habits may be affecting your micronutrient sufficiency levels, we want you to look at Table 4.5 on the next page and place a check (✓) in the Tabulations column for every day of the week that you might take part in one of these lifestyle EMDs. If, for example, you determine that you exercise 3 days a week, then you should give yourself three checks. Make sure to follow the directions at the top of the category. You need to tabulate your usage of each EMD in the chart.

Step 2: Fill in Table 4.6 on page 114. This is your current Everyday Micronutrient Depleters Lifestyle Habits Chart. Using the checks you entered in Table 4.5, calculate how many times each micronutrient might be affected. For example, if you had three checks next to exercise, then you will need to put three points next to each vitamin and mineral that exercise depletes. This means that you will write the number 3 next to vitamins A, B_2, C, and E; iron; magnesium; manganese; potassium; selenium; zinc; alpha-lipoic acid; and CoQ10. Mark down your total for each EMD in every micronutrient it depletes. You will hit some micronutrients more than once. When you do this, simply mark the second number to the right of the first. For example, you could end up with something like this:

Calcium: 11 6 27 5 3

Step 3: Total the numbers listed for each micronutrient. For example:

Calcium: 11 + 6 + 27 + 5 + 3 + = 52

Step 4: It's time to analyze your data. Are you a bit surprised at how micronutrient-depleting your diet and lifestyle actually are? Even your healthy habits, like exercise, may unknowingly be putting you at risk of depletions that could lead to further health issues later on. Our goal is to make you aware of your deficiency so that you can hold yourself accountable for your actions and make the changes in your life that will lead to micronutrient sufficiency and, ultimately, optimal health. Take a look at which micronutrients your current lifestyle habits deplete in Table 4.6 on page 114. Then turn back to page 27 in Chapter 1 and revisit "Your Personal Micronutrient Deficiency List." Do the micronutrients you are depleting through your diet and lifestyle correlate with those on "Your Personal Micronutrient Deficiency List"? If the answer is yes, great! That means that just a few simple lifestyle changes could add up to big health improvements for you.

(continued on page 115)

TABLE 4.5

EVERYDAY MICRONUTRIENT DEPLETERS DUE TO LIFESTYLE HABITS

DIETARY PROFILE (You may fit into more than one dietary profile.)	MICRONUTRIENTS COMMONLY FOUND DEFICIENT	TABULATIONS (Give yourself 7 points here, as your dietary profile stays the same each of the 7 days of the week.)
Vegan and vegetarian	A, B_3, B_9, B_{12}, D, calcium, chromium, copper, iodine, iron, magnesium, manganese, zinc, omega-3	
Gluten-free	A, B_1, B_2, B_3, B_5, B_6, B_7, B_9, B_{12}, D, calcium, copper, iron, magnesium, phosphorus, zinc	
Primal/Paleo	B_7, calcium, chromium	
Low fat	A, D, E, K, calcium, omega-3	
High protein	B_6	
Lactose-free	B_1, D, calcium	
Low carbohydrate	B_2, B_6, B_9, calcium, magnesium, potassium, iron	
High carbohydrate	B_3, D, calcium, chromium, copper, iron, magnesium, manganese, zinc	
Raw food	A, B_{12}, calcium, iron	
Low sodium	Iodine	
Low calorie	A, B_1, B_2, B_3, C, E	
Weight Watchers or similar	B_2, B_3, calcium, iron, magnesium, potassium, zinc	
Standard American diet (SAD)	A, D, E, K, calcium, iodine, magnesium, potassium, zinc, omega-3	

LIFESTYLE HABITS	MICRONUTRIENTS DEPLETED	TABULATIONS (one check for each day in a week)
Stress	A, B_1, B_2, B_3, B_5, B_6, B_7, B_9, B_{12}, choline, C, D, E, calcium, chromium, copper, iodine, iron, magnesium, potassium, selenium, zinc, omega-3, carnitine	
Exercise	A, B_2, C, E, iron, magnesium, manganese, potassium, selenium, zinc, alpha-lipoic acid, CoQ10	
Smoking	A, B_1, B_6, B_9, C, E, selenium, zinc, alpha-lipoic acid	
Pollution—living in a big city	A, C, D, E, copper, manganese, selenium, zinc, alpha-lipoic acid	

TABLE 4.5 (cont.)		
OTC DRUGS	**MICRONUTRIENTS DEPLETED**	**TABULATIONS** (one check for each time taken in a week)
NSAIDs: ibuprofen (Advil, Motrin), naproxen (Aleve, Midol)	B_9, C, iron, zinc	
Aspirin: Bufferin, St. Joseph, Bayer, Excedrin	B_9, C, K, iron, potassium, zinc	
Acetaminophen: Tylenol	B_9, C, iron, potassium, CoQ10	
Antacids: Gaviscon, Gelusil, Maalox, Mylanta	B_1, B_9, D, calcium, chromium, copper, iron, magnesium, manganese, phosphorus, zinc	
Laxatives: Carter's Little Pills, Correctol, Dulcolax, Feen-A-Mint	A, B_{12}, E, calcium, potassium	
H_2 inhibitors/ H_2 blockers: Axid, Pepcid, Mylanta, Tagamet, Zantac	B_1, B_9, B_{12}, D, calcium, copper, iron, magnesium, phosphorus, potassium, zinc	
Alli diet aid (Orlistat)	A, D, E, K, omega-3, omega-6	
TOXIC HEAVY METALS	**MICRONUTRIENTS DEPLETED**	**TABULATIONS** (one check for each time you come into contact with these sources per week)
Lead (see suspected sources on page 102)	B_1, B_6, C, E, calcium, iron, phosphorus, selenium, zinc, alpha-lipoic acid	
Mercury (see suspected sources on page 102)	C, E, selenium	
Arsenic (see suspected sources on page 102)	A, E, phosphorus, selenium	
HOUSEHOLD TOXINS	**MICRONUTRIENTS DEPLETED**	**TABULATIONS** (one check for each day you come into contact with any of these household toxins)
Currently purchasing household cleaners and personal care items without searching for nontoxic products (refer to "The Top 10 Terrific Tricks to Reduce Household Toxins" on page 103)	A, C, E, selenium, zinc, alpha-lipoic acid	

TABLE 4.5 (cont.)			
PRESCRIPTION MEDICATIONS	**INDICATION FOR USAGE**	**MICRONUTRIENTS DEPLETED**[54, 55, 56, 57]	**TABULATIONS** (one check for each time taken in a week)
Opiates: hydrocodone/ acetaminophen (Vicodin)	Pain relief	B_9, C, iron, potassium	
Statins: atorvastatin (Lipitor), ezetimibe (Zetia), fluvastatin (Lescol), lovastatin (Mevacor), pravastatin (Pravachol), rosuvastatin (Crestor), simvastatin (Zocor)	Lowering cholesterol	A, B_9, B_{12}, D, E, K, calcium, iron, magnesium, phosphorus, CoQ10	
Bile acid sequestrants (Questran, Colestid)	Lowering cholesterol	A, B_9, B_{12}, D, E, K, iron, phosphorus	
ACE inhibitors: lisinopril (Prinivil, Zestril), ramipril (Altace), quinapril (Accupril), enalapril (Vasotec)	High blood pressure	Phosphorus, zinc	
Thiazide diuretics: hydrochlorothiazide (Esidrix, Hydrodiuril, Oretic)	High blood pressure	D, calcium, magnesium, phosphorus, potassium, zinc, CoQ10	
Beta blockers: atenolol (Tenormin, Senorman), carvedilol (Coreg), nadolol (Corgard), metoprolol (Lopressor, Toprol XL)	High blood pressure; congestive heart failure	B_1, chromium, CoQ10, D	
Calcium channel blockers: amlodipine (Norvasc), felodipine (Plendil), nifedipine (Procardia, Adalat), nimodipine (Nimotop), nisoldipine (Sular)	High blood pressure	D	
Vasodilators: hydralazine (Apresoline)	High blood pressure	B_6, magnesium, CoQ10	
Antihypertensives: methyldopa (Aldomet)	High blood pressure	B_{12}	
Loop diuretics: bumetanide (Bumex, Burinex), ethacrynic acid (Edecrin), furosemide (Lasix), torsemide (Demadex)	High blood pressure; heart failure	B_1, B_6, B_9, C, calcium, chromium, iron, magnesium, phosphorus, potassium, zinc	
Potassium-sparing diuretics: amiloride (Midamor), spironolactone (Aldactone), triamterene (Maxzide, Dyazide, Dyrenium)	High blood pressure; heart failure	B_9, calcium, magnesium, phosphorus, potassium, zinc	

TABLE 4.5 (cont.)			
PRESCRIPTION MEDICATIONS	**INDICATION FOR USAGE**	**MICRONUTRIENTS DEPLETED**[54, 55, 56, 57]	**TABULATIONS** (one check for each time taken in a week)
Cardiac glycosides: digoxin (Lanoxicaps, Lanoxin)	Heart failure; arrhythmias	B_1, calcium, magnesium, phosphorus, potassium	
Anticoagulants: warfarin (Coumadin)	Heart: blood clots	K, iron	
Bisphosphonates: alendronate (Fosamax), risedronate (Actonel), ibandronate (Boniva), tiludronate (Skelid)	Osteoporosis	Calcium, magnesium, phosphorus	
Proton-pump inhibitors: lansoprazole (Prevacid), omeprazole (Losec, Prilosec), rabeprazole (Aciphex), pantoprazole (Pantoloc, Protonix), Nexium	Gastroesophageal reflux disease (GERD); severe gastric ulceration	A, B_1, B_9, B_{12}, C, calcium, iron, magnesium, zinc	
Methylxanthines: theophylline (Accubron, Theobid, Elixicon)	Asthma; COPD (chronic obstructive pulmonary disease)	B_6	
Beta-2 adrenergic receptor agonists: albuterol (Salbutamol, Proventil, Ventolin), bitolterol (Tornalate), fluticasone/salmeterol (Advair), isoetharine (Bronkosol, Bronkometer), levalbuterol (Xopenex), metaproterenol (Alupent), pirbuterol (Maxair), salmeterol (Serevent), terbutaline (Brethine)	Asthma; COPD	Calcium, magnesium, phosphorus, potassium	
Corticosteroids: cortisone (Cortone), hydrocortisone (Cortef, Hydrocortone), prednisone (Deltasone, Meticorten, Orasone, Panasol-S), prednisolone (Delta-Cortef, Prelone, Pediapred), triamcinolone (Aristocort, Atolone, Kenacort), methylprednisolone (Medrol), fluticasone (Flonase, Cutivate, Veramyst), beclomethasone (Beconase, Qvar, Vancenase, Vanceril)	Severe inflammation; autoimmune disease; immune system suppression; asthma; allergic rhinitis	A, B_6, B_9, B_{12}, C, D, K, calcium, magnesium, phosphorus, potassium, selenium, zinc, amino acids (carnitine)	

TABLE 4.5 (cont.)			
PRESCRIPTION MEDICATIONS	**INDICATION FOR USAGE**	**MICRONUTRIENTS DEPLETED**[54, 55, 56, 57]	**TABULATIONS** (one check for each time taken in a week)
Sulfonylureas: glyburide (Diabeta, Glynase, Micronase), glipizide (Glucotrol), glimepiride (Amaryl), chlorpropamide (Diabinese, Insulase)	Diabetes	CoQ10	
Biguanides: metformin (Glucophage)	Diabetes; prediabetes	B_1, B_9, B_{12}, CoQ10	
Colchicine (Colcrys)	Gout	A, B_9, B_{12}, D, iron, potassium	
Probenecid	Gout	B_2	
Progestin: medroxyprogesterone (Depo-Provera, Provera, Amen, Curretab, Cycrin, Prodroxy)	Birth control	B_2	
Conjugated estrogens: estrogen replacement therapies (Alora, Cenestin, Climara, Estinyl, Estrace, Estraderm, Estratab, FemPatch, Menest, Ogen, Premarin, Premphase, Prempro, Vivelle); estrogen and progesterone–containing oral contraceptives (Ovral, Lo/Ovral, Low-Ogestrel)	Hormone replacement therapy; birth control	B_1, B_2, B_3, B_5, B_6, B_9, C, D, calcium, magnesium, manganese, zinc, amino acids (carnitine)	
Antimalarial medications: chloroquine, Primaquine	Malaria	B_2	
Antimycobacterials: isoniazid, ethambutol, pyrazinamide	Tuberculosis	B_3, B_6, D, K, zinc	
Nucleoside metabolic inhibitors: 5-fluoracil (Efudex, Adrucil, Carac, Fluoroplex)	Cancer	B_1	
Anticonvulsant barbiturates: carbamazepine (Carbatrol, Epitol, Equetro, Tegretol), primidone (Mysoline), phenytoin (Di-Phen, Dilantin, Phenytek)	Seizure medication	B_1, B_3, B_6, B_7, B_9, B_{12}, C, D, E, K, calcium	
Levothyroxine (Synthroid, Levoxyl, Levothroid, Unithroid)	Hypothyroidism	Calcium	
Human immunodeficiency virus nucleoside analog reverse-transcriptase inhibitors: azidothymidine (AZT), zidovudine (Retrovir)	HIV	Copper, zinc	

TABLE 4.5 (cont.)			
PRESCRIPTION MEDICATIONS	**INDICATION FOR USAGE**	**MICRONUTRIENTS DEPLETED**[54, 55, 56, 57]	**TABULATIONS** (one check for each time taken in a week)
Tricyclic antidepressants: amitriptyline (Elavil), doxepin (Silenor, Zonalon, Prudoxin), desipramine (Norpramin), imipramine (Tofranil, Tofranil-PM), amoxapine (Asendin), protriptyline (Vivactil)	Depression	B_2, CoQ10	
Psychoactive drugs: benzodiazepines (Valium, Xanax, Ativan, Klonopin); SSRIs (Celexa, Luvox, Lexapro, Prozac, Paxil)	Anxiety, depression	B_6, B_9, B_{12}, C, D, omega-3, omega-6, CoQ10, amino acids	
Atypical antipsychotics: clozapine (Clozaril, Fazaclo), aripiprazole (Abilify)	Schizophrenia	Selenium	
Phenothiazines: chlorpromazine, promethazine, thioridazine	Antipsychotic	B_2, CoQ10	
Sulfonamides, sulphonamides, or sulfa drugs: sulfadiazine, sulfamethizole (Thiosulfil Forte), sulfamethoxazole (Gantanol), sulfasalazine (Azulfidine), sulfisoxazole (Gantrisin)	Bacterial infection	B_1, B_2, B_7, B_9, B_{12}, C	
Macrolide antibiotics: amoxicillin (Amoxil, Trimox), erythromycin (Robimycin), azithromycin (Zithromax), clarithromycin (Biaxin)	Bacterial Infection	B_1, B_2, B_3, B_6, B_7, B_9, B_{12}, K	
Aminoglycoside antibiotics: gentamicin (Geromycin), neomycin (Mycifradin, Neo-Fradin, Neo-Tab)	Bacterial infection	A, B_6, B_{12}, K, calcium, iron, magnesium, potassium	
Fluoroquinolone antibiotics: ciprofloxacin (Cipro), enoxacin (Penetrex), gatifloxacin (Tequin), levofloxacin (Levaquin), lomefloxacin (Maxaquin), moxifloxacin (Avelox), norfloxacin (Noroxin), ofloxacin (Floxin), sparfloxacin (Zagam), trovafloxacin (Trovan)	Bacterial infection	B_1, B_2, B_3, B_6, B_7, B_9, B_{12}, K, calcium, iron, magnesium, zinc	

TABLE 4.6
EVERYDAY MICRONUTRIENT DEPLETERS LIFESTYLE HABIT CHART

MICRONUTRIENT	TABULATION TOTALS
Vitamin A	
Vitamin B$_1$ (thiamine)	
Vitamin B$_2$ (riboflavin)	
Vitamin B$_3$ (niacin)	
Vitamin B$_5$ (pantothenic acid)	
Vitamin B$_6$ (pyridoxine)	
Vitamin B$_7$ (biotin)	
Vitamin B$_9$ (folate)	
Vitamin B$_{12}$ (cobalamin)	
Choline	
Vitamin C	
Vitamin D	
Vitamin E	
Vitamin K	
Calcium	
Chromium	
Copper	
Iodine	
Iron	
Magnesium	
Manganese	
Phosphorus	
Potassium	
Selenium	
Zinc	
Omega-3	
Omega-6	
Alpha-lipoic acid	
Amino acids (carnitine)	
CoQ10	

The most important thing is that between your diet analysis (completed at the end of Chapter 3), your lifestyle analysis (completed in this chapter), and your Personal Micronutrient Deficiency List, you are now aware of the micronutrients you will want to focus on becoming sufficient in over your 28-day plan. Your health is in your hands, and the first step to improving it is to restock your pantry with Rich Food. So turn the page and let's go shopping!

5

SHOPPING SOLUTIONS:
More Micronutrient Bang in Every Bite!

YOU'VE HEARD IT AT least a hundred times before: "If you want to find the healthiest foods, it's best to shop the perimeter of the grocery store." Well, while this is a good starting point, in today's modern grocery stores, loaded with misleading packaging and confusing label claims, it's really only partially correct. The truth is that there are both Rich Foods and Poor Foods in every aisle of the grocery store, including the perimeter! While the majority of the foods you're going to be choosing from to build your 28-day Micronutrient Miracle menus will be found on your store's perimeter, as you will soon see, if your goal is to bring home the freshest, most micronutrient-packed Rich Foods, there is a lot more to learn than simply to steer clear of the aisles. But never fear, you're about to get a personal lesson in how to shop safe, shop smart, save time, and save money in every aisle of the grocery store. While there is no way we can give you all the information we packed into our book *Rich Food, Poor Food*, we are going to give you a crash course so that you have all the information you need to make your 28-day Micronutrient Miracle plan a resounding success. However, we highly recommend you pick up a copy of *Rich Food, Poor Food* as well. Believe us, it's a resource you will use again and again throughout your journey to micronutrient sufficiency.

It's Time to Shop!

Yay! You finally made it to the fun stuff. It's now time to switch gears and start replenishing your purged Poor Food products with Rich Foods. And that can mean only one thing—a shopping excursion. (And who doesn't *love* shopping?) In this chapter, we are going to take you on a guided tour of the grocery store, focusing on the produce, proteins, and other pantry staples that you are going to need for your Micronutrient Miracle menus. Remember, our definition of Rich Food is twofold. First, our mission is to locate the foods with the highest micronutrient density; second, we must strive to avoid any problematic ingredients or processing pitfalls that can put your health at risk along the way. Always keep in mind the Poor Foods you just purged. You will want to make sure none of the foods you bring back into the house have any of the purged ingredients in them, under any of their aliases. It is time to show you how to identify the Rich Foods that pack the biggest micronutrient punch, because those are the foods we want in your shopping cart!

Now, there is a good chance that this Rich Food shopping expedition is going to be a little different than what you are used to. So here are a few tips to ensure that it is a success. First, give yourself plenty of time. Most first-time Rich Food shoppers spend more time than usual reading labels and identifying the Rich Food choices available in their grocery store. A tight schedule will not make for an enjoyable or productive experience. Neither will a hungry belly or a cart full of restless kids, for that matter. So make sure to pick a day when your schedule is clear. The good news is that once you have located the Rich Foods you will be using over the next 28 days, your subsequent shopping excursions will be a snap. Second, stay relaxed. If you get into the store and start feeling a little overwhelmed, don't worry. The concepts and terminology we have been introducing you to will become more familiar. By the end of your 28-day Micronutrient Miracle plan, we bet that you will be sailing down the aisles, pointing out Poor Food ingredients to perfect strangers. This is a common trait of those who have recently converted to the Micronutrient Miracle lifestyle. And lastly, remember that no one expects you to be perfect—we know we're not. We are here to give you guidelines, not orders. Our goal is to show you how to choose the most micronutrient-dense Rich Foods possible; it is not to make you feel guilty if a Poor Food ends up in your cart now and then. Just do your best. Even small changes can add up to miraculous results. Well, with all this in mind, it looks like there is just one thing left to do; let's jump right in. Our first stop is the produce department!

Note: Throughout this chapter whenever you see an asterisk (*) next to a product, you can find a coupon for that product in our Micronutrient Miracle Resource Center at mymiraleplan.com. Additionally, these Rich Food Picks are only a few of the fabulous finds mentioned in *Rich Food, Poor Food*. For an extremely detailed list of all the brands and products we choose, make sure to check out our book *Rich Food, Poor Food*.

Produce

Don't you just love how more and more stores have really decked out their produce departments? Some use wooden crates and handwritten signs to make it feel more like a farmers' market, while others go all out with intermittent rain showers, complete with stormlike sound effects. But make no mistake about it; while the produce department can seem like a magical place filled with brightly colored fruits and vegetables, it is also home to some very dangerous Poor Foods, as well.

Let's begin with what we already learned about micronutrient values. Remember, produce (or any food that travels) loses its precious micronutrients every minute of every mile that it is exposed to air, heat, and light. So, you are going to want to look for fresh, local produce whenever possible—local meaning that the produce has been grown within a 100-mile radius.

Choosing local can really have an impact on the micronutrients in your produce. Research conducted at Pennsylvania State University on the micronutrient loss in spinach lends insight into just how impactful buying local can be. The study showed that when stored at a cool 68°F, it only took 4 days for spinach to lose 47 percent of its vitamin B$_9$ (folate) and carotenoid content. Think about the back of a container truck: It can get much hotter than 68°F, and the hotter it is, the faster micronutrient loss occurs. The researchers also found that even when the spinach was kept in a refrigerator at 39°F, perhaps similar to the temperature in a refrigerated shipping truck or a cooler at a grocery store or restaurant, it lost an average of 53 percent of its folate and carotenoid content in approximately 1 week.[1]

So the trick to making sure you get all the essential micronutrients your produce has to offer is to buy it and eat it as quickly as you can after it has been picked. While this would have been a lot easier to do 70 years ago, when many Americans had backyard gardens, depending on location and the current season, you may be better off getting out of the grocery store and purchasing your produce from a local grower. In fact, based on the countries of origin we have seen stamped on many of the food boxes being delivered to the countless grocery stores across America, the produce from your local farmer is likely delivering a lot more of the micronutrients you are looking for. Kids love to pile in the car and go to the farm, and it's a great way to teach them where food comes from and how it is grown. Bottom line: Local means more micronutrient dense, and that satisfies the first part of our Rich Food definition.

You've likely also heard that eating organic produce is "healthier." But does it satisfy our Micronutrient Miracle definition of "healthier"? Do organic foods supply more micronutrients as well? In other words, will you get more micronutrients by eating an organic orange, for example, than by eating a conventionally grown orange? While surprisingly few studies have looked at this incredibly important issue, the answer appears to be—yes.

In a study published in 2008 in the *Journal of the Science of Food and Agriculture*, a team of Spanish scientists grew conventional and organic mandarin oranges on the same farm, using the same irrigation methods and tree variety.[2] The study found few visual differences between the conventional and organic oranges, although the organic fruit was marginally smaller in size.

The study found, however, that these organically grown mandarin oranges produced juice that was more intensely colored, had a superior aroma and taste, contained higher levels of all eight minerals studied (in three cases, higher by 50 percent or more), had 13 percent more vitamin C, and had a 40 percent higher concentration of vitamin A (beta-carotene).

Additionally, in one of the most ambitious attempts so far to find an answer to this elusive question, research published in 2014 in the *British Journal of Nutrition* found "statistically significant, meaningful" differences between organic and conventional fruits and vegetables. The study, which was the most comprehensive scientific analysis to date, examined more than 340 studies evaluating the nutritional differences between organic and conventional produce and determined that organic fruits and vegetables deliver between 19 and 69 percent more health-promoting antioxidants, like flavonoids and carotenoids, than conventional fruits and vegetables.[3]

So, both organic and local are going to increase your micronutrient levels over the next 28 days. But how do you think they satisfy the other part of the Rich Food definition? How do they fare when it comes to steering you clear of problematic ingredients that can put your health at risk? Whether you're buying your produce from a local farmer or from your local grocer, there are three potential dangers you are going to want to evaluate before purchasing any product: pesticide residue, GMOs (genetically modified organisms), and irradiation.

PESTICIDE RESIDUE, GMOS, AND IRRADIATION

The first potential danger we are going to investigate is pesticide residue. This is a big issue that most people do not think about when purchasing produce for their families. So, how dangerous are pesticides? According to the Environmental Protection Agency (EPA), "laboratory studies show that pesticides can cause health problems, such as birth defects, nerve damage, cancer, and other effects that might occur over a long period of time. However, these effects depend on how toxic the pesticide is and how much of it is consumed. . . . Infants and children may be especially sensitive to health risks posed by pesticides for several reasons: their internal organs are still developing and maturing, [and] in relation to their body weight, infants and children eat and drink more than adults, possibly increasing their exposure to pesticides in food and water. . . . Pesticides may harm a developing child by blocking the absorption of important food nutrients necessary for normal healthy growth. Another way pesticides may cause harm is if a child's excretory system is not fully developed, the body may not fully remove pesticides. Also, there are 'critical periods' in human development when exposure to a toxin can permanently alter the way an individual's biological system operates."[4]

So, according to the EPA, pesticides are a concern for adults who are exposed over a long period of time, as well as for children, who are vulnerable to even short-term exposure. In fact, three long-term cohort studies now suggest that certain chemical pesticides can interfere with brain development in young children.[5] Additionally, from a micronutrient perspective, foods such as fruits and vegetables that have large amounts of pesticide residue not only open the door to direct toxic damage but also work to deplete your micronutrients. Don't forget that, as we discussed in Chapter 4, micronutrients are your body's natural detoxifiers. In order to remove toxins, your body must use its essential micronutrients, making them unable to perform other vital bodily functions.

However, here is some good news that should really illuminate how great organic produce is for your health. Australian research published in the journal *Environmental Research* showed that when study participants switched to eating a diet of at least 80 percent organic food for just 1 week, their urinary analyses revealed a dramatic 89 percent reduction in detectable levels of organophosphate pesticides. Lead investigator Dr. Liza Oates stated, "Our results show that people who switch to eating mainly organic food for just 1 week can dramatically reduce their exposure to pesticides, demonstrating that an organic diet has a key role to play in a precautionary approach to reducing pesticide exposure."[6]

So if these individuals were able to reduce detectable pesticide residue by 89 percent in just 1 week by eating a diet of at least 80 percent organic foods, just think about what you are going to be able to achieve by going organic or avoiding produce known to contain high amounts of pesticide residue over your 28-day Micronutrient Miracle plan. We think you will be surprised at just how much better you'll feel when you do.

Next up on our "avoid at all costs" list is GMOs. In the produce section, there are seven genetically modified crops you currently need to avoid. They are corn, Hawaiian papaya, soybeans (edamame), potatoes, zucchini, yellow crookneck squash, and apples (Arctic apple). Two of these seven, the potatoes and the apples, were approved this year alone, and more than 30 other crops are currently being tested in field trials. These include barley, bell peppers, cabbage, carrots, cauliflower, cherries, chile peppers, coffee, cranberries, cucumbers, flaxseed, grapefruit, kiwifruit, lentils, lettuce, melons, mustard, oats, olives, onions, peanuts, pears, peas, persimmons, pineapple, popcorn, radishes, strawberries, sugar cane, sunflowers, sweet potatoes, tomatoes, walnuts, and watercress. However, we don't just avoid these GMO crops because of the lack of long-term safety data. We also dodge them because they are mineral deficient due to being sprayed with dangerous glyphosate, aka Roundup.

There are also two more reasons to steer your cart away from GMOs. The first is just how unsafe they are from a toxic perspective. Laboratory and epidemiological studies confirm that Roundup poses serious health hazards, including endocrine (hormone) disruption, DNA damage, birth defects, neurological disorders, and cancer. Yes, even cancer. A 2015 study published in the *Lancet Oncology* performed by the International Agency for Research on Cancer (IARC) declared that glyphosate is a "probable human carcinogen." Some of these detrimental effects were found at "realistic" low levels, like those found as residues on food, on feed crops, and in contaminated water. This suggests that people who eat foods made from GMO crops could be ingesting potentially dangerous levels of Roundup residues. Glyphosate has been detected in the air, in rain, in groundwater, in people's urine, and even circulating in women's blood. And this is of particular concern, since glyphosate can cross the placental barrier and potentially harm an unborn fetus.

The final reason to avoid genetically modified produce circles back to the discussion on lectins. Remember that lectins, one of the Everyday Micronutrient Depleters (EMDs), are a plant's natural pest repellent. In Chapter 3, you learned how these horrible little obesogens rob us of vitamins and minerals, cause leaky gut, and also induce weight gain. Well, when scientists want to create GMO produce that is heartier than the natural version of the fruit or vegetable and that can withstand more sprays and fend off more pests, guess what they do? Yes, you guessed it. Scientists splice in lectins in order to enhance the GMO produce's "natural" pest and fungal resistance, thus enhancing its obesogenic effects.[7]

Okay, you are probably getting the picture here: Your goal during the 28-day Micronutrient Miracle plan is to reduce your exposure to pesticide residue and GMOs as much as possible, and while buying local produce can't ensure where the seeds came from or how they were sprayed, we think you can probably guess by now how to protect yourself. The answer comes down to two little words you are already familiar with: *Buy organic!* Organic produce protects you from toxic pesticide residue, and it also guarantees that your food is not genetically modified and has not lost its micronutrient value due to irradiation—the third and final pitfall you want to avoid when purchasing produce. In fact, according to the USDA's *Organic Production and Handling Standards,* the term *organic* requires that a food be free of potentially harmful or toxic pesticides, herbicides, chemical fertilizers, sewage sludge, and genetically modified organisms. It must also be free of artificial hormones (including recombinant bovine growth hormone—rBGH and rBST) and antibiotics, both of which will become important later in the chapter when we discuss how to choose micronutrient-rich proteins. And, like we said, the organic seal also guarantees that your food, both produce and proteins, has not been processed using irradiation, chemical food additives, or industrial solvents.

DON'T BREAK THE BANK:
THE FAB 14 AND TERRIBLE 20 SAFE SHOPPING GUIDE

Now, while organic may be king in the produce department, we don't have a royal bank account, and we are pretty sure that your money matters to you, too. So you are going to have to find a way to purchase safe, micronutrient-rich foods within a realistic budget. Wouldn't it be great to have a list of some kind that told you which fruits and vegetables were GMOs and which contained the most pesticide residue so you could better decide where to spend your hard-earned money?

Well, guess what? We've created just such a list, and it does both of those things. It's called the Fab 14 and Terrible 20 Safe Shopping Guide, and it will help you avoid *all* the GMOs in the produce department (they are marked with a dagger [†]) as well as identify which produce should be purchased organically, due to high pesticide residue. Additionally, it shows which produce items have very low pesticide residue and are safe to buy conventionally. In fact, by only purchasing the foods on the Fab 14 list conventionally and anything on the Terrible 20 list organically, **you can reduce your exposure to dangerous, micronutrient-depleting pesticide residue by 80 percent**. Amazing, right?

We created the Fab 14 and Terrible 20 lists as a way for everyone to identify safe produce in the grocery store as well as when dining out. And we've added a new category we are calling the Tweens. These are the fruits and vegetables that fall somewhere in the middle—not as Fab as they could be, but not that Terrible, either. We have listed them for you from least pesticide laden (i.e., honeydew melon was next on the Fab 14 list) to more pesticide laden (i.e., cherries were next on the Terrible 20 list). Take a moment to examine the foods on each list.

THE FAB 14 AND TERRIBLE 20 SAFE SHOPPING GUIDE

THE FAB 14: On a budget, choose these conventionally grown. They are listed from best (lowest pesticide content) to worst (highest pesticide content).

THE TWEENS: These are listed from best (lowest pesticide content) to worst (highest pesticide content).

THE TERRIBLE 20: Always buy these organic and avoid them at restaurants, unless specifically listed as organic (listed from highest pesticide content to lowest and includes GMO produce[†]).

FAB 14	TWEENS	TERRIBLE 20
Avocado	Honeydew melon	Apples[†]
Pineapples	Watermelon	Peaches
Cabbage	Tomatoes	Nectarines
Sweet peas	Oranges	Strawberries
Onions	Bananas	Grapes
Asparagus	Green onions	Celery
Mango	Broccoli	Spinach
Kiwifruit	Carrots	Sweet bell peppers
Eggplant	Tangerines	Cucumbers
Grapefruit	Winter squash	Cherry tomatoes
Cantaloupe	Raspberries	Snap peas
Cauliflower	Green beans	Soybeans (edamame)[†]
Sweet potatoes	Pears	Potatoes[†]
Mushrooms	Plums	Hot peppers
	Cherries	Kale/collard greens
		Blueberries
		Lettuce
		Summer squash (zucchini[†] or yellow crookneck[†])
		Hawaiian papaya[†]
		Sweet corn[†]

Are you surprised by all the foods on the Terrible 20 list that you may eat on a regular basis, such as spinach, lettuce, or zucchini? Isn't it shocking that many of the foods parents put into their children's lunch boxes—like apples, strawberries, and grapes—are some of the worst offenders? With the Tweens category, you have to use your best judgment. If your budget allows, we suggest going organic. However, it's nice to know that you have a few extra choices that are not too heavily sprayed and are free of GMOs. For the next 28 days, both at home and when dining out, if organic options are not available, we want you to choose produce from the Fab 14, say asparagus or a sweet potato, over those falling in the Tweens, such as broccoli or green beans. However, when nothing from the Fab 14 list is available, you should try to choose from the Tweens over the Terrible 20 list. Remember: When dining out, always assume the food is nonorganic unless it's specifically noted on the menu.

FROZEN AND CANNED

Looking to save some money? Who isn't? Here is a time- and money-saving tip: Don't forget that the produce section extends to canned and frozen produce, as well. We have found that while the fresh produce section may not have a wide variety of organic to choose from, the canned and frozen sections may give you a few more organic options—and at bargain prices. If you're worried about the micronutrient levels of these alternative options, here's some data to ease your mind: Research shows that canned and frozen produce is often picked closer to ripeness and then packaged very quickly, so most of the micronutrients are still intact. And don't let the micronutrient loss due to the canning and freezing processes dissuade you from purchasing these options. Data suggests that the micronutrient content is similar to that in the produce section because "fresh" produce likely took a few micronutrient-depleting days or weeks to arrive at the grocery store. The bottom line is that in terms of micronutrient value, if your produce is coming from a local farmer and you are eating it right away, you are better off buying it fresh. But if your grocer's "fresh" produce is coming from someplace far away, then canned or frozen options may be just as micronutrient dense.

A few words of warning, though. First, canned produce can be a little tricky because many of the cans found in grocery stores today are still lined with BPA, although some brands—such as Eden, Natural Value, Native Forest, and Muir Glen—have gone BPA-free. Just to be safe, always check to make sure your can is labeled "BPA-free" before purchasing. Additionally, read the ingredient lists on canned and frozen produce carefully to make sure the manufacturers didn't sneak in any Poor Food ingredients. Many contain sugar (an EMD) and refined salt (which you should avoid when possible). We will cover the health benefits of unrefined salt, one of our favorite things to top our Rich Food vegetables, later in this chapter. Also, make sure all of your imported frozen produce is

Planning a trip to the farmers' market or local farm to collect your produce? Here are the top five questions to make sure to ask.

1. "Who grew this food?" or "Did you grow this food yourself?" While the market may feel "local," the produce sold in it may have been shipped in from other states or even other countries. By asking this question first, you establish that the food you're buying really is local.

2. "Is this food certified organic?" Look, we know a lot of local farms can't afford to get organically certified, as it is often cost prohibitive. This is not a deal-breaker. However, if they answer yes, ask to see their certification.

3. "If it is not certified, then how was this produce grown?" This is where you want to allow producers to go into detail about how they eliminate pests, where they get their seeds, and how they control weeds. Allow them time to explain, but be careful and keep pushing, as there is no one checking to see that their "no-spray," "chemical-free," "natural," or "grown using organic methods" claims are true—except you!

4. "Can I visit your farm?" If there is any trace of hesitation, then step away from the table. The farmers should be proud of what they are selling and how they are growing it.

5. And finally, "Are you an imposter?" No, you can't actually ask that question. However, there are a few tell-tale signs that the farmer is false. First, are the fruits and vegetables in season, or is this farmer the only one selling the out-of-season, obviously imported produce? Additionally, if he says he doesn't spray or he has a "no-spray" farm, make sure he can tell you how he is handling weeds and pests. And finally, ask if the farmer knows what OMRI means. If the farmer is trying to follow best organic practices, even without certification, he should know that OMRI stands for the Organic Materials Review Institute. This organization provides organic certifiers, growers, manufacturers, and suppliers with an independent review of products intended for use in certified organic production, handling, and processing. Most farmers trying to grow in a truly organic manner should know what this means.

Our Good, Better, and Best for Produce

Over your 28-day Micronutrient Miracle plan, we want you to implement our Good, Better, Best strategy when choosing all of your fresh, frozen, and canned produce.

GOOD: Conventionally grown, as local as possible. Make sure to eliminate any foods from the Terrible 20 list (page 123) unless you are able to purchase organic versions.

BETTER: Organic for the Tweens and Terrible 20 lists and conventional if on the Fab 14 list. Always purchase local when available.

BEST: Purchase all local and organic produce when available.

STEER CLEAR: Presliced produce and frozen and canned foods that contain sugar, citric acid, maltodextrin, dextrose, and refined salt.

OUR RICH FOOD PICKS: Cascadian Farms frozen produce, Safeway O Organics frozen vegetables, Native Forest organic canned vegetables,* Eden Organics, Natural Value Organic,* Muir Glen Organic, Bubbies pickles and sauerkraut

(For an extremely detailed list of all the brands and products we choose for fresh, frozen, and canned produce, make sure to check out our book *Rich Food, Poor Food*.)

organic. Why? Studies from Australia and Denmark showed disturbingly high pesticide contents in imported frozen fruits and vegetables.[8, 9] Some Chilean produce even tested positive for DDT, one of the most dangerous carcinogenic pesticides ever created. This makes choosing organic in the frozen food department even more important.

Picking Perfect Proteins

Well, we've covered everything you're going to need to know to pick the most micronutrient-rich produce. Next, we will continue around the perimeter of the store and show you how to pick the perfect proteins for your Micronutrient Miracle menu. Now while our vegan-based nutrivores will be getting protein through their produce selections, sprouted nuts and seeds, and plant-based protein powders, the majority of you will be including some form of animal-based protein in your menus. And just like in the produce department, there is a lot more to learn about choosing the most micronutrient-packed protein than you might think. For example, what is the difference between grass-fed and grass-finished beef, cage-free and pasture-raised poultry or eggs, organic and conventional dairy, or wild-caught and farm-raised fish? The information we are going to share with you here in the protein department is going to be just as important as what you just learned in the produce department, in terms of getting the micronutrients you need in order to successfully achieve and sustain a micronutrient-sufficient state. Let's get started.

It wasn't really that long ago that people personally knew the butcher, milkman, or fishermen they bought their meat, dairy, or fish from. But today, for the vast majority of us at least, this is sadly not the case. Just like we encouraged you to get to know your local farmer earlier in this chapter, we also suggest you get to know the names of the butchers and fishmongers in your local grocery store. These individuals can help you choose the best cuts of meats and the freshest seafood. However, when it comes to choosing the healthiest, most micronutrient-rich source of protein, that's where we come in. To do this, we are going to use the same Good, Better, Best system we introduced in the produce section, but you'll use it for purchasing beef, pork, lamb, poultry, seafood, dairy, eggs, and the ultrahealthy bits, like hearts and livers. (Don't worry, you won't even know you are eating them!)

THE BEST FROM THE BUTCHER

Let's start in the meat section, which covers beef, bison, lamb, venison, and goat. No, you do not have to eat goat or bison while on the Micronutrient Miracle plan if you don't want to. However, it's not a bad idea to expand your horizons a bit, either. Who knows, you may actually like lamb chops! The fact is, whether you like to be creative in the kitchen or stick to old favorites, all these meats have one thing in common: They are all from *ruminants,* or animals that eat plant-based diets and digest them through a process known as rumination, which involves chewing, regurgitation, and rechewing cud to stimulate digestion. Throughout human history, the natural "grass-fed" diets of these ruminants provided our ancestors with delicious, micronutrient-rich steaks and ribs. However, as we discovered in Chapter 1, most of the meats found in grocery stores today are from factory farms, also known as CAFOs (concentrated animal feeding operations). These factory farms no longer allow animals to graze freely on grass and roam open pasture; instead, they confine the animals to feeding pens where they are given a diet of GMO grains (including corn and soy) filled with antibiotics and growth hormones. Not only is this *not* the way our ancestors' meats were raised, but this is not the meat of our ancestors in terms of micronutrient value, either.

So how do we make sure that the meats we are choosing are raised humanely and have the highest micronutrient values possible? Well, if you love animals, like we do, you can start by looking for one of the industry watchdog logos on your package (shown below), which ensures that the animals were treated humanely. The good news is that the happier and more humanely treated animals are, the healthier and more micronutrient-rich they grow up to be. Funny how that works, isn't it? This is a win-win for everyone involved.

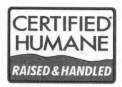   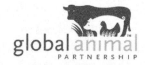

Certified Humane
A certification and label program developed by Humane Farm Animal Care and endorsed by the ASPCA and many other humane organizations.

Animal Welfare Approved
A program of the American Humane Association.

Animal Welfare Certified Run by the Animal Welfare Institute; the newest and currently the strictest certification and labeling program.

Global Animal Partnership
A five-tiered program used by Whole Foods Market that aims to improve the welfare of animals in agriculture.

However, the big game changer when it comes to the micronutrient value of your meats—and dairy products, for that matter—is whether or not they were grass-fed. The USDA requires that if a package is labeled "grass-fed," the animals must have been raised on a lifetime diet of 100 percent grass and forage (with the exception of the milk consumed prior to weaning). Research shows that the traditional grass-fed diet is far superior to a grain-fed diet in terms of essential micronutrients. For example, a joint research study between the USDA and Clemson University found that compared to grain-fed beef, grass-fed beef has higher amounts of calcium, magnesium, thiamine, riboflavin, and potassium; has over 400 percent more vitamin A and vitamin E; and is up to four times richer in heart-healthy omega-3 fatty acids. Additionally, the grass-fed beef was found to contain a healthier ratio of omega-3 to omega-6 fatty acids (i.e., higher amounts of omega-3s and lower amounts of omega-6s) and 300 to 400 percent more conjugated linoleic acid (CLA), a healthy fat that has been shown to have both anticancer and fat-metabolizing effects. However, don't be fooled by deceptive packaging. Some manufacturers stick a picture of a cow eating green grass on their packages to make you think the meat or dairy was grass-fed, or they use words like *pastured*. While "pasture-raised" is what you want to see on your egg and pork packages, as well as your chicken packaging (more on this coming up), where ruminants are concerned, we want "grass-fed" on the label. Look for the grass-fed symbols shown below to be sure your meat and dairy was truly grass-fed.

USDA Process Verified Sheild Verifies animals were raised on a lifetime diet of 100 percent grass and forage.

Food Alliance Verifies animals were raised on a lifetime diet of 100 percent grass and forage. Additionally, meats carrying this symbol are certified for not using antibiotics or hormones.

American Grassfed Verifies animals were raised on a lifetime diet of 100 percent grass and forage without onfinement, antibiotics, or hormones.

These symbols will also ensure that your meat was "grass finished," meaning that the cattle were fed grass right up through processing. Some farms "grain finish" to improve the taste and texture and to speed up the harvesting process. However, grain finishing dramatically reduces the amount of CLA and omega-3s found in the meat compared to grass-finishing, and it opens the door for GMOs.

Which brings us to the option of organic meat and dairy. Purchasing organic beef and dairy products guarantees that they are free of GMOs, antibiotics, and hormones. It also ensures that the animals have been put to pasture and allowed to eat some grass, but the time that is mandated is minimal (120 days) and the vast majority of what they eat (up to 70 percent) is permitted to come from non-GMO grains that are difficult for the animals to digest. The bottom line is that while purchasing organic meat and dairy products minimizes your toxic load, it does not guarantee the greater micronutrient levels of grass-fed beef and dairy. To get the best of both worlds, look for an option that is both grass-fed and organic.

Now, we know you may be thinking: "This is going to get expensive" or "My local grocery store doesn't carry any organic, grass-fed meats or dairy items." We completely understand; our goal is to show you the path to micronutrient sufficiency and make you aware of the safest, most micronutrient-rich choices throughout the grocery store. We are sensitive to budgetary restrictions as well as the fact that many grocery stores are not yet stocking high-quality grass-fed, organic meats and dairy items. However, Costco, Sam's Club, and other wholesale food clubs; Target; and even Walmart now carry organic and grass-fed options. This is where you have to weigh the choices and use your best judgment. We often find that people are satisfied with smaller portions of higher-quality, micronutrient-rich meats. This is because, the desire to eat more food often comes not from the fact that we did not ingest enough calories but rather from the hidden hunger for essential micronutrients. As this higher-quality, more micronutrient-rich food fills the body's requirements for micronutrients faster, less food or smaller portions satiate more fully. Keep that in mind over your 28-day Micronutrient Miracle plan and see if it isn't true for you. Additionally, don't forget to add up the cost of all the food items you may typically put into your cart on a weekly basis that are now either eliminated or restricted on your Micronutrient Miracle menu plan, including snacks, cereals, sodas, juices, store-bought desserts, pasta, wine, beer, chips, and bread. Many

Our Good, Better, and Best for Ruminants and Pork

Over your 28-day Micronutrient Miracle plan, we want you to implement our Good, Better, and Best strategy when choosing your beef, pork, and other proteins.

GOOD: Humanely raised meat free of hormones and antibiotics. Choose organic when available.

BETTER: Choose certified grass-fed/grass-finished meat or pasture-raised pork.

BEST: Choose organic, grass-fed/grass-finished meat or pasture-raised pork.

STEER CLEAR: Synthetic nitrates, dextrose, sugar, "flavoring" (as it is usually sugar and MSG), and the likely carcinogenic preservatives BHA/BHT.

OUR RICH FOOD PICKS: White Oak Pastures, Organic Prairie, Jones Creek Beef, Thousand Hills Cattle Company, Applegate (look for its organic line, as opposed to the naturals line), Atkins Ranch lamb, Pete's Paleo bacon,* and Becker Lane Organic pork. Better yet, visit mymiracleplan.com to shop online and have your high quality proteins delivered to your door from our favorite companies: US Wellness Meats, Wild Things Seafood, and Vital Choice.

(For an extremely detailed list of all of the brands and products we choose for pork, lamb, and beef, make sure to check out our book *Rich Food, Poor Food*.)

Request Rich Foods When They Aren't Sufficiently Stocked

If your local grocery store doesn't currently offer organic or grass-fed options, request them. We have created a free Rich Food request list just for you in our Micronutrient Miracle Motivation and Resource Center at mymiracleplan.com. The Rich Food request list includes all of our current Rich Food options along with their USP codes to make it easy for your grocery store manager to locate and order them. Make sure you check out the Rich Food Resources as well, including Rich Food coupons; our Fab 14 and Terrible 20 wallet guide; Rich Food video recipes; and even a Rich Food locator to help you find Rich Food farms, restaurants, and providers of raw dairy and grass-fed meat in your area. In fact, going direct for your grass-fed meats and dairy items can be a less expensive way to procure micronutrient-rich protein sources for you family. We go to local farmers who allow us to purchase high-quality, organic, grass-fed/pasture-raised meats, dairy items, and eggs at just a fraction of the price you'd pay at the grocery store. As long as you have extra freezer space, this is the most cost-effective option we have found.

times, the money you save on these items can more than make up for the difference in price between the conventional beef and dairy products and the grass-fed, organic options.

DIGGING A LITTLE DEEPER WITH DAIRY

You may have noticed that we have been referencing dairy throughout the protein department so far. Why? Well, when you think about it, dairy comes from cows and even goats, sometimes. So the rules of the meat department hold true in the dairy section, as well. This means that organic and grass-fed are still to be prioritized. However, here in the dairy section, there are a few new processing pitfalls that we need to address.

Many people have been told that they may have a dairy allergy. While there is a small percentage of people for whom this may be true, more often than not, we find that most people are actually sensitive to the two modern processing practices: pasteurization and homogenization. Pasteurization is a heating technique that "cleans" the milk, and while pasteurization kills any potentially dangerous bacteria that may be in the milk, it also kills the friendly, beneficial bacteria (like probiotics) and greatly depletes the natural micronutrient content of milk. The fact is, milk in its "natural," unpasteurized state is chock-full of micronutrients, including vitamins A, B_6, B_{12}, D, K_2, calcium, phosphorus, omega-3, and CLA. Compared to conventional pasteurized milk, natural, grass-fed raw milk has:

1. As much as 60 percent more vitamin B_1 (thiamine) and B_6
2. As much as 100 percent more B_{12}
3. As much as 30 percent more vitamin B_9 (folate)
4. Increased amounts of both calcium and phosphorus
5. Vitamin K_2 and greater amounts of CLA and anti-inflammatory omega-3s

The process of pasteurization, and especially ultra-pasteurization, denatures, or alters, the original molecular structure of the proteins in the milk itself. It flattens milk's protein molecules, allowing them to pass easily into the bloodstream, which causes an increasingly common health condition called leaky gut syndrome. When these denatured proteins get into the intestinal tract, where they do not belong, they are seen as foreign bodies, and the body initiates an immune response. Over time, this can result in reduced micronutrient absorption, an overstressed immune system, chronic fatigue, and gastrointestinal issues. Additionally, pasteurization also destroys something else: the natural lactase found in raw milk, which is the enzyme needed to digest lactose—a type of sugar naturally found in milk. So before you chalk yourself up to having a dairy intolerance, you may want to try a nonpasteurized dairy product or, at the very least, try either a lactose-free milk or goat's milk (which contains less lactose than cow's milk).

Homogenization is another problematic process for dairy products. Homogenization uses high pressure to force milk through tiny holes to break up or denature the naturally large fat particles and produce abnormally small fat particles. This is done so that the cream, which normally rises to the top of the milk container, stays suspended within the milk itself. However, this process completely changes the way the body digests and absorbs the fat and protein in milk, making it quicker and easier for the smaller fat particles to cross the gut wall, which in some people may cause allergic reactions.

While it may be difficult (and in most states impossible) to find unpasteurized milk in the grocery stores, nonhomogenized dairy products are more readily available. If you are lucky enough to procure raw dairy, be assured that unpasteurized products are always nonhomogenized. Luckily, it is much easier to find raw cheese than it is other forms of raw dairy in most grocery

Our Good, Better, and Best for Dairy

Over your 28-day Micronutrient Miracle plan, we want you to implement our Good, Better, and Best strategy when choosing your dairy products.

GOOD: Conventional, antibiotic- and hormone-free (look for rBGH- or rBST-free) dairy

BETTER: Conventional, antibiotic- and hormone-free (look for rBGH- or rBST-free) dairy from grass-fed animals

BEST: Organic, grass-fed, nonhomogenized dairy. Purchase unpasteurized (raw) milk and dairy products when available.

STEER CLEAR: Clear containers; BPA plastics; sugar; fruit fillings; carrageenan; maltodextrin; artificial colors, flavors, and sweeteners; vegetable oils; trans fats; shredded cheese that likely contains cellulose powder and natamycin

OUR RICH FOOD PICKS: Organic Valley Grassmilk, Traders Point Creamery, Natural by Nature, Meyenberg goat milk,* Kalona SuperNatural,* Nancy's, Stonyfield Organic Greek yogurt, Maple Hill Creamery yogurt, Lifeway unsweetened kefir,* Green Valley Organics plain kefir,* Rumiano Cheese Company,* Smjor Icelandic butter, Kerrygold pure Irish butter and cheeses

(For an extremely detailed list of all of the brands and products we choose for milk, cream, butter, yogurt, sour cream, cheese, and all other types of dairy, make sure to check out our book *Rich Food, Poor Food*.)

stores. However, your best bet for finding raw milk, cream, and yogurt is still your local dairy farm. Visit the Micronutrient Miracle Motivation Center at mymiracleplan.com to find a farm in your area. The good news is that natural, raw dairy is rich in essential micronutrients, tastes amazing, and solves the milk miseries for most people.

Which Came First: The Chicken or the Egg?

When looking for the most micronutrient-rich poultry and eggs, you will be following much of the same logic used with ruminants; however, because chickens and turkeys are omnivores, instead of the term *grass-fed*, you want to look for the term *pasture-raised*. Your goal is to find an animal that was allowed to roam free in the pasture, was exposed to sunshine (higher vitamin D levels), and was able to eat fresh grass and insects. However, even pasture-raised poultry still get as much as 50 percent of their food from feed mixes, which can include soybeans, corn, alfalfa, clover, and oats. This, of course, still leaves you exposed to GMOs, which is why purchasing organic poultry and eggs is so important. Organic poultry is also free of arsenic. You read that right, arsenic! Nonorganic poultry can be fed this poison to increase the pink color of its flesh. But, USDA certified organic poultry is always arsenic-free.

Don't be confused by the terms *cage-free, free range,* and *pasture-raised*. While *cage-free* means the chickens are not kept in cages and have continuous access to food and water, they generally have no access to the outdoors or the sunshine, fresh grass, and insects we want them to have. *Free range* is only slightly better in that the USDA requires 5 minutes of open-air access per day to receive this status, but open air can still mean confined in a concrete pen.

Our Good, Better, and Best for Poultry and Eggs

Over your 28-day Micronutrient Miracle plan, we want you to implement our Good, Better, and Best strategy when choosing your poultry and eggs.

GOOD: Antibiotic-free or cage-free and organic when available

BETTER: Antibiotic-free, free range, or pasture-raised and organic when available

BEST: Organic and free range or pasture-raised

STEER CLEAR: Pasteurized eggs (this is not the same as *pasture-raised or pastured*), powdered eggs, egg white–only cartons (most of the micronutrients are in the yolks!), "flavored" chicken products, and BHA/BHT in processed chicken

OUR RICH FOOD PICKS: Vital Farms eggs; Alfresco Farms eggs; The Country Hen; Organic Valley; Eggland's Best organic, cage-free eggs; Petaluma Poultry "Rosie" organic, free-range chicken; Mary's organic, free-range chickens and turkeys; Bell & Evans organic, free-range chickens. Here too we created a one-stop protein shop to deliver to your door. Visit mymiracleplan.com to check out these heavily discounted, high-quality proteins.

(For an extremely detailed list of all of the brands and products we choose for eggs, chickens, and turkeys, make sure to check out our book *Rich Food, Poor Food.*)

The term *pasture-raised* is unregulated. It implies that the chickens were raised receiving at least some roaming time in pastures, but without regulations no one knows for how long.

Additionally, you want to make sure your poultry and eggs are free of antibiotics. Don't worry about seeing "hormone-free" on the label; US law prohibits the use of growth hormones in poultry, and the USDA has never approved any hormone products for egg production.

SERVE UP SOME SEAFOOD

The next protein category we are going to cover is seafood. By focusing on incorporating seafood—such as shrimp, scallops, crab, salmon, rainbow trout, or catfish—into your Micronutrient Miracle menu, you can really increase your micronutrient levels, especially when it comes to your essential omega-3s. Additionally, omega-3s from fish contain two unique components not found in plant-based omega-3s, called EPA and DHA, which have well-documented anti-inflammatory effects and have been shown to reduce the risk of arthritis, psoriasis, Parkinson's disease, Alzheimer's disease, cancer, and heart disease. Some studies have even found that omega-3s are as effective for treating major depression as the prescription drug Prozac.

However, on the other side of the coin, you're probably aware that much of our modern seafood has been contaminated with heavy metals (such as mercury), industrial chemicals (such as PCBs and dioxins), and pesticides (such as DDT) that have found their way into our waters. The good news is that many experts feel the benefits of eating seafood outweigh the risks. Having said this, we urge you to err on the side of caution by choosing fish with the highest omega-3 values and the lowest likelihood of toxic exposure.

Additionally, your micronutrient levels may offer a protective benefit when it comes to eating seafood. Remember, micronutrients are your body's natural detoxifiers.[10] It turns out that the micronutrient selenium, as well as other powerful antioxidants, such as vitamins C and E, can offer protection from the toxic effects of mercury by inhibiting the absorption of it in the gut. These micronutrients bind to and draw out this toxic heavy metal, thus mitigating any toxic damage caused by mercury. So by creating a micronutrient-sufficient state, you are protecting yourself from any possible dangers of seafood.

Now when it comes to choosing the best fish, the term we want you to look for is *wild-caught*. Like the terms *grass-fed* and *pasture-raised*, *wild-caught* ensures that the fish you are going to serve your family lived its life in its natural environment, swimming the open waters and eating a natural diet. This is in sharp contrast to the term *farm-raised*, which we see more and more these days, both in the grocery store as well as in restaurants. In fact, 40 percent of the seafood eaten globally is farmed, and in America that number is closer to 50 percent. Unfortunately, while aqua farming may sound like a good idea, we are making the same mistakes with our aqua-based factory farms as we have with our land-based factory farms, such as overcrowding, using unnatural feed, creating an unnatural environment, and even genetic engineering. Instead of carnivorous long-distance swimmers like salmon being able to swim the thousands of miles that each generation of salmon has swam before them and eat a diet of other fish, farmed salmon are being crowded into small cagelike pens and are being fed food pellets containing GMO corn and soy. The result is unhealthy fish that often need antibiotics and other medications to deal with illness and sea lice that infect farmed fish, and perhaps the worst part is that these fish deliver less overall micronutrient value to us.

To make matters worse, a company called AquaBounty Technologies is seeking FDA approval for a genetically modified salmon (branded as AquAdvantage) that has been genetically modified to grow 11 times faster than wild salmon and reproduce in less than 2 years. If approved, this will be the first genetically modified animal to enter the US food supply.[11] While Whole Foods and other grocery store chains throughout America have announced that they would not offer the GMO AquAdvantage salmon, make sure you steer clear of this shady salmon at restaurants and your local grocery store. Does this mean all farm-raised seafood is off the Micronutrient Miracle menu? No, because it turns out some seafood favorites actually do quite well in an aqua

---

Seriously Smart Seafood That Contains
High Levels of Omega-3s with Low Toxin Levels

- Wild, fatty cold-water fish: Alaskan salmon, anchovies, herring, sardines
- Wild rainbow trout (Lake Superior preferred)
- Wild, small, line-caught albacore tuna
- Line-caught haddock
- Atlantic mackerel
- Alaskan king, Dungeness, Kona, and Florida stone crab
- Wild catfish
- Mussels
- Wild spiny lobster
- Pacific oysters
- Squid
- Wild shrimp

farm environment, particularly sedentary mollusks, such as mussels, clams, oysters, and scallops. Additionally, they are not fed GMO-based food pellets and have actually been shown to be environmentally friendly, helping to clean the water surrounding the aqua farm.

And, of course, as with any other protein, it is important to ensure that the wild fish are being caught in a responsible, sustainable way. By purchasing fish from companies that do not use radical fishing methods that exploit fish stocks and destroy the marine environment, we can help to ensure that the next generation of little nutrivores can enjoy the health benefits of wild-caught, micronutrient-rich fish. Look for the blue Certified Sustainable Seafood label from the Marine Stewardship Council (MSC) on your wild-caught selections, including BPA-free canned seafood.

Remember, working fish into your Micronutrient Miracle menu at least twice a week can have some real long-term brain-building benefits. A 2014 study published in the *American Journal of Preventive Medicine* found that weekly

Our Good, Better, and Best for Seafood

Over your 28-day Micronutrient Miracle plan, we want you to implement our Good, Better, and Best strategy when choosing seafood.

GOOD: Wild-caught fish. (Give priority to those in the "Seriously Smart Seafood That Contains High Levels of Omega-3s with Low Toxin Levels" box, opposite.)

BETTER: Wild fish that has been troll, pole, or line caught

BEST: Wild fish that has been troll, pole, or line caught and identified as sustainable by the Marine Stewardship Council (MSC)

STEER CLEAR: Fish packed in oil (it drains the omega-3s from the fish), BPA cans, GMO fish, farmed fish, bluefin tuna, swordfish, shark, orange roughy, marlin, Chilean sea bass, tilapia, Asian-imported fish, and sugars and artificial colors in smoked salmon products

OUR RICH FOOD PICKS: Natural Sea, Crown Prince,* Wild Planet, American Tuna, and Echo Falls smoked salmon. There is a ton of reasonably priced frozen, wild-caught seafood in grocery stores and big box stores today. Better yet, visit mymiracleplan.com to shop online and have your wild-caught seafood delivered to your door from our favorite companies: US Wellness Meats, Wild Things Seafood, and Vital Choice.

(For an extremely detailed list of all of the brands and products we choose for seafood, make sure to check out our book *Rich Food, Poor Food*.)

consumption of fish was positively associated with larger gray matter volumes in the brain. Researchers believe that weekly fish consumption starting at an early age could improve brain health later in life and may even prevent potential onset of dementia or cognitive decline leading to Alzheimer's disease.[12]

PICKING THE PERFECT PROTEIN POWDER

Now, while designing your Micronutrient Miracle menu, you are certainly welcome to create your meals using the vast array of wonderful, micronutrient-rich protein sources we just went over. However, sometimes you may find that it's faster and easier to make a quick and delicious smoothie rather than a full meal. In fact, that is what we do every day for two of our four meals. We make these high-protein smoothies because protein is an essential component of the blood, bones, muscles, nerves, and organs, and even the immune system. It is needed by just about every major system of the body. Throughout the course of the day, your body tissue breaks down and must be repaired or replaced. In order to accomplish this important task, your body needs a steady supply of high-quality protein. (If it is not there, your health may suffer.)

A quality protein powder delivers more than just essential protein; it also delivers another class of essential micronutrients called amino acids, which act as building blocks of protein. There are 22 standard amino acids, nine of which are essential amino acids: histidine, isoleucine, leucine, lysine, methionine, phenylalanine, threonine, tryptophan, and valine. They are called essential amino acids because our bodies cannot manufacture them, so we need to get a sufficient amount of each one every day, just like we need to get a sufficient amount of each essential vitamin, mineral, and essential fatty acid daily if we are going to achieve optimal health. Failure to get enough of even one of the essential amino acids can have serious health implications. Just like your body will rob micronutrients such as calcium from your bones when you do not get enough of it through your diet, your body will also begin to break down muscle and other protein-based structures to obtain the essential amino acids it needs when they are not obtained through your diet. And just like water-soluble vitamins, the body does not store excess amino acids for later use, so you must get all your essential amino acids through food or a supplement each day.

But don't worry; getting enough essential amino acids during your Micronutrient Miracle plan is as simple as it is delicious. Later, in Chapter 7, we will show you how to incorporate a quality whey protein powder into your menu plan so that you can get all of its scientifically proven health

Bone Broth: Great for Collagen, Not So Great for Calcium

Don't throw out your beef, chicken, or fish bones. Making a bone broth is a great way to protect your bones from osteoporosis, but perhaps not for the reason you may think. It might surprise you to learn that research conducted by the Weston A. Price Foundation has confirmed that bone broth is *not* a good source of the bone-building mineral calcium. According to analysis reports from Covance Laboratories in Madison, Wisconsin, bone broth contains a mere 4.25 milligrams of calcium per cup, compared to 291 milligrams of calcium per cup of whole milk. While it may not be rich in calcium, it still is a *soup-er food* with great bone benefits. It turns out that bone broth contains key amino acids, such as glycine and proline, that are needed to manufacture another important component of healthy bones: collagen. If you are suffering from osteopenia or osteoporosis or want to prevent these debilitating conditions, drinking bone broth or using supplemental collagen has been shown to reduce the loss of bone mass and the likelihood of bone fractures significantly.[13] Just make sure to always make your bone broth from organic grass-fed/pasture-raised/wild-caught bones. Our Rich Food pick for best premade broth: Pete's Paleo.*

benefits—such as lowered stress and improved mood, protection against cognitive decline, decreased risk of cardiovascular disease, lowered risk of type 2 diabetes, increased lean body mass, boosted beneficial gut bacteria, and even inhibited growth of cancer cells.[14, 15, 16, 17, 18, 19, 20, 21, 22, 23] For example, in a 2014 study published in the journal *Neurology*, researchers found that for every 20 grams of protein a person took in per day, they reduced their risk of stroke by 26 percent! The study also found that beyond lowering the risk of stroke, it also lowered blood pressure and significantly lowered triglycerides, total cholesterol, and non-high-density lipoproteins.[24] New research published in the journal *Clinical Lipidology* reveals that a complete protein source, such as a quality whey protein powder, may just be nature's equivalent to statins. Research shows that LDL cholesterol, commonly referred to as bad cholesterol is not a marker of heart disease at all but is instead a marker of a lack of the essential amino acid tryptophan.[25]

A study published in the *International Journal of Obesity* showed that protein shakes can safely produce significant and sustainable weight loss and improve weight-related risk factors of disease, and a related study found that women who increased their intake of whey protein lost twice as much visceral fat as women who skipped whey protein.[26, 27]

Additionally, whey protein concentrate may be just what more than 29 million Americans with diabetes have been looking for to eliminate dangerous after-meal sugar spikes, which have been linked to cardiovascular disease, cancer, Alzheimer's disease, kidney failure, and retinal damage. A 2014 study conducted at Tel Aviv University and published in *Diabetologia* found that whey protein concentrate taken 30 minutes prior to meals worked as well as or even better than antidiabetic drugs at improving the body's insulin response and reducing blood glucose spikes after meals in people with type 2 diabetes. In fact, the results were so powerful that leading researchers stated "the consumption of whey protein before meals may even keep diabetics' need for insulin treatment at bay."[28]

Much like in the meat and dairy departments, there are a few terms that you must look for when choosing a high-quality whey protein powder. First, because whey protein is derived from milk, all the same rules apply. This means that organic and grass-fed proteins are preferred. However, when considering the two types of whey protein powder, isolates and concentrates, there is a new processing pitfall to consider. When isolates are created, they undergo processing to "isolate" the fat from the protein. This is problematic because it also strips many key beneficial immunological components. However, protein powder concentrates don't undergo this fat- and benefit-stripping process. Concentrates keep the fat and protein intact, and because of this, you get all the immune-building benefits. But the real key benefit of

Low-Carb Dieters Pay Attention!

Many dieters choose a low-carb diet to help reduce blood sugar/insulin spikes and reverse diabetes. We've heard grumblings from this community that protein shakes provide too much protein and should therefore be avoided. We are going to ask you to rethink this as we move forward. The Micronutrient Miracle plan will show you how to incorporate the right amount of fat and protein in easy and delicious protein shakes and treats that will actually help you control insulin spikes, increase satiety, and reduce weight, if needed.

protein concentrates lies in the fact that they still contain critical bioactive cofactors such as *bovine serum albumin,* which contains glutamylcysteine, a rare molecule that is known for its affinity for converting to glutathione, as well as other glutathione-boosting health-promoting cofactors, such as immuno-globulins, lactoferrin, and alpha-lactalbumin.

What is so special about glutathione? Glutathione is your body's most powerful antioxidant and one of the greatest predictors of overall health. In fact, a study published in the top British medical journal the *Lancet* found that individuals with the highest levels of glutathione were the healthiest and those with the lowest levels were the sickest and often hospitalized.[29] In fact, there are nearly 90,000 medical articles written about this one disease-preventing micronutrient alone because it is so important to your ability to achieve optimal health. The good news is that the absolute best food source for this powerful antioxidant is organic, grass-fed whey protein concentrate.

Glutathione protects your cells from oxidative damage and helps to:
- Build a strong immune system[30]
- Reduce inflammation[31, 32]
- Optimize your central nervous system[33]
- Fight infections[34]
- Prevent cancer[35]
- Treat AIDS[36]
- Detoxify your body[37]
- Protect your body from alcohol damage[38]
- Promote heart health[39, 40, 41]
- Increase strength and endurance[42]
- Shift metabolism from fat producing to muscle building[43]
- Flush out heavy metals, including mercury[44, 45]
- Promote longevity and protect from chronic illness[46]

Now, if you are one of our vegetarian or vegan nutrivores, don't think that we forgot about you. You too are encouraged to use a protein powder during your program. However, it can be a little harder to get all of your essential amino acids. As we outlined in Chapter 3, soy, the most common plant-based protein, is likely GMO, is goitrogenic (reduces iodine intake), and mimics the female hormone estrogen. These are just a few of the many reasons soy protein is not recommended by most health professionals. Because of this, it is best for you to use a pea, rice, or hemp protein, or better yet, our IN.POWER organic plant protein that combines plant-based proteins to create a complete amino acid profile. A word of warning on plant proteins, though: In a 2002 study featured in the *Journal of Epidemiology*, a decrease in bone density in female participants correlated with an increase in plant-based protein intake, and this same study showed an increase in bone density in participants preferring animal-based proteins.[47] Lastly, if you just can't tolerate dairy and are looking for an alternative to whey that still has a complete amino acid profile, egg protein may be just the thing. Egg is a highly absorbable form of protein that tastes great and can be substituted for whey protein in our Micronutrient Miracle recipes.

Our Good, Better, and Best for Protein Powder

Over your 28-day Micronutrient Miracle plan, we will be suggesting you include protein powder. Follow these guidelines.

HEAVY METAL ALERT: Regardless of the type of protein powder you choose, make sure to ask for the manufacturer's heavy metal toxicity report. High levels of cadmium, lead, mercury, and arsenic have been found in many protein powder products currently on the market.

GOOD: A good-quality whey concentrate, egg, pea, rice, or hemp protein powder

BETTER: A high-quality grass-fed whey concentrate, egg, pea, rice, or hemp protein powder that has been tested for heavy metals and shown to have safe levels

BEST: An organic, non-GMO-verified grass-fed whey concentrate, egg, pea, rice, or hemp protein powder that has been tested for heavy metals and shown to have safe levels

STEER CLEAR: Artificial colors, artificial flavors, and artificial sweeteners, sugar, soy lecithin, maltodextrin, and carrageenan. Avoid products that do not show you the lab analysis for heavy metals. Additionally, if you are planning to use protein powder for the Micronutrient Miracle plan, choose one that does not contain added vitamins and minerals (more on why in Chapter 7).

OUR RICH FOOD PICKS: IN.POWER organic whey protein,* IN.POWER organic plant protein,* Gifted Earth Originals plain organic egg protein, NutriBiotic organic rice protein plain, Nutiva organic hemp protein

Our favorite protein powder is our IN.POWER whey protein. It is certified 100 percent organic, grass-fed with year-round access to pasture; Non-GMO Project Verified; and American Humane Certified. And not only does our whey protein concentrate taste delicious (like fresh cream), it contains healthy fats, like CLA and omega-3s, as well as all of the other health-enhancing cofactors.

Pantry Staples

Well, now that you know how to pick the healthiest, most micronutrient-packed produce and proteins, it's time to head down the aisles and fill your cart with family-favorite staples and must-have ingredients that you will be using in your Micronutrient Miracle menus. In this section, we will be offering our Good, Better, Best system for healthy oils, and then offering some Rich Food picks for spices, salt, condiments, salad dressings, flour and sugar alternatives, and beverages. There is an old culinary saying that goes, "No fat, no salt—no flavor." And it's true, both fat and salt really add flavor and dimension to a dish, but we want to make sure you are using the right fats and spices during your Micronutrient Miracle plan so let's start this pantry restock by first examining healthy oils.

HEALTHY OILS

There seems to be a ton of oils, margarines, and shortenings claiming to be healthy alternatives to saturated fats, such as butter, ghee, lard, tallow, duck fat, cream, palm oil, and coconut oil. Well, we are here to tell you that with the exception of the sparing use of organic extra-virgin olive oil, avocado oil, macadamia nut oil, flaxseed oil, and chia oil, none of them are included in the Micronutrient Miracle plan. When using fat (and we *love* fat) for cooking, marinades, or salad dressings, we want you to use those saturated fats your ancestors used. Do you think your grandparents cooked their eggs and bacon in a hydrogenated or partially hydrogenated, highly processed, oxidized, trans-fat-containing fat, like soybean oil, margarine, or genetically modified corn oil? Of course not, and we don't want you to either. Now, we still want you to go the extra distance, especially with the dairy- and protein-based fats—such as butter, ghee, cream, lard, tallow, duck fat, or chicken fat—and get the organic, grass-fed/pasture-raised options when available. And while palm oil, coconut oil, olive oil, avocado oil, macadamia oil, flaxseed oil, and chia oil are not currently genetically modified, we want you to purchase organic, extra-virgin, cold-pressed forms if available.

Now before we move on from the healthy oils section to the other pantry staples, we want to introduce you to SKINNYFat, a very special oil that, along with nutreince (our multivitamin) and IN.POWER (our organic, grass-fed whey protein concentrate), makes up our three Micronutrient Miracle foundational products. SKINNYFat brings the health benefits of some of the healthiest oils in the world—including organic virgin coconut oil, medium-chain triglycerides (MCTs), and organic extra-virgin olive oil—into your kitchen, making it easy to avoid highly processed, genetically modified oils, such as corn, canola, and soybean. We've found a way, through our patent-pending formulations, to optimize the unique benefits of these health-enhancing oils, while solving the individual challenges of each, so that you can easily integrate them into your favorite recipes and start improving your health today.

You've probably already heard about the scientifically proven, heart-healthy, cholesterol-normalizing, immune-supportive, thyroid-boosting, antibacterial, antiviral, and antiprotozoal properties of organic virgin coconut oil.[48, 49, 50, 51,52, 53, 54, 55] However, there is a problem with using coconut oil in your favorite recipes; it makes everything you prepare taste like coconuts. Additionally, because coconut oil is solid at room temp (76°F), it can be hard to work with in the kitchen.

If you haven't heard about MCT oil yet, you're going to love this: MCT simply stands for medium-chain triglycerides, specialized fats that have been naturally extracted from coconut or palm oil. Not only is it nearly impossible for your body to store MCT oil as body fat (more on this later), but peer-reviewed published research also shows that MCT oil increases metabolism, reduces body fat, and improves insulin sensitivity and glucose tolerance.[56, 57, 58] However, just like coconut oil, there is a problem with MCT oil, too. When used on its own, it has been known to cause stomach upset, making it unpopular outside high-performance athletic and scientific circles.

And finally, there is olive oil. Quality organic extra-virgin olive oil has long been recognized for its beneficial health properties (i.e., enhanced micronutrient absorption), but it too has a drawback. Olive oil is very high in omega-6 fatty acids, a type of fatty acid known by medical science to cause inflammation, a precursor to many of today's most deadly health conditions and diseases. A little omega-6 is good, but too much may have a negative effect.

SKINNYFat is a unique proprietary blend of MCT oil and organic virgin coconut oil, and SKINNYFat Olive starts with our original formulation and adds in just the right amount of organic extra-virgin olive oil for a completely new flavor dimension. By blending these beneficial oils together in just the right ratios, SKINNYFat solves the individual problems of all three fats. First,

SKINNYFat has solved the challenges of cooking with coconut oil by eliminating the distinct coconut taste, making it compatible with any dish. Additionally, SKINNYFat is liquid at room temperature and even stays liquid when refrigerated.

Next, SKINNYFat all but eliminates the stomach upset that can occur when using MCT oil on its own. And last but not least, SKINNYFat Olive successfully and deliciously delivers the full Mediterranean flavor of organic extra-virgin olive oil while reducing the omega-6 levels of traditional olive oil by 85 percent, allowing you to enjoy the health benefits with significantly less risk of inflammation. This makes SKINNYFat and SKINNYFat Olive the perfect choices to use in your favorite Micronutrient Miracle recipes found in Chapter 9. They are great for salad dressings, sauces, soups, spreads, smoothies, or anywhere you want to add a shot of fat-burning, energy-enhancing goodness!

How Does SKINNYFat Work?

One of the most amazing things about SKINNYFat is that it is nearly impossible to store as body fat. Which makes SKINNYFat perfect for anyone wanting to lose weight, control hunger, and naturally increase energy. Here is how it works: The majority of the fat in SKINNYFat is from MCTs, which do not require bile for digestion, like regular fat, and instead are rapidly metabolized by the liver, producing something called ketones. Ketones are an alternative form of energy that can be used by both your body and brain.

Ketones provide energy like a carbohydrate, but they do not spike blood sugar or stimulate the release of the fat storage hormone insulin the way carbohydrates do.[59, 60, 61] Instead, ketones increase your energy levels, rev up fat burning, and enhance mental focus. Clients who have used SKINNYFat during the 28-day Micronutrient Miracle plan tell us that they feel more energetic and satisfied while experiencing reduced hunger and increased weight loss. In fact, research published in the *American Journal of Clinical Nutrition* found that individuals who consumed MCT oil as part of a 16-week weight-loss program lost more total weight, total fat mass, trunk fat mass, intra-abdominal adipose tissue, and subcutaneous abdominal adipose than the group that consumed plain olive oil.[62]

However, as you know, the Micronutrient Miracle plan is about a lot more than just burning fat; our goal is to help you achieve micronutrient sufficiency, and by enhancing your micronutrient absorption, SKINNYFat helps

Our Good, Better, and Best for Oils and Fats

Over your 28-day Micronutrient Miracle plan, we will be suggesting you use the following fats.

GOOD: Conventionally produced butter, ghee, lard, tallow, duck fat, cream, palm oil, and coconut oil

BETTER: Grass-fed/pasture-raised butter, ghee, lard, tallow, duck fat, and cream and cold-pressed palm oil and coconut oil

BEST: Organic, grass-fed/pasture-raised butter, ghee, lard, tallow, duck fat, and cream and organic, cold-pressed palm oil and coconut oil

USE SPARINGLY: Organic, cold-pressed extra-virgin olive oil; avocado oil; macadamia nut oil; flaxseed oil; MCT oil; and chia oil

STEER CLEAR: Highly processed, genetically modified oils, such as corn, canola, and soybean; margarine; hydrogenated or partially hydrogenated oils; trans fats

OUR RICH FOOD PICKS: SKINNYFat* and SKINNYFat* Olive, Pure Indian Foods organic grass-fed ghee, Tendergrass Farms organic lard, Kasadrinos Organic Olive Oil,* Artisana Organics coconut butter. (For dairy picks, visit the dairy section on page 133.)

with that, as well. Although the majority of the fat in our oil comes from MCTs, which bypass the normal process of digestion, SKINNYFat was specially formulated to contain just the right amount of long-chain triglycerides (LCTs) to stimulate the release of the bile acids needed for proper absorption and utilization of the fat-soluble vitamins A, D, E, and K, as well as other essential micronutrients, including carotenoids, calcium, and magnesium. Additionally, the ingredients in SKINNYFat have been shown to have a long list of other health- and performance-enhancing benefits, including improving cholesterol levels, optimizing hormones, regulating blood sugar levels, and improving digestive issues.

SPICES

The most important thing you want to remember when purchasing spices is to make sure they are not irradiated; some spices will say this right on the jar, but when in doubt, organic spices are always safe from irradiation.

OUR RICH FOOD PICKS: Simply Organic,* Frontier Organic,* Smith &

Truslow, Morton & Bassett Organic (they also have a line of nonorganic, nonirradiated spices)

SALT

When purchasing salt, steer clear of white refined salt (i.e., the kind that is most likely in your kitchen). In its natural (unrefined) state, salt is slightly grey, brown, or pink, not bright white. It is also jam-packed with more than 90 health-promoting minerals. Yes, health promoting. For decades, doctors have advised limiting our salt intake to reduce the risk of heart disease and stroke, but 2014 research in the *New England Journal of Medicine* confirmed that sodium has little to no effect on blood pressure levels. And for many women, getting far too little sodium can be damaging.[63] The right salt can help fight fatigue, adrenal and thyroid disorders, and headaches, and it can normalize your cholesterol and blood pressure. In fact, salt is the one "spice" that is actually essential to life. Watch out, though, as even some sea salts have been refined, and in some cases, dextrose (a form of sugar made from GMO corn) has also been introduced. Would you ever have expected sugar to be hiding in your salt?

OUR RICH FOOD PICKS: Himalayan sea salt or any unrefined salt. Our favorite is Redmond's Real Salt.* We just love the flavor it brings to every meal.

CONDIMENTS

Condiments are definitely a pantry staple. After all, what is a hamburger or hot dog without ketchup, mustard, or mayonnaise, or a stir-fry without soy sauce? But while on your 28-day Micronutrient Miracle plan, you need to toss out your sugar- and soy-laden standbys and find some new Rich Food favorites. When restocking your condiments, steer clear of anything that includes the following ingredients: sugar (in any form), vinegar (white vinegar is made from GMO corn; organic vinegar is fine), soy (in any form), maltodextrin (from GMO corn), canola oil (GMO), soybean oil (GMO), sunflower oil, or any oils other than those indicated above as a Rich Food pick for oil.

Unfortunately, there are not very many Rich Food condiments to be found in the modern grocery store. But we do have some simple and easy recipes to make your own Rich Food versions in Chapter 9.

OUR RICH FOOD PICKS:

Ketchup: Killer Ketchup That Won't Kill You! (page 292)

Mustard: Annie's Homegrown organic yellow mustard, Eden brown mustard, Publix organic mustards

Soy Sauce: Coconut Secret coconut aminos

Mayonnaise: 5-Minute SKINNYFat Mayonnaise (page 288)

Salsa: Rejuvenative Foods salsa,* Muir Glen organic salsa, Amy's Organic Fire Roasted Vegetable Salsa

Guacamole: Holy Moly Guacamole (page 291), organic Wholly Guacamole*

SALAD DRESSINGS

Okay, now we are going to talk about one of the most popular condiments that you likely use on a regular basis: salad dressing. Whether you use it on your salad, as a marinade for your meats, or to dip your chicken wings in, salad dressings are some of the worst Poor Food offenders in the grocery store. We literally do not have one Rich Food salad dressing we want you to purchase while on the Micronutrient Miracle plan. Instead, this will be another condiment you need to make from scratch. Don't worry—we have simple, delicious recipes and easy videos for you to follow. The fact is, store-bought salad dressings are full of sugar (EMD, GMO), vinegar (GMO), canola or soybean oil (both GMO), and a host of other Poor Food ingredients.

OUR RICH FOOD PICKS:

Really Creamy SKINNYFat Blue Cheese Dressing (or Dip) (page 289), Simple SKINNYFat Italian Dressing (page 288), SKINNYFat Parmesan-Peppercorn Dressing (page 289)

Check out our "Cooking with the Caltons" videos in the Micronutrient Miracle Motivation and Resource Center.

FLOUR AND SUGAR ALTERNATIVES

One of the very best things about the Micronutrient Miracle plan is that with just a little imagination, you can create almost any of your favorite meals. Want pancakes for breakfast? We have a recipe for that! Love Mexican fajitas? We have a recipe for that, too. How about a rustic flatbread pizza, hot out of the oven brownies, or a delicious piece of cheesecake? They're *all* included! However, without our next two pantry staples, the flour and sugar alternatives, these family favorites would never be possible. Remember in Chapter 3 when we asked you to sack the sugar and whack the wheat due to their adverse health consequences? Well, now it's time to replace these pantry staples with easy-to-find, great-tasting, Rich Food flour and sugar alternatives.

Flour Alternatives

Contrary to popular belief, you do not need wheat flour to make great-tasting breads, brownies, pancakes, or tortillas, but you do need a flour alternative, such as coconut flour, almond flour, buckwheat flour (buckwheat is a seed, not a wheat), or flax meal. In addition, protein powder, like IN.POWER, makes a great low-carb flour alternative as well. Depending on what your goals are during the 28-day Micronutrient Miracle plan, you may not be using these alternative flours very often. If you are following either the weight loss, ketogenic, or blood sugar regulation protocols, for instance, we recommend limiting your use of these products to just once a week. However, if you are at your desired weight and are trying to normalize your blood pressure, increase your bone density, etc., then you may find yourself using these products on a more frequent basis. Either way, here is a tip that took us a while to figure out: None of the alternative flours seem to work perfectly on their own. That is why you will often see several of these Rich Food flours in our Micronutrient Miracle recipes. Experiment by combining their unique textures and flavors to find the perfect Rich Food flour combination for your recipes.

OUR RICH FOOD PICKS: Coconut Secret organic, raw coconut flour; Blue Mountain organics, raw, sprouted buckwheat flour,* Flour of Life organic, raw, sprouted buckwheat flour; Sprout Revolution organic, sprouted ground flax; Bob's Red Mill organic selections

Sugar Alternatives

When people first hear the Micronutrient Miracle plan sacks all forms of sugar, they often start asking, "What will I use to sweeten my coffee or make my favorite desserts?" Well, never fear, because stevia is here. If you haven't yet heard of or tried stevia, then you are in for a real treat: Stevia is an all-natural sweetener that substitutes for sugar in almost any recipe. We actually grow stevia in our flower box just outside our kitchen window and use the little green leaves in various dishes to add a touch of sweetness.

However, watch out for the stevia products in most grocery stores; they are often mixed with some kind of sugar base, such as dextrose or maltodextrin. The full name for stevia is *Stevia rebaudiana.* If you see this as the only ingredient listed, you know that you are looking at the real thing. There are some "baking" stevias that have come on the market recently. While this type of stevia product may be convenient for baking, you need to read the ingredient list to make sure that it does not contain any hidden sugars or anything that could be a possible GMO. Stevia is fine for those with diabetes or even very low-carb dieters. In fact, some studies suggest that stevia can help reverse diabetes and metabolic syndrome and reduce hypertension. The stevia plant has been used in South America for more than 1,500 years and is widely used around the world as a safe, natural sweetener. It's our number-one Rich Food pick!

WARNING: If you are allergic to ragweed, stevia may not be for you since it is a close relative and can sometimes cause similar allergic reactions.

Our second-favorite sugar substitute is a sweetener called *loa han*. Loa han comes from the monk fruit, a prized Chinese medicinal fruit, and is very similar to stevia in that it is a natural sweetener with zero calories and zero glycemic index, meaning that it is good for everyone, including those with diabetes.

In addition to stevia and loa han, or as an alternative to them, you may also use sparing amounts of sugar alcohols, such as xylitol, erythritol, sorbitol, or mannitol. However, some people also report stomach upset and bloating after eating foods made with sugar alcohols, and because these sweeteners are often derived from corn, make sure the ones you choose are either certified non-GMO or organic. And lastly, while we do not recommend the use of either organic raw honey or organic coconut sugar for our nutrivores with diabetes or prediabetes (or for anyone trying to lose weight), these two natural sugars may be used sparingly (once a week) during your 28-day Micronutrient Miracle plan—if you cannot use stevia or loa han for any reason or if they are not available.

OUR RICH FOOD PICKS:

Stevia extract Pyure organic powder; best for drinks, like coffee or iced tea.

Pyure Organic All-Purpose Sweetener (stevia-erythritol blend).

Stevita Simply-Stevia powder, Stevita flavored drops and crystals (perfect to flavor nutreince Natural).

Stevita Delight chocolate drink mix. (It's so good! We use it to make numerous chocolaty Triple Threat recipes.)

SweetLeaf stevia extract powders and drops; made from organic stevia extract.

Lakanto non-GMO loa han/erythritol sweetener. (It's in the dessert recipes!)

Big Tree Farms, Organic coconut plus stevia.
Coconut Secret organic coconut nectar or crystals.

HEALTHY BEVERAGES

The last pantry staples we are going to discuss are healthy beverages, including coffee, tea, wine, beer, spirits, waters, juice, and soda. Earlier we talked about the micronutrient-depleting effects coffee, tea, wine, and spirits can have on you, but, as you may remember, we are not asking you to give up your favorite caffeine- or alcohol-based libations, just to limit them. However, we do want you to get the highest quality you can find and go organic across the board for the next 28 days.

Coffee and Tea

No more Starbucks, Dunkin' Donuts, or McDonald's coffee; we want you to really make the effort to find organic coffee or tea. Why? Even with the antioxidant benefits that coffee and tea can deliver, coffee may be the most heavily chemically treated food commodity in the world, and according to a 2014 report by Greenpeace, tea isn't far behind. The report examined tea being grown by some of the leading brands—including Tetley, Lipton, and Twinings—and found a total of 34 different pesticide/insecticide residues in packaged tea purchased from the market, including 23 that were not even registered for use in the cultivation of tea, including DDT. Researchers stated that practically all the samples contained residues of at least one pesticide and more than half of them contained "cocktails" of more than 10 different pesticides, with one sample containing 20 different pesticides. Of these samples, 60 percent contained residues above the Maximum Residue Levels (MRL) set by the EU, with almost 40 percent of the tea samples exceeding the MRL levels by more than 50 percent.[64] Choosing organic coffee and tea over conventional options protects you from the long-term toxic effects of these micronutrient-depleting pesticides/insecticides, and it also reduces the global use of synthetic, petroleum-based fertilizers commonly used in coffee production that can destroy soil fertility and contaminate local water supplies.

Go the extra mile and look for coffee and tea with the "fair trade" label and coffee that has been "shade grown." The fair trade label requires a certification process, and it indicates that the laborers received fair wages for their hard work. While fair trade coffee and tea may be a bit more expensive, isn't it worth it to know that you are supporting fair wages for workers in developing countries? Additionally, coffee trees naturally grow in the shade of a dense rain forest. To increase productivity and keep up with the growing demand for coffee, nearly 70 percent of the world's coffee production now comes from sun-resistant coffee tree hybrids. This can lead to deforestation as growers make way for more sun-resistant coffee trees. Most quality organic coffee is shade grown, which is just another good reason to go organic!

OUR RICH FOOD PICKS: Camano Island organic coffee, Publix GreenWise Market organic coffee, Caffe Sanora Organic coffees,* Arbor Teas, Guayaki organic unsweetened yerba mate

Wine, Beer, and Spirits

When it comes to wine, beer, and spirits, it's time to start doing a little investigative work to find out what organic brands are available at your local grocery store as well as at your favorite restaurants and sports bars. We think you will be surprised by the selection you have to choose from. For wine, the key is to find organic or biodynamic wines, which are similar to organic but also take into account things such as astrological influences and lunar cycles. This will protect you from all the potentially dangerous synthetic chemicals and added sulfites found in conventional wine.

For beer drinkers, you have a whole world of adventure awaiting you. We want you to not only go organic, but also gluten-free! Yes, this will likely mean changing beers, but remember, change is good. There are so many great organic, gluten-free beers on the market now that you should have no problem at all finding a new favorite. Lastly, for you spirit lovers, your mission is to find an organic vodka, gin, rum, whiskey, cognac, or tequila. This, again, will likely mean a switch from your favorite brand, but the benefits of avoiding GMOs and residue from synthetic fertilizers, pesticides, and herbicides in your alcoholic beverages will yield huge health dividends over time.

For the 28 days of the plan, steer clear of sweet liqueurs, such as Frangelico or Baileys, as these are filled with sugar. Also, make sure any cocktails you order are made only with fresh lime, lemon, or olive juices—no syrups; Rose's lime juice; or neon blue, red, or green stuff! Additionally, skip the sodas and juice mixers and stick with ordering your drinks either on the rocks (ice only) or with flat or sparkling water. When out, we like to order vodka sodas and then top them off with a few Stevita vanilla drops that Mira carries in her purse.

OUR RICH FOOD PICKS:

Wine: Hall Wines (highly rated and delicious), Bonterra organic wines, Frey organic wines, Handley Cellars, Domaine Carneros wines and sparkling wines (our favorite organic champagne!)

Beer: Redbridge organic, gluten-free beer; Green's Discovery organic, gluten-free beer

Spirits: Ocean vodka, Prairie organic gin and vodka, 4 Copas tequila

All-Day Drinkables

Lastly, let's quickly go over the waters, juices, and sodas that we want you to restock your pantry with. Your children or your significant other may protest a bit at first, but, here again, quality is a major concern when choosing your waters, juicelike drinks, and sodas.

Here are our five fast tips for choosing your all-day drinkable options.

1. **Always purchase all-day drinkables in glass.** Pitch the plastics to say bye-bye to that BPA.

2. **Sparking water and coconut water make nice soda substitutes.** Create your own zero-calorie stevia sodas by adding flavored stevia drops to sparkling water. The options are endless, and our clients quit the soda habit in days. **OUR RICH FOOD PICKS:** San Pellegrino; Mountain Valley Spring Water; Perrier sparkling waters (comes in a variety of great flavors); Harmless Harvest organic, raw coconut water; Vita Coco pure coconut water (unflavored only)

3. **Forgo the fancy fakes.** Stay away from vitamin-enhanced waters, sports drinks, energy drinks, and flavored waters with added sugar and artificial colors and sweeteners. They are full of micronutrient-depleting ingredients, and you will learn to supplement smart rather than fall for their misleading marketing claims.

4. **Juices are out, but fermented beverages are fine.** The insulin spike and fat storage just isn't worth the juicing. We will discuss fruit intake when reviewing the Micronutrient Miracle protocol. Look for fermented beverages that start with a small amount of juice as their base, as they contain probiotics that can help your gut flora. **OUR RICH FOOD PICKS:** Kevita Coconut Sparkling Probiotic Drinks, LIVE Soda Kombucha (in soda pop flavors)

5. **Say so long to your soda habit.** All sodas sweetened with sugar or sinister sugar substitutes are out, but we have found a GMO-free, stevia-sweetened soda that really hits the spot. **OUR RICH FOODS PICK:** Zevia GMO-free, all natural soda—Mountain Zevia flavor*

Now that you have successfully restocked your home with health-enhancing Rich Foods and nontoxic personal care items and home goods, it's time to explore our third and final step to becoming micronutrient sufficient: smart supplementation. As you have seen, there is a lot of micronutrient depletion going on throughout a typical day. Step 3 offers you a way to tilt the micronutrient-sufficiency scales in your favor. Chapter 6 is actually one of our favorite chapters! If you currently take a multivitamin, get ready to have your mind blown. We are going to show you exactly how and why we reinvented the multivitamin.

6

Smart Supplementation

YOU PROBABLY KNOW THE saying, "It is always darkest before the dawn." It means that things can get pretty gloomy before they get better. It teaches us that there is hope even when all the facts make us think we are fighting a losing battle. Well, things are looking pretty dark right now where micronutrient sufficiency is concerned, wouldn't you say? We have taken quite a journey together thus far. Unfortunately, what we have discovered has been mostly bad news for your micronutrient sufficiency levels. Let's review a few of the facts.

1. We have seen that the soil is no longer the mineral-rich dirt that generations before us enjoyed, and this mineral-poor soil is in turn producing plants with reduced micronutrient content.

2. We have analyzed peer-reviewed studies on popular diet plans and found that no diet supplies enough micronutrients to meet minimum Reference Daily Intake (RDI) levels—regardless of dietary philosophy.

3. We have identified a multitude of Everyday Micronutrient Depleters (EMDs) that further reduce our micronutrient levels—even after we have eaten. Some are found in the foods and drinks we take in—such as oxalic acid, lectins, and tannins—while others are willfully included in our lives, such as exercise, medications, and toxins from household and personal care products.

Not to mix metaphors, but it sure looks like these three strikes might just knock out your ability to reach micronutrient sufficiency and achieve the optimal health that you desire. But remember, after the dark comes the dawn, and the dawn in our micronutrient sufficiency tale is the third and final step to living the nutrivore lifestyle. It is learning to supplement smart to account for the shortage of micronutrient-dense foods in your diet as well as the EMDs you will encounter every day.

Supplementation:
The Light at the End of the Tunnel

Let's think about it this way: Do you have a dog? If you do, you know that the dog likes to drink water from his water bowl. When you see that the water level is low, what do you do? You fill it up again. That is the smart thing to do so that the dog doesn't go thirsty, right? Well, imagine that the water in that bowl represents the micronutrients you need every day to reach sufficiency. You eat healthy, micronutrient-rich foods, which fills your "water bowl" with essential vitamins and minerals, but then you use up some of that fresh, cool water (micronutrients) by drinking too much coffee or tea or vigorously working out at the gym. These dietary and lifestyle habits drain the bowl. And what should you do when you see the level of water in the bowl getting low? Wouldn't it be smart to fill it back up? Of course it would.

That is the goal of sufficiency. We want to keep our micronutrients at that "full" level so we can protect ourselves from the lifestyle diseases that too many people globally are currently suffering from, as well as live extraordinary lives with all the energy and vitality needed to achieve our greatest dreams. Daily supplements do just that. They ensure that we stay sufficient. However, they are not a substitute for a good diet (Step 1 of being a nutrivore). You are still obligated to try to eat the healthiest Rich Food diet you can. However, because we are not perfect and life throws all sorts of curveballs at us, we need to supplement in today's modern age, and the easiest way to do this is to take a well-formulated multivitamin.

The Multivitamin—Myth or Miracle?

We know what you may be thinking. You've read the newspaper reports and seen news networks trash multivitamins. You may have even asked your doctor about multivitamins only to be told that taking one is like throwing good money down the toilet. Guess what? We agree. Well, we agree that *most* of the multivitamins on the market are, for the most part, a waste of money. They won't refill the "water bowl" or raise your micronutrient levels to the sufficiency line. They may fill it up a little, but in the long run, your body will not function at the optimal level you deserve. It took us years to figure out why. If you consider a multivitamin to be the sum of all its ingredients, then the multivitamin should be the most powerful disease-fighting and health-enhancing tool available. After all, we know that each individual micronutrient has been identified as being essential to our health in some way and can prevent or reverse specific health conditions. For example, vitamin C prevents and reverses scurvy, vitamin D does the same with rickets, and vitamin K is necessary for blood clotting. However, research has shown that when all the individual micronutrients are combined into a single multivitamin, the individual micronutrients fail to perform their incredible tasks. Why? This was the question that we wanted to answer, the riddle we needed to solve.

Remember, our study on the intricate relationships between individual micronutrients and multivitamin supplementation began with our attempts to reverse Mira's osteoporosis. We knew we needed to find out how to harness the benefits of each micronutrient if we were going to have any chance at preventing further bone loss or reversing Mira's debilitating condition, and so we began examining every detail of the multivitamin—from its invention right down to each decision made during the formulation process.

THE MULTIVITAMIN: IN ITS INFANCY

How long ago do you think the multivitamin was created? Would you be surprised to learn that McDonald's, robots, electronic shavers, and car stereos all existed before the multivitamin? It's true. Multivitamins are just in their infancy, and like our investigation into micronutrients was born out of a necessity to reverse Mira's osteoporosis, the creation of the first multivitamin was also born out of a necessity, of sorts. Imagine what you might do if you found yourself living abroad in a time of political unrest when fresh food was scarce and disease was spreading. How would you protect your health? This was the situation that a man named Carl F. Rehnborg found himself in while selling Colgate in China from 1915 to 1927, a time when, due to political unrest in Shanghai, many people were forced into isolation for long periods of time.

During one of these periods, Rehnborg came up with the idea to use nutritional elements to protect himself and his friends from developing scurvy and beriberi, two of the already well-known and understood micronutrient deficiency diseases of his time. To accomplish this, he supplemented their daily soup with local herbs, grasses, vegetables, rusty nails (for iron), ground-up animal bones (for calcium), and limestone (for calcium and magnesium). He shared his homemade concoction with his friends. When the political tension finally ended months later, Rehnborg and his friends emerged from their confinement much healthier than those who had not eaten his soup. This was Rehnborg's "eureka moment." He decided to create a single pill that would contain all the known minerals and newly discovered vitamins in one easy-to-take product. Upon his return to the United States in 1934, Rehnborg developed California Vitamins, one of the world's first multivitamin and multimineral food supplements.

Are you surprised that it has only been 80 years since the multivitamin was first created? Would you be more surprised to learn that many of the individual vitamins we take for granted today were not identified until the mid-1930s? It's true; it has only been just over 100 years since the first vitamin was discovered (vitamin A was discovered in 1912), so it is no wonder that we are still learning so much about them. But with all we have learned, the multivitamin still remains pretty much the same as that first prototype created by Rehnborg—a mix of vitamins and minerals thrown into tablet form. Can you think of anything in your life that still uses technology from the 1930s, without a redesign? Probably not. *So, is it possible that the failure of the multivitamin may be from a lack of redesign and upgrading, rather than from a failure of the individual micronutrients themselves?*

Identifying the Four Major Flaws of the Multivitamin

How would a Ford Model T fare against a brand-new Ford Mustang? Or how would the capability of an early UNIVAC computer, which took up entire floors of an office building, compare to the smartphone you now carry around in your hand? Big difference, right? So it's really not that hard to imagine that a multivitamin that has not been updated and reformulated using the latest advances in supplemental science might not be living up to its ultimate potential. But this is great news because if this is true, it means that by simply identifying the outdated design flaws and updating the way we formulate the multivitamin, we should be able to improve the efficacy of the multivitamin itself.

In this chapter, you will learn the four flaws that we identified through our numerous years of research on the interactions of specific micronutrients. Remember, like the instruments in an orchestra, micronutrients all have subtle differences in how they perform, and you will need each and every essential micronutrient to be properly absorbed and utilized by your body to create the harmony equal to living a healthy, vivacious, strong, and abundant life.

The truth is, it can take many years of study to fully understand the science behind each micronutrient, and we definitely do not want to turn this into a course in biochemistry, so we decided to make the information we are about to share with you as easy and straightforward as possible. In order to easily explain the four flaws of the multivitamin, we created a simple acronym and accompanying guidelines so that you can stop wasting money on products still being created using 80-year-old technology and identify an updated multivitamin that will enhance your health. While the acronym may appear elementary, we don't want you to underestimate its importance. The vital, cutting-edge information you are about to learn will change the way you supplement forever and may finally unlock the full power and potential of the multivitamin.

THE ABCS OF OPTIMAL SUPPLEMENTATION GUIDELINES

The acronym is easy. In fact, it is as easy as the ABCs—because it is the ABCs. We call it the ABCs of Optimal Supplementation Guidelines; and the *A*, *B*, *C*, and *s* stand for the four flaws we identified. These flaws are easy to overcome. You just have to know what to look for.

Prefer videos? You can learn all about the ABCs of Optimal Supplementation Guidelines online at ABCsofSupplementation.com.

A Stands for Absorption

Have you ever wondered why many physicians state that multivitamins are no better than flushing money down the toilet? Well, the truth is that most of the time they are right. Many of the multivitamins on the market do end up in the sewers or backing up your septic tank, and if they end up down there, then there is little chance that they were effective in improving your health. As it turns out, the process of absorbing micronutrients isn't as easy as one might think; and if your body can't absorb the vitamins and minerals found in your daily multivitamin capsule or tablet, then they simply pass right through it. This makes absorption a huge issue and the first flaw we identified in most multivitamins.

When discussing micronutrient absorption, the delivery system is key. Some delivery systems simply have better absorption rates. It isn't so difficult to understand why, either. Pills or capsules, when ingested, must first disintegrate, or break down, in order to make the vitamins and minerals available. According to Raimar Löbenberg, PhD, lead researcher in a study published in the *Journal of Pharmacy and Pharmaceutical Sciences,* "active ingredients [micronutrients] can only be absorbed if they are released into solution from the dosage form. Disintegration is the first step in this process. . . . If a mineral has to be absorbed within an absorption window but the dosage form does not release its content in a timely manner, the therapy might be compromised or fail." Dr. Löbenberg conducted a study to identify just how problematic poor disintegration might be when it comes to multivitamins. He examined 49 well-known commercially available multivitamins that were in either capsule or tablet (pill) form to determine if they would disintegrate and release their contained vitamins and minerals within a 20-minute time period—the time necessary for potential absorption. The results showed that out of the 49 multivitamins studied, 25 (or 51 percent) did not disintegrate within the allotted 20-minute window. The worst performers were Kirkland Signature formula (Costco brand), Nu-Life Ultimate One for Men, Trophic, SISU Only One, Super Swiss One, and GNC Mega Men—all of which failed to disintegrate at all![1]

Incredible, right? More than 50 percent of the well-known store-brand multivitamins using capsules and tablets as their delivery system did not disintegrate within the allotted time frame. And as disintegration is the first step in absorption, if you were taking one of these popular store-bought multivitamin brands, your ability to absorb the essential micronutrients contained within these multivitamins would be poor at best. So your doctor is right; based on Dr. Löbenberg's research, you have about a 50/50 shot of choosing a multivitamin capsule or tablet that will allow absorption to take place by properly disintegrating. This is something a physician is taught early on. Have you ever heard of the *PDR*? Well, it stands for *Physicians' Desk Reference,* and you've probably seen one in your doctor's office. This pharmaceutical guide to all things prescribed indicates that the contents of both capsules and pills, which make up the majority of multivitamin sales, are only 10 to 20 percent absorbed by the body. No wonder physicians feel that there is little value to multivitamins; they are constantly being reminded of their inability to disintegrate.

However, the *PDR* does recognize a delivery system that allows for nearly perfect absorption. It states that liquid formulas are the most absorbable, at up to 98 percent. This means that it is super simple to avoid this first flaw we found in modern multivitamin formulation. Not only will taking your multivitamins in a liquid form increase absorption, as there is no need for disintegration to occur, but it is also easier for a great number of people. First of all, small children can't take pills, and according to a nationwide survey conducted by Harris Interactive, a global market research firm (they conduct the Harris poll), 40 percent of all adults surveyed also admitted to having difficulty taking pills. Bariatric patients and individuals suffering from irritable bowel syndrome, hiatal hernias, and diverticulitis also have particular difficulty when taking their supplements in pill or capsule form. This makes taking a liquid multivitamin easier and smarter, as this delivery system bypasses disintegration completely and greatly increases the potential absorption and utilization of each micronutrient.

The Problems with Liquid Delivery Systems

While a liquid delivery system for your multivitamin is better in terms of the potential absorption of each of its micronutrients, there are still problems we want you to be aware of when it comes to liquid multivitamins. Remember that just because the multivitamin is going to be *taken* in liquid form doesn't mean it is necessarily *sold* as a liquid. It could be a powder, as well. However, simply purchasing a large bottle of a liquid multivitamin or a multiple-serving canister of a powdered multivitamin may not be the best answer either. To begin with, remember how we told you earlier that your food loses micronutrients when it comes into contact with light, air, and heat while traveling to your table? Well, the same is true of the micronutrients in your multivitamin. So, if you purchase a premade liquid multivitamin or a vitamin beverage that may have been exposed to heat during its long journey to the store in the back of a container truck and that has been sitting on the store shelf exposed to fluorescent lighting, there is a good chance the micronutrients have been degraded to some extent. Making matters worse, as these micronutrients degrade, they release antagonistic (or competitive) elements that further degrade other micronutrients in the same formula. For example, vitamin B_{12} in a liquid solution can break down and release a cobalt ion. This cobalt ion can then contribute to the destruction of vitamins B_1 and B_6.

Powdered multivitamins in a tub or canister also have their own unique problems. Not only can they become oxidized every time the canister is opened, but this delivery system makes it virtually impossible to guarantee which micronutrients will be distributed in each daily serving. You see, some vitamins are light and fluffy, while some minerals are dense and heavy. Over time, the heavier micronutrients will naturally sink to the bottom of the canister, so you just don't know which ones you are scooping into your daily multivitamin drink. This can be problematic, as the last few scoops full of heavy minerals waiting for you at the bottom of your canister can cause stomach upset, and the imbalance in micronutrients might leave your micronutrient orchestra playing a very off-key musical concerto.

Unwanted Ingredients Can Hinder Absorption

An additional problem with many of the powdered and liquid multivitamins, as well as those that come in pills and capsules, is unwanted add-ins. Have you ever noticed that women's multivitamins are sometimes pink and that men's are sometime blue? Is that really necessary? Or have you noticed that the chewable children's multivitamins are available in a rainbow of fruit colors and flavors? Do the potentially carcinogenic artificial colors really add to the benefits your child will receive? Unscrupulous vitamin manufacturers use artificial colors— such as Blue 1, Blue 2, Yellow 5, Yellow 6, and Red 40—to make their products more attractive to the consumer, but these potentially dangerous artificial colors have no place in a health-promoting product and should definitely be avoided.

Ingredients That Inhibit Proper Absorption

- All artificial sweeteners
- Artificial flavors
- BHA or BHT
- Blue 1 or 2
- Cane sugar
- Cellulose
- Corn syrup, cornstarch, or solids
- Croscarmellose sodium
- Crospovidone
- Disodium hydrogen phosphate
- Fructose
- Gelatin
- Gellan gum
- High fructose corn syrup
- Hydroxypropyl cellulose
- Hypromellose
- Magnesium or calcium stearate
- Maltodextrin
- Methylcellulose
- Microcrystalline cellulose
- Polyvinyl alcohol
- Red 40
- Shellac
- Silica
- Sodium benzoate
- Sodium starch glycolate
- Stearic acid
- Sucrose
- Sugar
- Talc
- Tapioca syrup
- Wax
- Yellow 5 or 6

And those fruit flavors we just referred to: How are they making the vitamins and minerals taste so good? As you learned in the pantry purge, both sugar and artificial flavors (often containing MSG) are EMDs, which reduce the absorption of the very micronutrients that your child's multivitamin is promising to deliver. So, when considering the A for absorption, sugar, high fructose corn syrup, artificial colors, artificial flavors, and all of the sugar substitutes are potential roadblocks to achieving micronutrient sufficiency.

On the opposite page, there's a brief list of many of the absorption-inhibiting ingredients that act as binders, fillers, excipients, sweeteners, flow agents, flavors, and preservatives. Check to make sure these do not appear on the labels of your supplements.

Fixing Flaw 1: Absorption

We identified disintegration as a key problem in the absorption of micronutrients and have proven that tablets and capsules just don't cut it if you want to make sure your multivitamin (aka, your micronutrient health insurance policy) is able to do its job. And while liquids and powders are superior, as they don't require disintegration, those delivered as premade liquids and powders in multiple-serving bottles or canisters are not the best choice either. This is because many of the micronutrients can be degraded, and it is difficult to determine accurate daily doses with powders. Additionally, we have warned you about unhealthy add-ins that can impact absorption. To help you avoid all of these absorption issues, we've included a quick checklist in Table 6.1 on page 164 that you can use when purchasing your supplements. By using the A part of our ABCs of Optimal Supplementation Guidelines, you will be able to successfully overcome the multivitamins first flaw—inhibited absorption.

B Stands for Beneficial Quantities and Forms

The second flaw we discovered is represented by the letter B in our ABCs of Optimal Supplementation Guidelines and has two parts that are equally important when trying to harness the miraculous nature of the multivitamin's individual micronutrients. The letter B stands for beneficial quantities and beneficial forms, and when examining products on the market, you will find that most fall short in both categories.

So how much of each micronutrient is beneficial? Luckily, you don't have to figure out any of that. The RDI, or Reference Daily Intake, is the amount of each micronutrient that will keep you from getting a micronutrient deficiency disease. Is it optimal? Will you thrive from this amount? Probably not. However,

TABLE 6.1
IDENTIFYING IF YOUR SUPPLEMENT FOLLOWS THE RULES FOR ABSORPTION

MAKE SURE YOUR MULTIVITAMIN . . .	CHECK IF YES
Is delivered in powdered form in single-serving packets	
Does not contain sugar under any name, such as sucrose, maltodextrin, fructose, corn syrup solids, high fructose corn syrup, cane sugar, tapioca syrup, or corn syrup, to name but a few	
Does not contain the preservatives sodium benzoate, BHA, or BHT	
Does not contain any binders, fillers, or flow agents, such as cellulose, disodium hydrogen phosphate, talc, polyvinyl alcohol, cornstarch, sodium starch glycolate, microcrystalline cellulose, crospovidone, croscarmellose sodium, gelatin, or gellan gum	
Is not coated with shellac, wax, hydroxypropyl methylcellulose, magnesium or calcium stearate, hypromellose, silica, or stearic acid	
Does not contain any artificial colors or flavors	

because you will already be eating a micronutrient-rich diet during your 28-day Micronutrient Miracle plan, you will be receiving a good portion of your essential vitamins and minerals through your food. Even after you take into account the micronutrient-leaching EMDs you may have identified in your life—such as oxalic acid, stress, pollution, and perhaps alcohol or medications—your smart supplementation will get you above the sufficiency line every time, *if* the supplement you choose contains the beneficial quantities and forms of the individual micronutrients your body needs.

Mathematically speaking:

Your Rich Food Diet—EMDs + Smart Supplementation = Micronutrient Sufficiency

Now when we say beneficial quantities, we are not implying that you need to megadose. In our opinion, more is rarely better when it comes to achieving and maintaining micronutrient sufficiency. After all, when would our ancestors have taken in 25 milligrams of vitamin B_1 (thiamine) or vitamin B_2 (riboflavin), the amount often found in popular multivitamin brands? In order to ingest these megadoses by eating real food, our ancestors would have had to consume 100 cups of asparagus (one of the richest sources of thiamine) or 100 eggs (one of the richest sources of riboflavin) each and every day. We doubt this was the case. These megadoses are not what nature intended, nor what we suggest. However, there is one micronutrient that we, and most other health professionals, feel should be taken at levels higher than RDI. We are talking about vitamin D, and, again, to be fair, let's consider our ancestors. Long before Prada and Gucci, our distant relatives simply weren't impressed by labels. In fact, how could they have been? They didn't even have any clothes. That's right, instead they trekked and worked for hours under the sun, and that sunshine kept them full of vitamin D. We currently recommend 2,000 IU of vitamin D in your multivitamin, which is 500 percent of the Daily Value (DV). (The RDI is used to determine the DV of foods, which is printed on nutrition facts labels in the United States. The DV tells you what percentage of the RDI is delivered.) While 500 percent may seem like a lot, imagine how much more the human body is acclimated to receiving. For example, a fair-skinned individual in Miami would probably need about 6 minutes of exposure to the sun in summer and 15 minutes in winter to make 10,000 IU of vitamin D. Our guess is that generations upon generations of men and women have been outside for more than 6 minutes at a time, thus manufacturing far greater amounts than even 10,000 IU of vitamin D. And rest assured that while 2,000 IU is 500 percent of the RDI, it is definitely not enough to raise safety concerns.

While manufacturers often add in too much of some micronutrients, like the inexpensive B vitamins, more often than not, the problem is one of too little. Calcium and magnesium are often the minerals that manufacturers skimp on most. This is because they are bulky and expensive and don't fit neatly into just a few capsules or tablets. Manufacturers don't want to deter you from taking their products, so they actually leave out essential micronutrients from their formulas so they can keep the number of pills you have to take each day as low as possible. It's true. Here is a direct quote from a representative from Thorne Research, a well-respected supplement manufacturer, on this very topic. "ThorneFX believes that taking three capsules in the morning and three capsules in the evening is practical for most people. . . . We could have suggested four capsules in the morning and four capsules in the evening, but at a certain point even the most committed individuals can get tired of taking too many pills."[2] Wow! So, as you just read, some multivitamin manufacturers actually make the decision to put only what they can into a predetermined amount of pills, regardless of whether or not the RDI for each essential micronutrient has been met. You can see the flaw here, right?

In our case, we needed a multivitamin that contained beneficial quantities of each essential vitamin and mineral so that Mira could rebuild her bones. Unfortunately, not a single multivitamin we found was formulated to include this basic requirement. So what are the consequences of multivitamin manufacturers formulating products that do not contain beneficial quantities? Believe it or not, it's more pills! Without adequate calcium and magnesium, for example, there is a good chance you may get high blood pressure. Then, you will need to add in an additional daily pill, this time a prescription medication that can further deplete the body of its essential micronutrients. So you see, leaving out beneficial quantities of each specific micronutrient is a flaw that can lead to potentially dangerous levels of micronutrient depletion, even in those believing that they are protecting themselves through supplementation.

Time Is of the Essence

What would happen if you only ate once a day? Our guess is that you would probably feel pretty tired and depleted by midafternoon. This is because your body requires fuel all day long to help it with the thousands of functions it performs throughout the day. Not only do these functions require adequate amounts of macronutrients (carbohydrates, protein, and fat) for energy, but they also require your essential micronutrients to be there at the exact time the biological function needs to be performed. Do you remember when we told you about the two families of vitamins—water-soluble and fat-soluble? The water-soluble vitamins move through your system very quickly and are often absorbed by the body and excreted within a 12-hour window. Can you see the problem? If you take your multivitamin at 7 a.m., then your water-soluble vitamins, like the B vitamins and vitamin C, might not be there to perform the functions necessary at 9 p.m. This is why many physicians and nutritionists, including Dr. Oz, suggest taking several of the water-soluble micronutrients in multiple doses.

"You want to give your body the right amount of fuel for when you need it," says Dr. Oz. "Vitamins have water-soluble elements to them, so they are quickly moved through your system." He recommends splitting your multivitamin into a.m. and p.m. doses because "by taking half your multivitamin in the morning and half in the evening, you're guaranteeing that your body can absorb all the nutrients it can."[3]

Another reason that some micronutrients need to be taken multiple times a day is their limited absorption capacity. For example, while the RDI recommends that healthy adults take in 1,000 milligrams of calcium a day and women over the age of 50 take in 1,200 milligrams, science suggests that calcium can only be absorbed at increments of no more than 600 milligrams at one time. In order to assure the RDI is met, one would have to take calcium multiple times during the day, either in supplement form or through food. So, the beneficial quantities part of the equation makes it clear that if we are to reach a sufficient state, we must choose a supplement that is taken multiple times during the day and that delivers the RDI levels (or in the case of calcium only 600 milligrams) without megadosing or leaving out essential vitamins and minerals.

B Also Stands for Beneficial Forms

Wouldn't you be angry if you thought you purchased a Porsche but were delivered a Yugo? That kind of bait and switch is common in the multivitamin world. You see, for each and every micronutrient, there are numerous forms that a manufacturer can choose from to include in its formula. And, like cars, some offer high performance at a higher price tag to the manufacturer, while others are less expensive and less effective. Including these inferior forms increases the manufacturer's profits. But unless you know which is which, you may be purchasing the multivitamin equivalent of the Yugo with a Porsche price tag.

There are approximately 20 to 30 vitamins and minerals included in the formulation of a typical multivitamin. Here are some of the essential micronutrients and their beneficial forms, along with brief explanations as to why we prefer these forms in your smart supplementation (see Table 6.2, below).

TABLE 6.2
BENEFICIAL FORMS OF SPECIFIC MICRONUTRIENTS [4, 5, 6, 7, 8, 9, 10, 11, 12]

ESSENTIAL MICRONUTRIENT	BENEFICIAL FORM(S)	WHY IS THIS SUPERIOR?
Vitamin A	5,000 IU, or 100% Daily Value, of mixed vitamin A from palmitate and beta-carotene	Some multivitamins only contain beta-carotene, an inactive form of vitamin A (provitamin A), which must be converted in the body to retinal (preformed), an active form (conversion rate of 21:1). Due to the poor conversion rate of beta-carotene, a supplement should be formulated to include at least 2,500 IU of preformed vitamin A (retinyl acetate or palmitate).
Lutein	6 mg lutein (often omitted)	Most multivitamins do not contain lutein at all, but we recommend 6 mg of lutein because this is the amount that is recommended to prevent/reverse age-related macular degeneration.
Vitamin B_2 (riboflavin)	1.7 mg of riboflavin-5-phosphate	While many products contain riboflavin HCl, it is inferior to riboflavin-5-phosphate because it is not the bioactive form of vitamin B_2. Riboflavin HCl needs to be converted in the liver to the active form.

TABLE 6.2 (cont.)		
ESSENTIAL MICRONUTRIENT	**BENEFICIAL FORM(S)**	**WHY IS THIS SUPERIOR?**
Vitamin B_3 (niacin)	20 mg of niacin and niacinamide	Most multivitamins only contain niacinamide. However, the two forms of vitamin B_3 perform completely different functions in your body. Niacinamide controls blood sugar, but only niacin has been shown to lower LDL (bad cholesterol) and raise HDL (good cholesterol). It is best to include both forms to cover all bases.
Vitamin B_6	2 mg of pyridoxal-5-phosphate	The bioactive form is pyridoxal-5-phosphate. However, many inferior products use pyridoxine HCl, which is not the active form of this B vitamin.
Vitamin B_9 (folate)	400 mcg of 5-MTHF (methyltetrahydro-folate)	Research published in the *American Journal of Epidemiology* shows that more than 34% of the US population may have a genetic enzyme defect, known as MTHFR mutation, that makes it difficult for them to convert folic acid into biologically active 5-MTHF, and new estimates suggest that up to 60% of the population may be affected. For these individuals and many others, 5-MTHF may be a more effective method of folate supplementation. 5-MTHF is a breakthrough in supplemental science.
Vitamin B_{12}	6 mcg of methylcobalamin	The standard source of B_{12}, cyanocobalamin, is not a natural source. In fact, it's not found anywhere in nature and must be converted by the liver into methylcobalamin in order to be usable by humans (and all other animals). Cyanocobalamin is typically found in inexpensive products offered in grocery stores. Methylcobalamin is the form of vitamin B_{12} active in the central nervous system. It is essential for cell growth and replication.
Vitamin D	2,000 IU of vitamin D_3	There are two forms of vitamin D available in supplements: vitamin D_2 (ergocalciferol) and vitamin D_3 (cholecalciferol). D_3 is the form that is produced in our skin when we are exposed to sunlight and is more biologically superior for supplementation. In fact, research published in the *American Journal of Clinical Nutrition*, found that vitamin D_2 supplementation actually caused a reduction in overall serum concentrations of vitamin D [25(OH)D] over 28 days, with serum levels actually falling below baseline (starting) levels! The researchers concluded that vitamin D_2 should no longer be regarded as a nutrient appropriate for supplementation or fortification of foods.

TABLE 6.2 (cont.)		
ESSENTIAL MICRONUTRIENT	**BENEFICIAL FORM(S)**	**WHY IS THIS SUPERIOR?**
Vitamin E	30 IU of mixed tocopherols and mixed tocotrienols	Vitamin E is split into two families: the tocopherols and the tocotrienols, each containing four unique derivatives (alpha, beta, gamma, and delta). Smart supplements contain the full spectrum of each. Look on the label for "full spectrum d-tocopherols and d-tocotrienols." University of California studied the two families and found that tocotrienols are 40–60% more effective as antioxidants. New research suggests that delta-tocotrienol can completely prevent the erosion of the bone surface and also be effective in increasing bone formation and preventing bone reabsorption. Additionally, avoid the synthetic form of this vitamin, which starts with a dl-. According to a study published in the *American Journal of Clinical Nutrition*, researchers found that levels of natural vitamin E (d-tocopherol) in the blood and in the organs were double that of synthetic vitamin E (dl-tocopherol) when compared, showing natural vitamin E is better retained and more biologically active than synthetic.
Vitamin K	80 mcg of vitamin K_1 and vitamin K_2 (MK-4 and MK-7)	Vitamin K is all too often omitted from multivitamin formulations, but it is essential for bone strength and heart health. It is important for a supplement to include both K_1 and K_2 and even more superior and rare if it also includes both forms of vitamin K_2 (MK-4 and MK-7). Vitamin K_1 plays a role in blood clotting, while K_2 is a more important inducer of bone mineralization in human osteoblasts (bone-building cells). Vitamin K_2 has been proven in studies to be as effective as prescription drugs in reducing the incidence of bone fractures. Additionally, because K_2 directs calcium out of the arteries and into the bones, where it is needed, K_2 is essential for the prevention of coronary heart disease.
Calcium	600 mg *Pills and capsules:* calcium citrate or malate *Liquids and powders:* Same as above or calcium carbonate + citric acid (non-GMO)	Choose a supplement that delivers the maximum amount of calcium that can be absorbed by the body at one time (600 mg). This is the only micronutrient that should be less than 100% RDI. While pills and capsules should use calcium citrate or malate as they are more absorbable, liquids and powders have an additional option: Combining calcium carbonate with non-GMO citric acid stimulates the conversion of the calcium carbonate to calcium citrate in water, thus supplying the best absorption in a liquid form.

TABLE 6.2 (cont.)		
ESSENTIAL MICRONUTRIENT	**BENEFICIAL FORM(S)**	**WHY IS THIS SUPERIOR?**
Copper	Should not be included in supplement	Taking a multivitamin with copper is generally not recommended because too much can hinder your body's ability to destroy the proteins that form the plaques found in the brains of Alzheimer's patients. Many Alzheimer's patients have elevated levels of copper, and in studies, it was determined that many of those affected took multivitamins with copper. Additionally, pregnant women should avoid copper in multivitamins because copper levels can nearly double during pregnancy, making toxicity a concern. Cramps, abdominal pain, vomiting, nausea, and diarrhea are all common when taking supplements that include copper.
Iron	Should not be included in supplement	Iron is a vital mineral your body needs to function normally. However, the National Institutes of Health's Office of Dietary Supplements has indicated that too much iron can cause serious health complications. Because of this, you may want to take an iron-free multivitamin to avoid iron overload, a medical condition that causes excess iron to be stored in vital organs, such as the liver and heart. Too much iron may be toxic—and even fatal. In general, iron supplementation is not recommended for adult males and postmenopausal women. If you are a premenopausal woman, an athlete that works out for more than 6 hours a week, or a strict vegan/vegetarian, you may want to consider iron supplementation. *(In the "C Stands for Micronutrient Competitions and S Stands for Synergies" section, you will uncover another reason iron should be omitted from multivitamin formulations.)*
Magnesium	400 mg *Pills and capsules:* magnesium citrate, glycinate, or L-Thronate *Liquids and powders:* Same as above or magnesium carbonate + citric acid (non-GMO)	Most multivitamins supply small amounts of magnesium because of its bulky size. Locate supplements that supply 400 mg of magnesium, a micronutrient responsible for over 300 essential metabolic reactions in the body as well as controlling sugar cravings. Similar to calcium, magnesium carbonate is converted to magnesium citrate, one of the most bioavailable forms, through ionic conversion using non-GMO citric acid and water.
Selenium	70 mcg selenomethionine	This is a superior bioavailable form.

Fixing Flaw 2: Beneficial Quantities and Forms

Can you now see how important it is to take supplements that are formulated with both the beneficial quantities and beneficial forms of each micronutrient? Your money could really be wasted otherwise. This information on beneficial quantities and forms goes a long way toward explaining why many of the studies on multivitamins have been unsuccessful at providing health benefits. After all, how could a multivitamin with insufficient quantities of calcium and no vitamin K_2 promote bone health? Below is another quick, little checklist we want you to use when evaluating a multivitamin; this one covers all of the B aspects of our ABCs of Optimal Supplementation Guidelines.

TABLE 6.3
IDENTIFYING IF YOUR SUPPLEMENT FOLLOWS THE RULES FOR BENEFICIAL QUANTITIES AND FORMS

MAKE SURE YOUR MULTIVITAMIN . . .	CHECK IF YES
Is taken twice a day	
Does contain 500–600 mg of calcium	
Does contain 400 mg of magnesium	
Does contain 2,000 IU of vitamin D_3	
Does not contain more than 100% DV of any micronutrients (vitamin D excluded)	
Does contain 100% of the DV for all micronutrients (vitamin D and calcium excluded)	
Does contain methylcobalamin for B_{12}	
Does contain selenomethionine for selenium	
Does contain both niacin and niacinamide	
Does contain at least 2,500 IU of vitamin A as retinyl acetate or palmitate	
Does contain vitamin K_1, vitamin K_2 (MK-4), and vitamin K_2 (MK-7)	
Does contain L-5-MTHF and not folic acid	
Does contain all eight forms of vitamin E (mixed tocopherols and tocotrienols) and does not use dl- forms (synthetic)	
Does not contain copper	
Does not contain iron	
Does contain at least 425 mg of choline	
Does contain 6 mg of lutein	
Does contain riboflavin-5-phosphate for vitamin B_2	
Does contain pyridoxal-5-phosphate for vitamin B_6	
Does contain any of the following beneficial but nonessential micronutrients: grape seed extract, quercetin, CoQ10, alpha-lipoic acid, or L-carnitine	

C Stands for Micronutrient Competitions and S Stands for Synergies

While the A and the B in the ABCs are really important to increase the overall benefits your multivitamin can deliver, the C and the s are really the game changers! To understand C and s let's use our orchestra analogy again. Imagine that all the musicians in the orchestra arrive at the concert hall to perform a piece of music. All the essential instruments needed for the piece are there. However, for this performance, the musicians decide to toss away their sheet music and just play randomly all at once; they aren't waiting for their parts in the musical piece before beginning. What do you think that might sound like? A big jumble, right? The sound of each instrument would compete with the others for your ear. The loud, deep blasts of the tubas would drown out the delicate sound of the flutes, and the crash of the cymbals would completely negate the sound of the harps. You would not get the balance and beautiful harmony that could be achieved if the same instruments were to play the piece of music as properly composed. In fact, you wouldn't end up with music at all; you would end up with chaos.

Now here is the amazing part: The same is true of your micronutrients. Remember, each micronutrient has a unique function (or sound) in the body, and, like instruments, some harmonize well and others do not. A typical multivitamin is a lot like the musicians in the orchestra all playing at the same time without any properly composed sheet music (or formulation). Instead of the micronutrients working together as a synergistic unit, they all compete with one another for absorption pathways and utilization.

This brings us to the third, and potentially the biggest, flaw we discovered in the multivitamin: C stands for micronutrient competition. Our research uncovered numerous peer-reviewed scientific studies clearly demonstrating that certain micronutrients, when delivered at the same time (like within a multivitamin), greatly reduced or eliminated the ability of other micronutrients to be absorbed or utilized. This is a big problem if your goal is to create a multinutrient product that will successfully deliver all the vitamins and minerals your body needs each and every day. In fact, we believe that micronutrient competitions are the main reason multivitamin research has fared as poorly as it has compared to research using individual or small groupings of micronutrients, in terms of overall benefits. An example of this is when copper and zinc are taken at the same time; they will duke it out for domination of the receptor site. These receptor sites, or absorption pathways, act as docking locations for specific micronutrients and are found throughout the entire gastrointestinal tract. Of course, micronutrient competition is not as simple as one micronutrient blocking another. There are actually four types of micronutrient competitions that can take place when taking a typical multivitamin: chemical competition, biochemical competition, physiological competition, and finally clinical competition. Let's take a moment to look closer at each.

Chemical competition occurs during the manufacturing of all nutritional supplements, including multivitamins. When manufacturers combine competing micronutrients in one formulation, a chemical battle can ensue within the formulation itself, leaving the competing micronutrients unable to be absorbed. For example, vitamin B_9 (folate) forms an insoluble complex with zinc when they are put together in a nutritional supplement or multivitamin. When this happens, the absorption of both is compromised.

Biochemical competition happens after ingestion but before the micronutrients have been absorbed. Here the micronutrients compete for a common receptor site, or absorption pathway, like in the example we gave earlier with zinc and copper, but this also occurs between many other micronutrients as well, such as lutein and beta-carotene.

Physiological competition happens after micronutrient absorption when one or more micronutrients cause decreased utilization of competing micronutrients. For instance, in some studies, copper has been shown to reduce the activity of vitamin B_5 (pantothenic acid).

Clinical competition is when the presence of one micronutrient masks the deficiency of another, making it difficult for even trained health professionals to detect a deficiency. The classic example here is vitamin B_9 (folate) and vitamin B_{12}. Folate can mask B_{12} anemia, a condition of inadequate red blood cells that can lead to depression, dementia, and the inability to carry oxygen throughout the body.

Now don't worry, we are not going to ask you to memorize these micronutrient competitions. We have listed them here just so you can see how many times competition can occur from the beginning of a micronutrient's journey at manufacturing all the way through to utilization. In fact, when you draw out all the competitions that can occur between 34 of the micronutrients most often included in a multivitamin supplement, it looks like a big spiderweb. In all, our research has identified 48 competitions that can occur between those 34 micronutrients, with 30 of the 34 (88 percent) having at least one competition, 15 of the 34 (44 percent) having at least three competitions, and one micronutrient, iron, having competitions with 10 other micronutrients.

Shocking, right? We thought so, too; we couldn't believe how many people in the supplement industry were aware of micronutrient competitions, but even more shocking to us was the fact that no one seemed to be doing anything about it.

It wasn't until we stumbled across the topic of micronutrient competition on the Wal-Mart Web site, of all places, that we started to understand the problem. Here is how Wal-Mart described the topic of micronutrient competition to their customers: "Another area of controversy is whether all of the nutrients in a multiple would be better utilized if they were taken separately. While certain nutrients compete with each other for absorption, this is also the case when the nutrients are supplied in food. For example, magnesium, zinc, and calcium compete; copper and zinc also compete. However, the body is designed to cope with this competition, which should not be a problem if multiples are spread out over the day."[13]

Did you catch that? First they agreed with us regarding *beneficial quantities* by telling their consumers to take their multivitamins multiple times throughout the day. They also supported the fact that micronutrient competitions exist and even gave a few great examples. However, then they simply disregarded the problem, stating that because competitions take place when you eat certain foods, they are not really a problem with your supplementation. This is completely misleading and, in our opinion, incorrect. If the goal of taking a multivitamin is to achieve micronutrient sufficiency by filling in the vitamin- and mineral-deficiency gaps in one's Rich Food diet, then wouldn't it seem self-sabotaging to take a multivitamin whose formulation contains micronutrients that are known to compete with others for absorption and utilization?

Instead of simply throwing up our hands and saying, "Well, the competitions take place in food, so we have kept them in our multivitamin," we felt that by reviewing the science concerning micronutrient competitions and carefully separating the known competitors, we could formulate a multivitamin that would have as few competitions as possible and thus enhanced absorption and utilization potential.

The fact is, we don't know from day to day which micronutrients our Rich Food diet is going to leave us deficient in. So it is the job of a well-formulated multivitamin to cover the bases and do everything it can to ensure you absorb and utilize as many micronutrients as possible. Does that make sense? If you know that a certain micronutrient will reduce or eliminate the ability of one or more micronutrients, then by eliminating that competitive micronutrient from the formulation, you have, by definition, enhanced the absorption and utilization potential for the micronutrients that would have been affected.

While we knew the science behind our new theory of Anti-Competition Technology was strong, we needed to see if it would work in practical application. So we started searching the medical and nutrition journals for any studies that would support our theory. After all, we knew that if we were going to have any success reversing Mira's osteoporosis, we would have to overcome this third flaw in multivitamin formulation. During our research, our faith was strengthened by two studies that seemed to prove our anti-competition theory. The first was published back in 1998 in the *American Journal of Clinical Nutrition*; in it, researchers showed that "lutein negatively affected beta-carotene absorption when the two were given simultaneously."[14] So science had determined that lutein and beta-carotene compete, but could separating these competitive micronutrients make any real difference? In 2002, the TOZAL study on age-related macular degeneration (AMD), an eye condition that leads to blindness and affects over 2 million people over the age of 50, gave us the answer we were looking for when researchers used this information to successfully prevent and even reverse the progression of AMD. For years, scientists had known that both lutein and beta-carotene individually had beneficial effects on patients with AMD. However, in the TOZAL study when, for the first time, the competition between lutein and beta-carotene was accounted for, supplementation was able to either improve or stabilize vision in 76.7 percent of patients. The study's developer, Edward Paul, OD, PhD, of the International Academy of Low Vision Specialists, called the discovery "ground shaking," stating that this information "will really turn the way we look at nutrition on its ear." According to Dr. Paul, this new understanding of micronutrient competition represents a "huge paradigm shift when you consider that we had been recommending lutein be combined with other antioxidants, which is a reasonable thing to recommend. But when these two nutrients are competing for the same receptor site, they're only neutralizing one another."[15]

Incredible, right? This was exactly the type of evidence we were looking for. When the competing micronutrients were separated, the beneficial effects of both micronutrients were finally realized. With as many as 48 micronutrient competitions in a typical multivitamin, it seemed to us that there were numerous potential benefits currently being unrealized by most multivitamin takers. We knew that our idea of separating competing micronutrients to enhance absorption and utilization was truly innovative, but, amazingly, we discovered something else along the way that enhanced micronutrient absorption and utilization even more when paired with our anti-competition theory. It's called *micronutrient synergy*, and it's represented by the s in the ABCs of Optimal Supplementation Guidelines.

Opening the Door for Synergy

It turns out that micronutrient synergy is like a mirror image of micronutrient competition. While micronutrient competitions can reduce or eliminate the beneficial effects of certain micronutrients, micronutrient synergies can enhance the beneficial effects of certain micronutrients. However, and this is important, micronutrient synergies cannot reverse or eliminate the effects of micronutrient competitions on their own; they can only offer enhanced absorption and utilization if all of the micronutrient competitions that could affect their absorption have been eliminated.

You can think of micronutrient synergy as the icing on the ABCs of Optimal Supplementation cake. Assuming that A, B, and C have all been accounted for, micronutrient synergy works to enhance overall results. That is why the s for synergy is lowercase in the ABCs; it is an aspect of proper formulation, but one that can only be realized if A, B, and C are in place.

Using our orchestra analogy once again, we can see that if our musicians stopped playing their instruments over one another and started following the sheet music again (i.e., the micronutrient competitions were accounted for), then the composer's intentional synergistic pairing of certain instruments could be appreciated. In other words, if the tuba was no longer drowning out the melody of the flute and the cymbals were no longer masking the sound of the harp, then when the flute and harp were played together as the composer intended, the synergistic harmony created would enhance the musical piece. Even if the flute and harp were both synergistically playing the musical piece exactly as the composer had intended, if all the other instruments, including the tuba and cymbals, were all still randomly playing (i.e., the competitions were not accounted for), then the synergy between the flute and harp would not be realized. In short, the benefits of synergistic micronutrients can only be realized when the competitions are eliminated.

Just like there are four types of micronutrient competitions, there are also four types of micronutrient synergies.

Chemical synergy is the opposite of chemical competition. It occurs in the nutritional supplement itself, prior to ingestion, when two micronutrients are put into the same multivitamin to form an advantageous complex that can help increase the absorption of one or both micronutrients. Vitamin B_2 (riboflavin) and zinc share such a relationship.

Biochemical synergy is the opposite of biochemical competition. Here, rather than competing for a receptor site, or absorption pathway, one micronutrient aids in the absorption of the other. An example is when vitamin D enhances the absorption of calcium.

Physiological synergy is the opposite of physiological competition. Instead of two micronutrients decreasing each other's utilization, one micronutrient aids in the performance of a second micronutrient. This can happen when one micronutrient needs to perform a specific function in order for a second micronutrient to do its job. For example, vitamin K_2 is required to direct calcium out of the blood and into the bone, where it is needed.

Clinical synergy is the opposite of clinical competition. Clinical synergy occurs when two or more micronutrients work together to create an observable yet unexpected beneficial change in the body. For example, when vitamins B_6, B_9 (folate), and B_{12} are all present in adequate quantities, they have been shown to lower homocysteine levels, a known marker of coronary disease, by converting homocysteine into cysteine and methionine.

Fixing Flaws 3 and 4: Micronutrient Competitions and Synergies

Like absorption and beneficial quantities and forms (flaws 1 and 2), you can see how important it is to take a multivitamin formulated using Anti-Competition Technology, which separates the known micronutrient competitions and pairs the synergistic micronutrients. Again, understanding micronutrient competitions and synergies can help us understand why many of the benefits often associated with individual micronutrients are often unrealized when those same micronutrients are paired randomly within a typical multivitamin formulation. When evaluating your multivitamin, use Table 6.4, below, to see how your multivitamin stacks up regarding the C and s of our ABCs of Optimal Supplementation Guidelines.

TABLE 6.4
IDENTIFYING IF YOUR SUPPLEMENT FOLLOWS THE RULES FOR COMPETITIONS AND SYNERGIES

MAKE SURE YOUR MULTIVITAMIN . . .	CHECK IF YES
Does not contain both vitamin B_9 (folate) and zinc in the same dose	
Does not contain both lutein and beta-carotene in the same dose	
Does not contain both vitamin B_5 and copper in the same dose	
Does not contain both vitamin A and vitamin D in the same dose	
Does not contain both zinc and copper in the same dose	
Does not contain both vitamin B_5 (pantothenic acid) and B_7 (biotin) in the same dose	
Does not contain iron at all	
Does contain and claim Anti-Competition Technology on packaging to account for all competitions and synergies	

Putting the ABCs Together

After evaluating the modern multivitamin and identifying the four flaws reducing its overall effectiveness, we were left with our ABCs of Optimal Supplementation Guidelines. And while our guidelines were originally developed to evaluate the multivitamin, they can really help increase the absorption and utilization potential of any nutritional supplement. When we put the ABCs of Optimal Supplementation Guidelines together, it revealed that the most effective multivitamin would be a single-serving, powdered formula delivered in liquid form free of binders, fillers, excipients, artificial flavors and colors, and sugars. It would contain beneficial quantities (approximately 100 percent of the RDI) of each micronutrient, with two exceptions: calcium would be lower than the RDI (around 600 milligrams) and vitamin D would be higher than the RDI (around 2,000 IU). Additionally, where applicable, the multivitamin would also contain a full spectrum of beneficial forms for each micronutrient and be formulated using Anti-Competition Technology, which completely separates known competitive micronutrients to enhance absorption and utilization. This would require that it contain at least two completely different formulations to be taken at two different times during the day. And lastly, synergistic micronutrients would be paired in each formula to enhance the potential health benefits of each micronutrient.

Our Reinvention of the Multivitamin: nutreince

Our ABCs of Optimal Supplementation Guidelines had certainly painted a very different picture of what a properly formulated multivitamin should look like. We searched high and low to find a multivitamin that would offer superior absorption and that contained the beneficial quantities and forms we were looking for. Sadly, there wasn't one. Beyond that, none of the multivitamins we found were formulated using Anti-Competition Technology or anything like it. Sure, the synergies were there, but remember that without getting rid of the micronutrient competitions, the synergies are all but useless.

So, we did the only thing we could do: We started from scratch and began to piece together a multivitamin of our own. Because we believed that eliminating the micronutrient competitions would be essential to Mira's healing, we focused on that aspect of our ABCs to start with and began by purchasing each micronutrient separately and taking them in small groupings before and after each of our four meals, eight times throughout the day. Two or three pills before breakfast, three or four after, and so on, until the 30-plus pills we had to take each day were gone. We attempted to open and pour some of the capsules into water to help with the absorption, but most were just not palatable in this way and had to be taken as capsules. Not only was this method hugely expensive, costing nearly $300 for each of us per month, it also became a seemingly never-ending chore of choking down pills every time we turned around. Even Mira, who didn't have a hard time swallowing pills in the beginning, developed an aversion to them about a year in and 10,000-plus pills later.

But in the end, our Anti-Competition Technology worked! The proof was in the DEXA scan, and after witnessing Mira's incredible recovery, we were excited to share this knowledge with others. Soon all of our clients, including Mabel, whom you read about in Chapter 2, started on the same regimen, and client after client saw their health improve, as well. However, it wasn't long before our clients started to complain about our anti-competition, pill-stacking method. From the busy moms to the high-level executives, they all wanted something simple and convenient. "Why can't you just create something that we can take a couple times a day?" they would ask. So we decided to do just that.

We wanted to create a multivitamin that followed the ABCs of Optimal Supplementation Guidelines to the letter—a single-serving, powdered multivitamin that would once and for all get rid of the handfuls of pills we, and our clients, were forced to take every day. A complete multivitamin that would eliminate all four of the flaws we had identified in the modern multivitamin that we felt were reducing its overall effectiveness. We knew that the hard part would be following our own guidelines and ending up with something palatable and affordable. Manufacturer after manufacturer looked at our formulation and told us that it was impossible. "It will taste horrible," they said. And to be honest, we almost gave up several times. The truth is, if there had been even one other multivitamin, anywhere in the world, that met the ABCs of Optimal Supplementation Guidelines, we would have been thrilled to use it (and would likely be suggesting it to you right now). But there wasn't one. So after 6 years of countless formulation attempts and more than 3 years of working with the US Patent and Trademark Office to validate and patent our invention of Anti-Competition Technology, we finally introduced our patented multivitamin—nutreince (pronounced "nutrients")—to the world in 2012.

We share this story with you because we want you to know how and why we created nutreince and that we didn't just haphazardly decide to throw together and sell a multivitamin to make money. A properly formulated multivitamin like nutreince is absolutely essential in order to achieve optimal health, which is why we felt so strongly about spending the time, energy, and money to search out one of the most highly respected, FDA-regulated, NSF-certified US manufacturers to help us develop nutreince and bring it to market. Over the last 3 years, nutreince has grown wildly in popularity and has received praise from some of the most respected figures in the health and wellness world. nutreince is now available worldwide, and nothing makes us happier than receiving e-mail testimonials regarding the health successes of our global customers.

We take nutreince twice daily and instruct our private clients to do the same in order to get the maximum benefits from their Micronutrient Miracle plans. While we cannot require you to choose nutreince as your multivitamin, we highly recommend that you do so. For those who opt to search for their own multivitamin among the plethora of products lining store shelves from respected manufacturers like Garden of Life, NOW, and Thorne Research, we strongly suggest you take our ABCs of Optimal Supplementation Stack Up Quiz (MultivitaminStackUpQuiz.com). We cannot stress enough the importance of this extremely thorough and free analysis. After filling in some specific information about the multivitamin you've chosen, we will give you a fair and objective score and an in-depth, multipage evaluation of its strengths and weaknesses. Remember, the entire objective of the Micronutrient Miracle plan is to help you achieve micronutrient sufficiency, and supplementing with a properly formulated multivitamin, one that is able to eliminate all four major flaws in supplementation, is the essential third step to achieving that goal.

Okay, well that's smart supplementation in a nutshell. We hope you have learned a nugget or two of great information that will help you choose a smart supplement. In the next chapter, we are going to put it all together and introduce you to the 10 Golden Rules of the Micronutrient Miracle plan. We are even going to show you two completely mind-blowing exercise techniques that we developed exclusively for our private clients. They will have you burning fat and building muscle faster than ever before!

7

The Signature 28-Day Micronutrient Miracle Plan

CONGRATULATIONS! YOU HAVE DONE the hard work and are ready to begin your 28-day Micronutrient Miracle plan. You've stocked your home full of Rich Foods and nontoxic home goods and personal care items, taken responsibility for your micronutrient-depleting actions, and gathered the smart supplement staples you are going to be using during your 28-day plan. There is nothing left to do but jump right in.

In this chapter, we will get down to brass tacks. In Part 1, we will review the three-step plan and give you the Micronutrient Miracle's 10 Golden Rules to follow for the next 28 days. Then, in Part 2, we will delve into the dining options. You will learn which foods you need to limit, which foods we want you to focus on, and how to schedule your meals. Finally, you will get a 28-day menu plan that will show you just how varied and delicious your diet will be. And because each and every person is unique, so is each Micronutrient Miracle plan. While the Signature 28-day Micronutrient Miracle plan in this chapter is perfect for all people looking to improve their diets and overall health while creating a state of micronutrient sufficiency in their bodies, this book goes one step further in the next chapter and offers modifications designed for specific health conditions. However, regardless of your goals and how you plan on personalizing this plan, the information in this chapter is necessary for your success.

Part 1: Introducing the Micronutrient Miracle's 10 Golden Rules

Each Micronutrient Miracle plan is based on our core belief that micronutrient sufficiency is the foundation of optimal health and can be achieved by following the 10 Golden Rules defined by our simple three-step approach.

STEP 1:
Choose Micronutrient-Rich Foods—Learn Your Rich Food Rules

Over the next 28 days, we want you to follow these four golden rules when choosing your Rich Foods. We don't have much more to add to this first step, as it is well outlined in the previous chapters. Additionally, you will find that we have taken care of a lot of this work for you. For example, none of the recipes in the menu section contain any sugar, wheat, or soy products. Additionally, the recipes follow the proper preparation techniques for reducing the Everyday Micronutrient Depleters (EMDs). For example, you will only find spinach (which contains oxalic acid) cooked in the daily plans. We've made the plan easy for you to follow.

GOLDEN RULE #1 Pass on These Poor Food Perpetrators

You must completely eliminate the following three foods, as well as all of their aliases.

Sugar	Wheat	Soy

GOLDEN RULE #2 Oust the Obesogens

Do your best to eliminate these obesogens that you come into contact with on a daily basis.

MSG	BPA	Phthalates

GOLDEN RULE #3 Reduce the EMDs Found in Foods and Beverages

Use proper preparation to minimize micronutrient loss or eliminate all together.

Phytates	Trypsin inhibitors	Caffeine
Oxalates	Phosphoric acid	Tannins
Lectins	Alcohol	

GOLDEN RULE #4 Shop Using our Good, Better, Best System and our Rich Food Picks

We went down the aisles and demonstrated how you can get the most micronutrient bang in every bite for all the foods we want you to put in your grocery cart over the next 28 days. Follow our guidelines and use our Rich Food picks in each of the following categories.

Produce	Oils and fats	Sugar alternatives
Ruminants and pork	Spices	Coffee and tea
Dairy	Salt	Alcohol
Poultry and eggs	Condiments	All-day drinkables
Seafood	Salad dressing	
Protein powder	Flour alternatives	

STEP 2:
Drive Down Depletion—Learn Your Lifestyle Rules

While we want to reiterate that many of the lifestyle EMDs that we covered in Chapter 4 cannot and should not be entirely eliminated, over the next 28 days we want you to focus on driving down depletion in the three areas that we believe can make the greatest positive impact on your health.

Stress	Exercise	Toxins

GOLDEN RULE #5 Reduce Stress

No, we aren't telling you that your life will somehow become miraculously easier. Your children aren't getting a nanny, and your job won't suddenly become less taxing. However, for the next 28 days, we want you to find a stress-reduction technique that works for you. This is a very personal choice. For example, meditation stresses Mira out, and dancing around the room will not soothe Jayson's stress. Additionally, not every stress-reduction technique we share will work in every stressful situation. Perhaps, at the office, tuning in to your body would be preferable to blaring tunes and moving to the music. You will have the opportunity to learn more about each of these techniques in our Micronutrient Miracle Motivation and Resource Center when you join our community online at mymiracleplan.com. We have prepared a variety of videos outlining techniques that you can use daily to relieve stress and counteract the depletions caused by it.

Use one or more of the techniques below when stress hits. If time permits, you can use these techniques in the morning and before bed, to center yourself. After all, even as little as 5 minutes can help. Aren't you worth it?

1. **Meditate with a mantra.** Centering can be so simple. Reciting a mantra in rhythm with your breathing can help to calm you in times of stress. This is a great technique when you are in your office, as well as both in the a.m. to center you and in the p.m. to ready you for sleep.

2. **Become aware of your body.** This is one of Mira's favorite techniques before bed. From the tips of your toes all the way to the crown of your head, pay attention to any pains, aches, and stress being held throughout your body. This is key to self-awareness and de-stressing. You quite literally release tension one muscle at a time.

3. **Dance till stress levels drop.** How can you be anxious with your favorite tune playing in your ears? This one might not be great for public periods of panic, but letting loose and moving your body freely allows the tunes to turn off your tension—and the boost in metabolism doesn't hurt, either.

4. **Practice focused breathing.** Breathing is the body's natural relaxation response, so it makes sense that practicing proper breathing techniques has been shown to elicit a physical state of deep rest that decreases heart

rate, blood pressure, respiratory rate, and muscle tension. This is perfect for when you are in public faced with scary or stressful circumstances.

5. **Move it to lose it.** That's right! With exercise, you literally sweat out the stress, all the while helping your body to achieve the strength, weight regulation, and heart health you deserve. While you may not always be able to drop and give us 20 pushups, you might be surprised by how much stress you can relieve with just 1 minute of jumping jacks.

GOLDEN RULE #6 Exercise Smarter, Not Longer

Imagine you are taking a road trip. You type the address of your final destination into your GPS and hit enter. Your handy-dandy trip planner then offers you two routes. The first will take you about 25 minutes. The second will take you a lot longer, about 3 hours, and it will cost you a lot more in gas. Which would you choose: the longer journey that takes the indirect route for hours, or the direct route that uses less energy—saving you both time and money? The shorter one, right? You would want to use your time effectively and reach your destination as quickly as possible.

Isn't exercise the same way? Your goal is a healthy body, built of strong muscle and solid bones. While you may enjoy exercise, chances are that you would give anything to make your workouts more efficient in a shorter amount of time, right? Well, say goodbye to hours on the treadmill. No more spinning your wheels on the stationary bike, not getting anywhere fast in your fitness goals. We are going to teach you how to work out wisely, getting maximum results with less effort and less time. For the next 28 days, we want you to burn fat and build muscle faster using our trademark *Zero Movement Training (ZMT)* for cardiovascular fitness and *One Set To Failure (1-STF)* for weight training.

Zero Movement Training

Now, you are likely wondering how we can promise you an effective cardiovascular workout without movement, but truth be told, you will still have to move. In fact, you are going to move harder and faster than you ever thought possible. The good news is, however, that you won't be moving *at all* most of the time. In fact, in a 20-minute workout, which is all we ask of you 3 or 4 days a week, you'll be sitting or standing completely still for 12½ of the minutes, and 3 of the minutes will be a slow and comfortable warmup. This means that you only have 4½ *minutes* of strong, intense, and dedicated hard work. That is less than 20 minutes of intense cardiovascular work in an entire week. Doesn't that sound incredible? And what is more incredible is that this workout style will actually make you a better fat-burner with a stronger aerobic capacity and a more "youthful" body, all while sparing your muscles so that your metabolism can soar 24–7.

Make sure to join our Micronutrient Miracle Motivation and Resource Center to view Zero Movement Training (ZMT) workout videos created for all fitness levels, from beginner to advanced. We'll share how you can use ZMT in the gym, outdoors, and even in your living room or a hotel room (with no gym equipment) to make your body a fat-burning machine.

Here are five benefits, *above and beyond time efficiency* that you will reap from Zero Movement Training (ZMT).

1. **You will improve your cardiovascular (aerobic) capacity.** A 2011 study presented at the American College of Sports Medicine's Annual Meeting found that just 2 weeks of high-intensity interval training, like ZMT, improved participants' aerobic capacity as much as 6 to 8 weeks of endurance training. Aerobic capacity refers to the functional capacity of your heart, lungs, and blood vessels. More simply put, the higher the aerobic capacity, the greater the level of aerobic fitness, and the better shape your heart will be in. Talk about quick improvements![1]

2. **You will increase calorie burn and fat metabolization.** ZMT makes you a fat-burning machine—even long after your brief workout is over. There is a 2-hour period following a workout that is referred to in the world of exercise science as EPOC (excess post-exercise oxygen consumption). It is the period when the body works to restore itself to preworkout levels. And this uses a lot of energy (i.e., calories). According to the American College of Sports Medicine, when individuals participate in intense interval training, such as with ZMT, the EPOC lasts longer than after normal workouts; research by the organization suggests that you can burn up to 15 percent more calories

overall. So while you're watching your favorite television show or reading your new book, you are still burning calories because you exercised smarter—not longer.

3. **You will decrease fat production.** Not only will you be burning more fat with ZMT than with long, drawn-out cardio programs, but your body will also be simultaneously turning off its fat-producing mechanism. Researchers from the Norwegian University of Science and Technology reported that subjects with an increased risk of cardiovascular disease and diabetes who followed a 16-week intense interval program, like ZMT, had a 100 percent greater decrease in fatty acid synthase (a fat-producing enzyme), proving you can blunt your fat production while burning more fat.

4. **You will increase production of human growth hormone.** Human growth hormone (HGH) is produced by the pituitary gland—a pea-size structure at the base of the brain—to fuel childhood growth and help maintain bone, muscle, and organs throughout your life. The higher your levels of HGH, the healthier and stronger you will be. However, once you hit the age of 30, you enter what's called somatopause, at which point your levels of HGH begin to plummet. This dramatic decline drives the aging process, and it causes things like decreased muscle and bone mass.[2] Intense interval training, like ZMT, turns back the clock by stimulating your production of HGH by up to 450 percent during the 24 hours after you finish your workout.[3]

5. **Your joints, bones, and muscles will be spared.** Marathon runs on the treadmill cause mayhem for your knees and joints. These longer bouts of cardio also cause the body to utilize muscle as fuel, and when you want to lose weight, muscle is key to your metabolism. ZMT allows your body to spare the hard-earned muscle you will gain from weight training, while ensuring that your weight loss is fat loss.

The brevity of the ZMT workouts makes our system of training ideal if you are busy and have little time to train. It allows you to use the least amount of time to gain maximum results. Remember, the goal of exercise should always be to gain or retain muscle and lose fat (which is very different from losing weight). See Table 7.1 on page 188 to get an idea of what a 20-minute ZMT workout looks like. However, remember to sign up at mymiracleplan.com for access to our online community so you can work out with us! There are no excuses not to, when ZMT is so fast and easy.

TABLE 7.1

TIMELINE FOR A ZMT WORKOUT

TIME (IN MINUTES)	ACTIVITY (EXAMPLE: STATIONARY BIKE)
00:00–02:59	Warm up slowly. Keep the resistance and speed low, simply spinning and getting your legs ready for your first burst.
03:00–03:30	Hit it! Your muscles are fresh. Turn up the resistance and go, go, go! During each 30-second intense interval, you should work to your max—likely becoming quite out of breath.
03:31–04:59	Ooh, Zero Movement Training allows you to stop completely after your intense activity. Some stationary bikes may require you to spin slowly, but take the resistance all the way down and do as little as you can. And if your machine allows, stop altogether. You will notice that when you stop, your heart rate soars even higher. Cool, right? No movement and your heart rate stays up, burning calories.
05:00–05:30	Hit it again! Turn up the resistance and turn up the intensity. Yes, it is harder than the first time. But it is only 30 seconds, so push through it. You should never leave your 30-second bout with energy to spare.
05:31–06:59	Bliss! Again, you have a minute and a half of *zero* movement. You will need this recovery period more and more as we near the 20-minute completion time.
07:00–07:30	Ok, go! Yes, it is tough to work at 100% effort, but when the entire workout is so brief, you know you can do it. You should be saying, "OMG, I don't know if I can do this anymore." Each revolution is work. Your chest will pound, and sweat should begin to pour out of you.
07:31–08:59	Breathe deeply during your breaks, and grab a sip of cold water when your heart stops pounding long enough to get it down. Remember, this is the time to psyche yourself up for your next intense spin.
09:00–09:30	Go time! Grit your teeth or swear in your own mind. Just do whatever you have to do to keep the bike cycling. Keep in mind the goal. At this point you may be slowing down. Some ZMT beginners find their muscles starting to give out after only 20 seconds. Do your best; you are halfway there.
09:31–10:59	Zero movement again (or minimal movement to keep the machine running).
11:00–11:30	Dig deep and push hard! This is intense exercise using every bit of muscle and heart you have. Each day you do this program, you will improve. Make sure to turn up the intensity any time you aren't feeling intense burn.
11:31–12:59	Zero movement time. Your brow is likely soaked no matter how in shape you currently are because you are working at 100% of your capacity.
13:00–13:30	Burst into action! You are getting so close to finishing your routine. Remember, work to your own level. It is not a competition. You should work as hard as you can for 30 seconds and watch how rapidly you improve.
13:31–14:59	Rest. Breathe and stop moving (a slow spin with zero resistance also works).

TABLE 7.1 (cont.)	
TIME (IN MINUTES)	**ACTIVITY (EXAMPLE: STATIONARY BIKE)**
15:00–15:30	Give it all you've got! Exhaustion may be felt, but you need to keep your goals in mind as you spin and push as hard as you can. This whole workout is only 20 minutes. Think about how great you will feel when you achieve your personal goals and how easy it will be to keep ZMT as part of your schedule.
15:31–16:59	Thank goodness for this rest. How crazy to be so tired in so little time. Remember, you are lighting the fat-burning fire for the rest of the day.
17:00–17:30	There is no playing around; it is time to push yourself! Each revolution is tough, even if it is only for 30 seconds. Think of the human growth hormone and how you are literally working to turn back the clock. Only one bout left and you've got this one in the bag!
17:31–18:59	Smile. You only have one intense, give-it-your-all, 30-second period left. You know you can do this. And you know how good it will feel to be finished. Get ready to hit it . . .
19:00–19:30	And go! Your legs are burning and so is your desire to achieve your goals. Drive it home harder and faster with each revolution. Even if you can barely turn the pedals, this time just push through it. You are not a quitter and this is the very last interval.
19:31–20:00	Zero movement, but stay seated to allow yourself recovery time. Drink water and breathe in. Again, your heart rate will increase just after stopping, so stay seated until it recovers. Smile and think to yourself, *you made it!* It was only 20 minutes and your whole day will be better because of it.

Remember, the more time you spend sweating in the gym, the more micronutrients your body depletes. ZMT is a perfect solution—minimizing your micronutrient loss while maximizing your fat-burning.

One Set to Failure Weight Training

You now have a great understanding of ZMT. You've learned how and why to perform this style of intense cardiovascular training three or four times a week. Remember, one of the benefits of ZMT is that it doesn't break down and destroy your muscles. That's right, ZMT is muscle-sparing. But, we have to make sure that you have enough muscle first. And don't think about weight training as just a way to get bigger. Let's blow up that myth right now. Ladies, you can breathe easy because you are not going to bulk up like Arnold Schwarzenegger; and for the men out there, we are sorry to tell you, but chances are that you will never build that kind of muscle mass either, even if you want to.

Think about this: When you were growing up, your body knew when to stop getting taller. You were "coded" to be a certain height. Well, your body also has been coded as to how much muscle it should have. It is called your genetic potential, and our One Set To Failure weight-training technique will allow your muscles to grow and gain strength quickly so that you can reach this potential. There are many obvious benefits to being strong. Of course, strength allows you to move and carry items with ease. However, the reasons to build strong muscles go far beyond moving furniture.

Here are four reasons above and beyond strength and muscle size that you should be lifting weights.

1. **Your bones will thank you.** Often, when your bones start hurting or you hear, as Mira did, that you have osteoporosis or osteopenia, you stop lifting weights because you worry that you're too frail. However, this is the opposite of what you should be doing. Aging brings about natural muscle and bone mass loss, and whether you're already losing bone mass or simply want to avoid any loss in the future, lifting weights can help. Your bones react to lifting weights much like your muscles do. When you lift, the muscles adapt to the stress by becoming bigger and stronger. Your bones also perceive stress, and because of this, your body will respond by building bone. Therefore, we want you to think about your weight training as both muscle building *and* bone building.

2. **You will reduce your diabetes risk.** According to a 2012 study published in the *Archives of Internal Medicine* (now *JAMA Internal Medicine*), men who lifted weights had a 34 percent lower risk of diabetes. But, the research gets even better: Those individuals who added in regular cardiovascular exercise (like our ZMT training) slashed risk by 59 percent.[4]

3. **Your heart will be happier.** Doing aerobic workouts isn't the only way to improve your cardiovascular health. In fact, a study out of Appalachian State University in Boone, North Carolina, found that there was up to a 20 percent decrease in blood pressure after a moderately intense weight-training session, which is the equivalent to (or slightly better than) the reduction experienced after taking antihypertensive drugs. This reduction in blood pressure continued for up to 24 hours in those who trained regularly a few times a week, which could eliminate the need for antihypertensive, micronutrient-depleting drugs altogether.[5]

4. **Your performance at work will improve.** With our One Set To Failure training protocol, you will learn to push hard, even when your brain tells you that you can't. This determination, this "I can do it" mentality,

will carry into your daily life, and you will be one of those go-to employees that employers know can be counted on when times get tough. Additionally, weight training will improve the muscles of your core and those that support your spine. This lessens any discomfort that you might feel sitting at your desk all day, and while you're not complaining about your back, you can be achieving success at the office.

Jayson Learns the Pro's Secret to Gaining Muscle Fast

What you likely don't know is that many, many years ago (did we just age ourselves?), even before we were a couple, Jayson was very interested in bodybuilding. It had been a major influence in his life since childhood, and one of the primary reasons he first became interested in nutrition. This wasn't just a hobby, either. In fact, Jayson won Mr. Orlando for his weight class—and he did it all naturally, competing at a shredded 154 pounds. However, because of his interest in science and human biology, Jayson was intrigued to see how much muscle he could add to his frame without the use of steroids (which are common in the bodybuilding world). He began training with the world's best bodybuilders in order to really push himself. Perhaps some of you might know one particular name, Dorian Yates, as he was named Mr. Olympia six consecutive times. Winning the Mr. Olympia competition is an equivalent accomplishment to being a Superbowl champion, so working out with and learning from this 300-pound muscle-bound legend was truly an exceptional hands-on training experience.

Dorian Yates shared with Jayson his personal secret to building muscle fast and revealed why most people never reach their full potential. Simply put, much like overtraining for hours on cardiovascular equipment, most people overtrain when lifting weights, as well. In order to understand why One Set To Failure is so effective, you need to understand how and why muscles grow. Let's imagine that your muscle is the ground. When you lift weights, you break down muscle tissue, the equivalent of digging a hole in the ground. Then, your muscle must recover from this breakdown. Using the dirt analogy, the hole must be filled in before any new dirt—new muscle—can be added on top.

Now, if you do a lot of lifting, what do you think happens? You dig a really deep hole, right? Well, it will take a long time to refill that hole, or to recover from that workout, and this gives you little opportunity to build new muscle on top of it. Doing a lot of sets, or repetitions, when lifting is actually counterproductive to building muscle. The smaller the hole, the bigger the pile of dirt you can lay on top of it, meaning the faster you get to muscle gain and the quicker you achieve your weight-training goals.

So, what do we mean by One Set To Failure? Too often when personal trainers at the gym write out weight-training programs, they take you around a Nautilus circuit, or something similar, and they choose a weight for each exercise. Then they recommend that you lift that weight for three or four sets of up to 20 repetitions, with breaks between each set. However, they will often choose a weight that is too light for you. How else would you be able to lift it so many times? This kind of lifting doesn't even dig a hole. This means that your body doesn't need to recover, and the whole process of digging, recovering, filling, and adding new dirt is a moot point.

On the other hand, if you choose something really heavy to lift many times for many sets, this is like digging and digging and digging some more. After the first set you are exhausted, you can hardly lift the weight again, and you get through it just to start another set. Following this system, your body will spend all of its time recovering, filling the deep hole you dug, and it won't have time to add muscle on top. For the 28-day Micronutrient Miracle plan, we don't want you to do either of these options. While they may build muscle over the long haul, you will not be efficient—we are after a muscle miracle, and One Set To Failure is the fix!

How It Works

When you do One Set to Failure, your entire workout only lasts about 20 minutes. Again, like with ZMT, this is an intense 20 minutes, but you will work at your level of intensity and it is safe and effective for all people of all ages, from elite athletes to those trying to rebuild after bouts of illness or osteoporosis. It is the same program that Jayson used back in the day to add an extra 100 pounds to his 5-foot-9 frame to reach his goal of 250 pounds. Now, don't worry, you aren't going to get huge through this weight-training program unless you really, really dedicate yourself to it like he did. Today, we both lift following the One Set To Failure principles, and this keeps us at our genetic potential for muscle with very little effort.

One Set to Failure means exactly what it says. You will do 1 set until you literally cannot do even one more repetition of that exercise. How long is your set? We want you to start off by shooting for 15 repetitions. If you can make all 15 reps, then your weight is too low. Take a short break, and then increase your weight until failure falls within the first 15 reps. Make sure you can at least get 6 reps using good form.

Also, it is imperative that you recognize that *failure* is the key word in this program. Your final rep should always take every bit of energy you can muster. Sometimes you will only be able to hit 9 reps at a new weight, and the 10th time you will only get the weight up 50 percent of the way. Other times, you may completely fail at the 14th rep. Your muscles will let you know when they can't go any further; don't allow your brain to decide for you. Ignore the internal voice that says, "Ooh, that last rep was hard, I can't get another. I will just stop now." That is not the voice we want you to listen to. Instead, you should be thinking, "I've got one more in me. I will just push and push . . . a bit more . . . almost there." We need you to give every last bit of effort on each repetition. You are only giving yourself 1 set, so allow yourself to fail. Failure is the goal. You need to push past mental failure to achieve physical failure. In the dirt-digging example, it is failure that allows you to push that shovel into the dirt to create a hole in such a short time. And because you created such a shallow little hole with the One Set To Failure technique, your body instantaneously starts to recover and add new soil to the earth, or new muscle to your body. Every time you reach your goal of 15 reps for a particular exercise, you increase the weight slightly the next week.

Tools You Can Use

For the first couple of workouts, it will take you a bit of time to identify your starting weights and chosen exercises. However, because we want you to record your weights and reps, this workout will be fast once you have the program down. You will find great tools online at our Micronutrient Miracle Motivation and Resource Center at mymiracleplan.com. We have an area where we put together some of our favorite One Set To Failure weight-training routines. You will also find downloadable exercise-tracking forms to keep your weights and routine organized. And for those of you who are new to lifting weights, you will also find videos teaching best form. (Our personal favorite is the video explaining what failure really looks like.) See you in video land!

Unlike many trainers, we do not want you going around a whole circuit every day that you hit the gym (or your home gym). This means that life just got even easier. You only work certain muscle groups on certain days. This gives the other muscles time to recover and build up in between workouts. This is also great because it means you only have to lift weights 4 days a week to reach your personal genetic potential for muscle.

		TABLE 7.2	
		MUSCLE-SPECIFIC WEEKLY SCHEDULE FOR ONE SET TO FAILURE WEIGHT TRAINING	
DAY	**MUSCLE GROUPS**	**BEGINNER (OR MAINTENANCE MODE) # OF EXERCISES PER MUSCLE GROUP**	**ADVANCED # OF EXERCISES PER MUSCLE GROUP**
Day 1	Chest	3	4
	Biceps	2	3
Day 2	Legs	4	6
Day 3	Rest and recover— This means no lifting		
Day 4	Shoulders	3	4
	Triceps	2	3
Day 5	Back	3	4
	Abdominals	2	3
Day 6	Rest and recover— This means no lifting		
Day 7	Rest and recover— This means no lifting		

Your Schedule

It doesn't matter if your Day 1 is a Monday or a Thursday. It just needs to fit your personal schedule in a way that allows you to put the time into your workouts. If you aren't sure which body parts require which machines or how to use free weights to work these specific muscle groups, don't worry. We are here to help with that as well. Just pop into the Micronutrient Miracle Motivation and Resource Center at mymiracleplan.com to get a list of which exercises are best for which days. A good trainer at a gym should also be able to show you how to appropriately work these body parts.

So, you now know that you will be exercising from two angles. First you will get a cardio workout with Zero Movement Training, and then you will weight train with One Set To Failure. You can choose to schedule these in whatever way works best for you. If you can fit a workout into your schedule 4 days a week, you should do weight training first and then do Zero Movement Training on those 4 days. However, if you prefer short bouts instead, you can choose to do ZMT on the days you are recovering from lifting weights. It is up to you. This may seem like a lot at the beginning, but when you compare our training techniques to jogging on a treadmill like a hamster for up to an hour or endless reps and sets around a full Nautilus circuit, you will see just how quick and easy our 20-minute workouts really are. And the results will speak for themselves. It is your body to live in—love it and it will love you in return! Remember, this is not all about weight loss, either; it is about building a strong structure that you can live in for many years to come and that moves easily through the world, allowing you to go places, try new things, and take chances with confidence in your own strength and agility.

To Weigh or Not to Weigh

There are quite a few opinions out there on whether or not you should weigh yourself, and if so, how often. Some people think that it stresses weight over health, and to some extent, we agree. Remember that our 28-day Micronutrient Miracle plan is not a weight-loss plan, per se. However, your body will find its "healthy," natural weight as a result of your micronutrient-sufficient state allowing all your systems to function properly. That being said, we know that many of you out there right now have a strong desire to lose weight. We can be sure of this because many of the clients we have worked with in the past also came to us with this very same goal. Luckily, the Micronutrient Miracle plan will allow your body to find its genetic potential for muscle, and when this level is reached, it is miraculous how quickly the weight can drop, because once muscle is maximized, fat loss is inevitable.

Unfortunately, many popular diets leave dieters with far less muscle than they started with. Have you ever watched *The Biggest Loser* on TV? How do you think the contestants can drop those huge numbers of pounds in only 1 week? Well, they aren't losing all fat, that's for sure. They are losing muscle, as well. Our goal for you while on this plan is to ensure that you keep as much muscle as possible and that your weight loss is almost exclusively from unhealthy body fat. We want to share with you a success story that reveals how all scales are not created equal and that unless you have all the data, you might not be seeing the whole truth.

A Micronutrient Miracle—Nelly

Nelly came to us with a desire to lose weight. Her starting weight was 216 pounds, and because of Nelly's attitude and determination, we had high hopes for her. However, when Nelly came in for her weekly examination after her first week on the plan, the scale still read 216 pounds. We don't have to tell you that Nelly was practically in tears. She had done everything right. She had supplemented, she had exercised, she had followed the dietary guidelines, and yet she lost no weight. Why? The why of this story is important to each and every one of you reading this right now. In fact, we are going to give you a small gem of information that you can keep with you, just in case this ever happens to you.

Here it is: *Scale weight means nothing.*

You see, when we took Nelly's body fat reading, we found out that not only had she lost fat, her real goal, but she had also gained much-needed muscle tissue. Let's look at Nelly's numbers a little closer:

	STARTING	WEEK 1	WEEK 2	WEEK 8	TODAY
Body weight	216	216	211.5	191	169
Body fat percentage	64.9%	58.8%	54.7%	45.2%	36.2%
Total fat in pounds	140.3	127.1	115.6	86.3	58.8
Total muscle in pounds	75.6	88.8	95.8	104.6	110.2

What we want you to look at is Nelly's starting muscle weight—75.6 pounds. Now, what you might not know is that an average, healthy woman of 5 feet 4 inches to 5 feet 6 inches is going to naturally have a genetic potential of approximately 100 to 110 pounds of muscle. Nelly, however, came to us after many failed diets with only 75.6 pounds of muscle. This is because the weight Nelly was losing on those other diets was muscle, not fat, which is common with most diets. She now needed to build back that very important muscle she had lost because muscle controls metabolism. So, the more muscle you have, the higher your metabolism will be. This is why when people lose weight in the form of muscle on most diets, they usually gain all the weight back—plus a little bit more. The little bit more is due to their newly acquired lower metabolism, in the form of lost muscle.

In Nelly's case, however, look at what happened to the pounds of fat she had on her body; she went from 140.3 pounds to 127.1 pounds in 1 week, meaning she had lost 13.2 pounds of pure fat. Had Nelly already had her 100 pounds of muscle, her fat loss would have been reflected in her scale weight. If she had weighed herself and seen 13.2 pounds off the first week, she would have been thrilled, but all she saw was a stalled scale.

By the second week, Nelly's scale weight finally started to move, but it still wasn't reflecting her true accomplishments. This is because she still had more muscle tissue to gain. We tell this story because so many people base all of their hope on the numbers on the scale. However, when you look at Nelly's overall 2-week performance, you can see that she was able to lose 24.7 pounds of fat and gain 20.2 pounds of lean muscle tissue—an unbelievable accomplishment for anyone. But Nelly almost gave up on Week 1, all because of scale weight.

Our goal for you is that you achieve your genetic potential for lean muscle tissue, lose your desired amount of fat, and achieve the disease-free body of your dreams. Don't simply look at numbers randomly and get discouraged. The plan works. Some of you will lose weight faster than others. But as long as you aren't losing muscle, you are doing the plan correctly. Stick with it and remember: *Scale weight means nothing.*

That being said, we are not "antiscale" people. In fact, we love our scale because it gives us all of the information we need to make informed, educated conclusions about our weights. Our scale can tell us what percentage body fat we have, how many pounds of muscle we have, and how much visceral (unhealthy) fat we carry around our bellies, and it even estimates our metabolic age, telling us if we are aging faster or slower than our real, or calendar, age. Most of our clients purchase similar scales before beginning this plan. This way, there is no devastation when the scale stalls. Most often, muscle is gained while fat is lost and they cancel each other out, just like they did for Nelly, until genetic potential is met. Similar scales are often available for use at gyms and through doctors' offices. If you don't have a body fat scale available, you might want to consider simply using your clothes to measure your success. Getting into an old pair of jeans might be just the encouragement you need.

> If you want suggestions on which body fat scale to purchase, simply visit our Micronutrient Miracle Motivation and Resource Center at mymiracleplan.com. We have chosen a few of our favorite models available at a wide variety of price points and listed them there.

Our point here is that making decisions with a lack of information will probably not benefit you in the long run. Our answer to the great scale debate is simple. ***Weigh wisely, or don't weigh yourself at all.***

GOLDEN RULE #7 Dump the Toxins—Get Out of the Toxic Soup

That's right! Just like a relationship gone sour, we hope that you will kick the unhealthy toxins in your life to the curb. You might still have fond memories of your favorite cologne or toothpaste, but it is time to face the facts—they just aren't good for you anymore. Now that you know their dirty little secrets, it is time to ditch them once and for all. Sure, you may get back together in the future, but let's try to make these next 28 days a cooling-off period, where you can see how easily they can be replaced by healthier, more supportive products.

We listed our Top 10 Terrific Tricks to Reduce Household Toxins back in Chapter 4, and we urge you to take this on if you can. You can choose to do all 10, or you can do as many as you feel you are able to try. You will be shocked to discover that there are a slew of alternative nontoxic products out there waiting for you to discover them. Manufacturers of these fantastic healthy alternatives spend their lives dedicated to creating the products they feel are missing from the marketplace. Remember, this is only our top 10 list. This doesn't mean that your exposure to toxins ends there. The world that we live in exposes us thousands of times each day to chemicals that science is now showing might have some very dangerous and unwanted side effects. While the government has stated that these chemicals are "safe," we do not yet know how they all interact with each other or the consequences of the cumulative exposure to them over a day, a week, a year, or even a lifetime. Today's children will be the first to fully live in this "toxic soup," and everything we can do to help them avoid this murky bath and limit their toxic exposure will help. Slowly but surely, we are fighting these chemical companies, and some of the big brands are realizing our desires to avoid obesogens and other hazardous chemical compounds. Because of this, companies are starting to create products with safer ingredients. Perhaps they are more difficult to find or cost a bit more, but over time, if we purchase them, other companies will follow and prices will drop as consumer demand increases.

While you may be attached to many of these household and beauty conveniences, take some time to really consider eliminating as many as you can. By doing so, you prevent your micronutrient levels from being depleted by your body's constant attempts to remove and flush these toxins. In turn, those micronutrients can then work toward your micronutrient sufficiency and, ultimately, your optimal health.

Purchase new nontoxic alternatives for as many of these products as you can.

Perfume/cologne	Detergent	Dryer sheets
Toothpaste	Shampoo and body wash	Makeup
Deodorant	Dish soap	Plastic storage containers
Nonstick pots and pans		

Step 3: Supplement Smart—Learn the ABCs and Beyond

Your goal over the next 28 days is to become sufficient in the essential micronutrients. And as long as you keep that goal in mind, you can follow any dietary philosophy that you would like while on the Micronutrient Miracle plan. However, as we discovered in Chapter 4, no diet can deliver the essential micronutrients you need every day from food alone. This makes smart supplementation the third and final essential step to achieving your goal of micronutrient sufficiency. You have three types of micronutrients you will need to be keenly aware of over the next 28 days; they are your vitamins and minerals (multivitamin), your amino acids (protein powder), and, finally, your essential fatty acids (omega-3s).

GOLDEN RULE #8 Supplement with a Properly Formulated Multivitamin Twice Daily

The first key supplement is your multivitamin. As we stated earlier, your body needs to be able to absorb and use the micronutrients delivered in a multivitamin, so they don't just get flushed down the toilet. We firmly believe that following our ABCs of Optimal Supplementation Guidelines will guarantee that your money is being well spent on a formulation that eliminates the common delivery flaws. We created our multivitamin, nutreince, for this specific reason, and we are confident that if you decide to use it, like thousands of clients before you, you will experience unparalleled benefits from this superior formulation. However, if you want, you can opt to choose an alternative multivitamin. In this case, we recommend that you use our ABCs of Optimal Supplementation Stack Up Quiz, which goes into minute detail to identify any flaws in the products you are considering (MultivitaminStackUpQuiz.com). Your multivitamin is your first priority when considering supplementation, and taking it consistently is key. Remember, multivitamins should be taken *with* a

Ironing Out the Need for Iron and Dealing with Digestion

Properly formulated multivitamins should not contain iron because it competes with 10 other micronutrients. This greatly inhibits the availability of many essential vitamins and minerals. However, iron supplementation is essential for certain demographics. If you are a premenopausal woman, pregnant, or breastfeeding; have kidney failure, ulcers, or gastrointestinal disorders; or work out intensely or follow a vegan or vegetarian diet, you should add a daily iron supplement to your regimen. Women should take 18 milligrams, and men should take 8 milligrams. Make sure the iron supplement is taken midday and apart from your multivitamin to ensure proper absorption and utilization.

There is one more supplement that we often suggest to our private clients, and that is digestive enzymes. Every function of every single cell in our body relies on enzymes. They also help to regulate the speed and efficiency of the body's metabolic functions. One of their primary responsibilities is to break food down to be properly utilized by the body. While they are present in raw, natural foods, food processing and cooking deplete the enzymes that allow for optimal absorption of both the macronutrients and micronutrients. While on the Signature 28-day Micronutrient Miracle plan, it is optional to add digestive enzymes to your supplementation schedule, but we highly recommend it for enhanced micronutrient absorption, especially for those suffering from digestive issues, including heartburn. Look for a product with amylase, protease, and lipase, as well as a variety of other digestive enzymes, such as bromelain, ox bile, pancreatin, papain, pepsin, and betaine HCL.

source of fat to increase absorption of the fat-soluble nutrients but *away* from meals to avoid any micronutrient competitions. Certain demographics should also consider adding in an iron supplement or digestive enzymes (to increase micronutrient absorption).

GOLDEN RULE #9 Consume Two Protein Shakes or Protein-Based Meal Replacements Daily

The second key supplement—which will supply your body with enough of the essential amino acids—will be your protein powder. We already explained all of the great benefits of adding protein to your daily routine and detailed the importance of muscle maintenance for weight loss. You will find that these shakes and treats make life really easy, keeping your body satiated and strong throughout the day. We highly suggest you follow our delicious Triple Threat recipes, as they will simplify your supplementation schedule.

Creating the Perfect Triple Threat Shake

Have you ever seen a Broadway musical or watched *The Wizard of Oz* or *The Sound of Music* on television? The stars of those highly entertaining shows are referred to in show business as triple threats. This means that they are incredibly strong and talented in three distinct disciplines: singing, dancing, and acting. We decided to call our daily micronutrient-dense, muscle-building, and fat-burning shake the Triple Threat, as well, because we felt it covered all the bases. It is everything you would want or need, all wrapped up in one great-tasting creamy beverage. It combines the vitamins and minerals from nutreince with the amino acids from IN.POWER protein, and the fat-metabolizing and brain-boosting power from SKINNYFat. Basically, it takes our three foundational products and creates two meals a day that are perfectly formulated for all-day energy and lasting micronutrient coverage.

Some clients ask if they can change out the protein or the fat in the Triple Threats, and here is our stance. First, our protein does not have any flavor or add-ins. The flavors of nutreince are created to be slightly intense so that they can mellow out nicely in the creamy Triple Threat Shakes. Unlike many of the protein powders on the market, our IN.POWER protein is also created without adding vitamins and minerals, which might compete with nutreince. Additionally, many of the plant-based proteins contain high levels of certain micronutrients, which would also create micronutrient competitions when adding nutreince to the shakes, so we don't recommend using them unless you are a strict vegan. So, if you are going to look for an alternative protein, make sure that you choose one that is free of unwanted ingredients and added micronutrients.

As for choosing an alternative fat source, here are a couple of issues we have encountered. Coconut oil will clump when it comes into contact with ice in the shake, leaving you with a rather waxy, fat globule–filled, unappetizing beverage. MCT (medium-chain triglyceride) oil alone will not aid in the absorption of the micronutrients as the body requires long-chain fats for absorption, and MCT does not have any. Most fish oils make for fishy shakes, which we don't suggest either. We have spent years creating the best meal-replacement shake possible, and our Triple Threat is something we look forward to every day, twice a day. While you can try to create your own meal-replacement shake by sourcing different ingredients, we stand behind the Triple Threat because we know that you are getting three of the absolute best products on the market in every delicious glass. The results we have seen—our clients' successes—are based on using our exact recipes, and they speak for themselves! There are some delicious recipes for Triple Threats in Chapter 9. Don't miss out on our delicious Triple Threat Shakes and other Triple Threat treats, including puddings and ice cream. They will have you asking, "How can anything so delicious be this good for you?" And when the puddings are premade and kept in the fridge, they're not only delicious but convenient, as well!

> **GOLDEN RULE #10** Make Sure You Are Getting Enough Omega-3s

Where your omega-3s are concerned, we are going to give you a couple of choices: You can eat 'em or take 'em. First, you can choose to eat a 4-ounce serving of fish two or three times a week to acquire your required EFAs (essential fatty acids). This is a preferred source if you are choosing *only* wild-caught fish that is free of BPA packaging. While it might seem like a small amount of fish, you should remember that you are also taking in omega-3s in your pastured eggs, grass-fed beef, and grass-fed butter. However, if you don't like fish or you can only find farm-raised fish, choose a fish oil supplement. One problem, however, with fish oil is that research has discovered that the beneficial components EPA and DHA compete with one another for absorption just like certain vitamins and minerals. Because of this, we created Origin Omega which is the first and only omega-3 product formulated using our patented Anti-Competition Technology to separate the EPA and DHA to eliminate the competition and greatly improve the absorption and utilization potential of both. If you decide to take an alternative fish oil, look for one that has more EPA than DHA (perhaps about 500 milligrams of EPA and 250 milligrams of DHA per serving), as EPA converts to DHA in the body. Make sure to refrigerate once opened to reduce oxidation from heat. Remember, your essential fatty acids are "essential," but eating a few servings of wild-caught fish per week is a perfectly delicious way to get them in!

Part 2: The "What to Eat" and "When to Eat"

Okay, so far you've learned the 10 Golden Rules of the 28-day Micronutrient Miracle plan, and by now you are probably wondering what and when exactly you are going to be eating. You already know that we aren't going to tell you which type of dietary philosophy to choose. That is up to you! You will choose the foods that you like and that meet your philosophical, ethical, religious, or medical needs.

Time to Set Some Daily Limits

However, just because we let you choose the philosophy, it doesn't mean that you just arrived at the all-you-can-eat Micronutrient Miracle buffet line. You will have some limitations, but as you will see, they are easy to follow for a lifetime of optimal health. It is time to learn the restrictions set on fruits, starches, nuts, seeds, alcohol, and caffeine for the Signature Micronutrient Miracle protocol.

FRUITS, OR SHOULD WE CALL THEM LITTLE SACKS OF SUGAR?

Do you want to know Mira's two favorite foods back when she had osteoporosis? They were honeydew melon and Swedish fish—both loaded with sugar. You might look at them and say to yourself that one is much healthier than the other. In truth, you would be correct. One is natural and the other is processed sugar along with chemicals and coloring agents. However, Mira's body didn't really care which she ate. Both made her want more "sweets" in her mouth. Both induced further cravings, and neither supplied any healthy fats or proteins that could satiate, boost metabolism, or improve her weak bones. Both will spike your insulin levels and cause fat storage, as well. When you think about it this way, neither of these "sugar sacks" are the foods we want to bombard our bodies with on a regular basis.

STEER CLEAR OF TOO MANY STARCHES, NUTS, AND SEEDS

Much like those sweet sugary sacks that we call fruit, some other foods have similar effects on the body. While there is nothing inherently wrong with eating a potato now and again or enjoying a handful of mixed nuts and seeds, when you start to consider the micronutrients per bite, you have better options. Remember, many of these starches, nuts, and seeds contain a great deal of antinutrients, as well. For example, why add in too many inflammation-causing, omega-6-intense nuts and seeds that are loaded with calories and contain a plethora of phytates and lectins when there are better foods that build micronutrient sufficiency and don't contain these depleting factors?

Limiting Fruits, Starches, Nuts, and Seeds

Want to hear some great news? We aren't going to tell you if you should or shouldn't eat fruits, starches, nuts, and seeds. Like most things on this plan, you'll get to choose. It is your plan and you can personalize it to suit your taste. However, while on the Signature 28-day Micronutrient Miracle plan, we do want you to *limit* your fruit, starch, nut, and seed intake to 2 servings a week *at most*. You can choose the foods that you like best, so you will never feel like you are missing out on your favorites. For example, you may choose fruit with your breakfast on Monday and a potato with your dinner on Thursday, or you might opt for wheat-free pasta twice in 1 week. This doesn't mean, however, that those 2 days can be loaded with restricted foods. *You are permitted 2 servings total in each of the 4 weeks.* Regardless of your sweet or salty tendencies, this allows you to really savor your favorite treats. You will also find that you will lose your cravings and reliance on them in only a short time. Individuals following health-specific protocols should always review the guidelines in Chapter 8 because in some protocols, like those for blood sugar regulation or weight loss, we have reduced or eliminated these foods altogether for the first 28 days to achieve the greatest results.

FRUITS		STARCHES AND OTHER LIMITED FOODS
While all fruits are available, those **bolded** are better options. *1 serving = 1 whole fruit or 1 cup berries*		All of the items below are considered starches and must be limited. Please make sure to check proper preparation guidelines to reduce antinutrients. *1 serving = up to 1 cup for women and up to 1½ cups for men*
Apples⁻	All dried fruit	Amaranth (sprouted)
Apricots	Bananas	Beans (sprouted)
Berries⁻	Dates	Beets
Cherries	Figs	Buckwheat (sprouted)
Coconut	Grapes	Corn (non-GMO)⁻
Dragon fruit	Lychee	Green peas⁺
Grapefruit⁺	Mangoes	Jicama
Melons⁺	Papayas	Nuts (sprouted)
Nectarines⁻	Pineapples	Oats (sprouted)
Oranges/tangerines	Raisins	Parsnips
Passion fruit	Watermelon	Potatoes (non-GMO)⁻
Peaches⁻		Quinoa (sprouted)
Pears		Rice (fermented or soaked)
Persimmons		Seeds (sprouted)
Plums		Squash (acorn, butternut, winter)
Pomegranates		Sweet potatoes/yams⁺
Prunes		Pastas, breads, or any other products made out of the ingredients above

+ Fabulous 14—Safe to buy conventional
– Terrible 20—Always purchase organic

ALCOHOL AND CAFFEINE LIMITATION—ENJOY EACH TWICE A DAY

You've already read about the micronutrient-depleting properties of both caffeine and alcohol, and you've also read about the health benefits they can deliver. It can be a tad confusing, right? Well, it seems that in the case of these two EMDs, there is a bit of a scientific "sweet spot" where you tip the scales from depletion and negative side effects to optimal benefits. For the next 28 days, we want you to hit that "sweet spot." This means you can enjoy up to two caffeinated beverages a day and two alcoholic beverages a day. This does not mean that you should start drinking coffee or wine if you don't already. It also doesn't mean that you should grab a super-vente or big gulp–size coffee so that you can convince yourself that 32 ounces is the right size for one of your servings. Be reasonable and responsible. And for those looking to trim their tummies, we suggest eliminating gluten-free beers from the plan until you reach your desired weight.

Now, when we are talking alcohol, we don't mean a sugary lemon drop or fruit-filled mango daiquiri. Remember, the no sugar rule is always in play. What you can enjoy is the following: wine, champagne, gluten-free beer, and hard alcohol alone or mixed with sparkling water and stevia drops for flavor. Cheers!

The same holds true for coffee. We aren't allowing those syrup-filled, frappucino-esque beverages on this plan. What we do suggest, however, is pairing your caffeinated drinks with healthy saturated fats—such as cream, SKINNYFat, or butter—to minimize the release of the caffeine. You can still create delicious flavored coffees, though, especially if you add in a few drops of stevia. Check out our Double Chocolate Mocha Triple Threat recipe on page 312.

For some of you, these alcohol limitations may prove a bit more difficult. For example, you may be one of those people who has a hard time stopping after two beers (gluten-free, of course) while watching Sunday football with friends, or perhaps on moms' night out, your two-glass limit might not seem like quite enough. Well, if you can see yourself in a similar scenario—not being able to stop yourself after 2 servings—then we suggest limiting the alcohol to one night a week to give yourself a bit more leeway. Why set yourself up for failure? Most of our clients find that this simple one-night-a-week option actually helps them to get their alcohol intake in check, even when they didn't think they were drinking in excess to begin with.

FOODS WE WANT TO FLOURISH!

With the restricted and limited foods defined, you are all set to discover the foods we really want you to focus on. From fabulous ferments to inflammation-fighting fish and unrestricted quantities of colorful vegetables, these are the fabulous finds we want you to fill your menus with.

Get Your Gut in Check! Focus on Ferment

Did you know that your brain and your gut are made from the same type of tissue? Today, science is discovering that more and more of the decisions about how healthy you will be are decided in your gut. It is thought that as much as 80 percent of your immune system is located in your digestive tract. The colonies that live in your gut are a complete ecosystem that influences all aspects of your health. There are both "good" and "bad" bacteria in your gut, and maintaining an optimal ratio between them is the key.

The 28-day Micronutrient Miracle plan gets your gut healthy by first eliminating some key factors that are known to throw off the optimal ratio of 85 percent good bacteria to 15 percent bad bacteria, including sugar, refined grains, antibacterial soaps, and pesticides. However, because your micronutrients are absorbed throughout your digestive tract, we want you to go one step further: We want you to add in extra "good" probiotic bacteria, as well. Here again, like with the EFAs, it is your choice: eat 'em or take 'em.

If you choose to eat your probiotics, then you have some options. You have kefir, yogurt, lassi, kombucha, kimchi, sauerkraut, and cheese curds. Try to find unpasteurized (raw) options, as pasteurization can injure the probiotic strains. If you choose to gobble up your good bacteria, you don't need much. Just one or two forkfuls or a few sips each day will keep the colony kicking!

Now, while we prefer trying to eat our probiotics, those of you who don't like fermented foods should be favoring your gut flora by taking a supplement. When choosing a probiotic, find one that delivers at least 5 billion to 7 billion viable organisms for adults and 1 billion for children. Select a brand with as many different types of probiotic species as possible (at least five), spanning both *Lactobacillus* and *Bifidobacterium* families.

Fish Fabulous Fish!

We discussed this in our coverage of proper protein picking in the supermarket shopping solution in Chapter 5, but we just want to make sure that this is clear, so we will say it again (just in case any of you were eager and jumped directly into this Micronutrient Miracle protocol chapter): We believe that wild-caught fish is a fantastic form of protein that can greatly reduce inflammation, and you should try to eat at least 2 or 3 servings a week. For those who aren't fond of fish, please at least try the recipes. We think you may change your mind when you see how flavorful and "un-fishy" they are!

Enjoy a Variety of Very Colorful Vegetables

Unlike fruits and starches, there are tons of great vegetables that we want to see on your plate. Here is a list of our go-to vegetables, which tend to be on the low-carbohydrate, high-fiber side. They won't cause that fat storage you are trying to avoid, and they are loaded with a variety of fabulous accessory nutrients that are not readily available in supplements. For the next 28 days, try to eat vegetables that deliver all the colors of the rainbow, because a vegetable's color can tell you a lot about what micronutrients it will deliver. The specific plant compounds that a vegetable contains determine the color of its skin. So choosing vegetables with varied colors delivers the greatest variety of benefits. (See Table 7.3 on page 208.)

CREATE YOUR PERFECT PERSONAL DINING SCHEDULE

Are you a stay-at-home parent who wakes early, runs errands all day, and rarely has time to grab a balanced meal? Does your work schedule dictate what time you get to eat each day? Do you prefer to sleep in and love a big breakfast on the weekends? Regardless of your personal schedule, the Micronutrient Miracle plan has a solution that will make your dining convenient for your lifestyle.

During your 28-day Micronutrient Miracle plan, you will be eating four times a day. Remember, though, that according to Golden Rule #9, two of these four meals will be in the form of shakes. For most of you, they will be Triple Threat Shakes—a combination of your essential micronutrients (nutreince multivitamin), essential amino acids (IN.POWER), and brain-boosting, energy-enhancing, and fat-metabolizing fats (SKINNYFat). These shakes really keep you mentally sharp and satisfied for hours due to the combination of all three foundational ingredients. The other two meals each day will be made up of your favorite selections from the numerous recipes in our menu plan. We also supply a nonmeal replacement alternative in The 28-Day Micronutrient Miracle Menu Plan Q&A on page 217, where we discuss eating three meals a day with a snack and taking nutreince (or an alternative multivitamin) alone twice daily for those individuals who either do not tolerate protein powder or who prefer eating only whole foods.

TABLE 7.3
LIST OF NONSTARCHY VEGETABLES TO ENJOY

(Yes, we know some are technically fruits.)
Serving size: Eat until satiated, not stuffed.

Artichokes	Hot peppers⁻
Asparagus⁺	Kale⁻*
Avocado⁺	Kohlrabi*
Bamboo shoots	Lettuce (all leaf varieties)⁻
Bell peppers (all colors)⁻	Mushrooms⁺*
Bok choy*	Okra
Broccoli*	Onions⁺
Brussels sprouts*	Pumpkin
Cabbage⁺*	Radishes*
Carrots	Snap/snow peas⁻
Cauliflower⁺*	Spaghetti squash
Celery⁻	Spinach⁻*
Cherry tomatoes⁻	Summer squash⁻
Collard greens⁻*	Swiss chard*
Cucumbers⁻	Tomatoes
Eggplant⁺	Water chestnuts
Green beans	Zucchini⁻

+Fabulous 14—Safe to buy conventional
−Terrible 20—Always purchase organic
*Always cook

When it comes to timing your meals, the Micronutrient Miracle protocol is to eat every 3 to 5 hours—4 being optimal. So, for example, if you wake up at 6:30 a.m., you might grab a cup of coffee and have a Triple Threat Shake at 7:00 a.m. Then at 11:30 a.m. you could have lunch, and at 3:00 p.m. you would make and enjoy another Triple Threat Shake or grab a Triple Threat pudding. Lastly, at around 7:00 p.m., you would enjoy dinner. That would be one example. However, most of us lead ever-changing lives with daily routines that are, well, anything but routine. This means that your schedule might vary from one day to another.

Here are six basic scheduling options.

Option 1: Shake—Meal 1—Shake—Meal 2

Option 2: Meal 1—Shake—Meal 2—Shake

Option 3: Meal 1– Shake—Shake—Meal 2

Option 4: Shake—Meal 1—Meal 2—Shake

Option 5: Meal 1—Meal 2—Shake—Shake

Option 6: Shake—Shake—Meal 1—Meal 2

Note: Options 4, 5, and 6 are perfect for individuals interested in intermittent fasting. While they may not be traditional intermittent fasts, as they contain protein, these options will help to reset your leptin levels, allowing you to feel better in the long run as well as lose weight faster, if that is your goal.

We will be providing you with our Signature 28-Day Micronutrient Miracle Menu Plan; however, should you want to make alterations to any of the days, feel free. Just remember to have two shakes a day and eat every 3 to 5 hours. Some busy individuals and those looking to try liquid cleanses even opt for more shakes. Some opt for three a day on busy days, while others choose to take all four of their meals as Triple Threat Shakes for a short period. If you find that your schedule gets hectic, an extra shake is always preferential to falling off the wagon and making poor dietary choices. However, if opting for more shakes per day, make sure that you only take two nutreince packets per day (one in the morning and one in the evening). You can either eliminate the multivitamin from the additional shakes or split up the packets. And don't forget that any time you see a Triple Threat Shake, you can use any of the Triple Threat recipes for shakes or treats.

> Those choosing alternative multivitamins or protein powder options should consume their meal-replacement shakes and their multivitamin supplements whenever they see "Triple Threat" in their schedules.

The Quick-Start Guide to the Signature 28-Day Micronutrient Miracle Plan

This plan is specifically designed for individuals who are looking to build an overall state of micronutrient sufficiency in their bodies. This protocol will help you increase energy, detoxify, build strength, manage weight, and prevent and reverse deficiency-related health conditions and diseases. Look for our condition-specific protocol adaptations in Chapter 8. Don't forget: Before beginning any of our Micronutrient Miracle protocols, make sure you have completed all the items on the "Your Micronutrient Miracle Program Planner" on pages 48–49. This will ensure you are set up to succeed and see amazing results.

The Signature Micronutrient Miracle Protocol Is Designed for Individuals Who Are:

- Working toward micronutrient sufficiency to improve all areas of their health
- Looking for a realistic and sustainable plan to achieve optimal health

Follow the 10 Golden Rules

1. Completely eliminate sugar, wheat, and soy and all of their aliases.
2. Try to eliminate the obesogens (MSG, BPA, and phthalates) that you come into contact with on a daily basis.
3. Reduce the EMDs found in foods and drinks (phytates, oxalates, lectins, trypsin inhibitors, phosphoric acid, alcohol, caffeine, and tannins).
4. When shopping, follow our Good, Better, Best system and use our Rich Food picks.
5. Reduce stress with one of our proven techniques.
6. Burn fat and build muscle with our Zero Movement Training 3 or 4 days a week and our One Set To Failure weight-training techniques 4 days a week.
7. Attempt to replace your beauty and home care products with nontoxic alternatives.

8. Take a properly formulated multivitamin, preferably nutreince, twice daily. Consider supplementing with iron or digestive enzymes (or both), as well.

9. Have two protein shakes a day. We highly suggest you follow our delicious recipes for Triple Threat Shakes and treats.

10. Take a 1-gram serving of omega-3 fish oil twice daily, or, alternatively, you can eat 2 or 3 servings per week of omega-3-rich, wild-caught fish. If using a supplement, opt for Origin Omega or look for a product that contains more EPA than DHA (perhaps about 500 milligrams of EPA and 250 milligrams of DHA per serving).

Know Your Daily Limits

Starches, fruits, nuts, and seeds: Choose 2 servings a week. This can be 2 servings of gluten-free starch *or* 2 servings of fruit *or* 2 servings of nuts/seeds *or* any combination (not to exceed 2 servings *total* per week).

Alcohol: Enjoy 2 servings per day

Caffeinated drinks: Enjoy 2 servings per day

Find Your Focus

Ferments: Have 2 or 3 forkfuls each day (preferably raw) or use probiotic supplementation.

Fish: Eat 2 or 3 servings per week or use omega-3 supplementation.

Fibrous vegetables: Eat these until satisfied, not stuffed.

Timing: Have four meals a day, eaten every 3 to 5 hours (4 is optimal). Two meals should be Triple Threat Shakes or treats.

The Signature 28-Day
Micronutrient Miracle Menu Plan

The foods that are limited are *italicized* so that you can see where they fit into your plan.

Don't forget to make and freeze as much of the Miracle Pestos and Miracle Butters as you can prior to starting; they make cooking on a time-crunch much more simple and tasty.

WEEK 1

DAY 1 (Sunday)

9:00 a.m. *Baked Apple à la Micronutrient Miracle Mode (page 332)* or *Greek Yogurt and Fruit Bowl (page 331)*

1:00 p.m. Traditional Triple Threat Shake (page 311)

5:00 p.m. Buffalo Chicken Chili (page 340) with optional Ridiculously Simple Wrap (page 353) for dipping

9:00 p.m. Triple Threat Pudding (page 313)

DAY 2 (Monday)

7:30 a.m. Cinnamon Spice Triple Threat Shake (page 312)

12:00 p.m. Leftover Buffalo Chicken Chili

3:30 p.m. Traditional Triple Threat Shake (page 311)

7:30 p.m. Salmon with green beans and choice of a Miracle Pesto or Miracle Butter (pages 314–318)

DAY 3 (Tuesday)

7:30 a.m. Triple Threat Cheesecake (page 314)

12:00 p.m. Big salad with leftover salmon and green beans and choice of SKINNYFat salad dressing (pages 321–322)

3:30 p.m. Traditional Triple Threat Shake (page 311)

7:30 p.m. Greek Chicken (page 337)

DAY 4 (Wednesday)

7:30 a.m. Traditional Triple Threat Shake (page 311)

12:00 p.m. Leftover Greek Chicken

3:30 p.m. Triple Threat Pudding (page 313)

7:30 p.m. Quick Tandoori Shrimp (page 336) with Cooling Cucumber Raita (page 320)

DAY 5 (Thursday)

7:30 a.m. Triple Threat Cheesecake (page 314)

12:00 p.m. Big salad with leftover Quick Tandoori Shrimp and choice of SKINNYFat dressing (pages 321–322)

3:30 p.m. Triple Threat Pudding (page 313)

7:30 p.m. Bun-less beef burger and Oven-Roasted Brussels Sprouts (page 352)

DAY 6 (Friday)

7:30 a.m. Traditional Triple Threat Shake (page 311)

12:00 p.m. Broccoli Cheese Soup (page 327)

3:30 p.m. Traditional Triple Threat Shake (page 311)

7:30 p.m. Grilled steak with choice of a Miracle Pesto (pages 314–318) and Cauliflower Mash (page 352)

DAY 7 (Saturday)

9:00 a.m. Speedy Salmon Cakes (page 329–330) and eggs any style

1:00 p.m. Traditional Triple Threat Shake (page 311)

5:00 p.m. *Fish and Chips (page 350)*

9:00 p.m. Chocolate Triple Threat Ice Cream (page 314)

WEEK 2

DAY 8 (Sunday)

9:00 a.m. French Onion Egg Tart (page 328)

1:00 p.m. Traditional Triple Threat Shake (page 311)

5:00 p.m. Zughetti pasta (page 345) with Mom's Beef Bolognese (page 324)

9:00 p.m. Triple Threat Pudding (page 313)

DAY 9 (Monday)

7:30 a.m. Traditional Triple Threat Shake (page 311)

12:00 p.m. *Grilled or broiled chicken thighs, choice of a Miracle Pesto or Miracle Butter (pages 315–318), and sweet potato*

3:30 p.m. Triple Threat Pudding (page 313)

7:30 p.m. Moqueca (aka Brazilian Fish Stew) (page 343)

DAY 10 (Tuesday)

7:30 a.m. Traditional Triple Threat Shake (page 311)

12:00 p.m. Leftover Moqueca

3:30 p.m. Traditional Triple Threat Shake (page 311)

7:30 p.m. Coq au Vin (page 347) served with Cauliflower Mash (page 352)

DAY 11 (Wednesday)

7:30 a.m. Traditional Triple Threat Shake (page 311)

12:00 p.m. Leftover Coq au Vin

3:30 p.m. Triple Threat Pudding (page 313)

7:30 p.m. Thai-Style Chopped Pork on greens (page 347–348)

DAY 12 (Thursday)

7:30 a.m. Traditional Triple Threat Shake (page 311)

12:00 p.m. Leftover Thai-Style Chopped Pork on a salad with choice of SKINNYFat dressing (pages 321–322)

3:30 p.m. Traditional Triple Threat Shake (page 311)

7:30 p.m. Scallops in Lemon Butter Sauce (page 334) with broccoli

DAY 13 (Friday)

7:30 a.m. Traditional Triple Threat Shake (page 311)

12:00 p.m. Mexican Chicken Wrap (page 338)

3:30 p.m. Traditional Triple Threat Shake (page 311)

7:30 p.m. Salad and Rustic Flatbread (page 346)

DAY 14 (Saturday)

9:00 a.m. *Carrot Cake Pancakes with Cream Cheese Frosting and chopped walnuts and raisins (page 333)*

1:00 p.m. Traditional Triple Threat Shake (page 311)

5:00 p.m. Micronutrient-Packed "Offaly" Tasty Meatloaf (page 348) and steamed vegetable with choice of a Miracle Pesto or Miracle Butter (pages 315–318)

9:00 p.m. Triple Threat Pudding (page 313)

WEEK 3

DAY 15 (Sunday)

9:00 a.m. Leftover meatloaf heated in a frying pan, topped with a fried egg, and covered in melted cheese

1:00 p.m. Traditional Triple Threat Shake (page 311)

5:00 p.m. *Camarão na Moranga (aka Brazilian Shrimp Stew in a Pumpkin) (page 335–336)*

9:00 p.m. Traditional Triple Threat Shake (page 311)

DAY 16 (Monday)

7:30 a.m. Traditional Triple Threat Shake (page 311)

12:00 p.m. Big salad with ½ can of tuna or salmon (bones in) and choice of SKINNYFat dressing (pages 321–322)

3:30 p.m. Traditional Triple Threat Shake (page 311)

7:30 p.m. Chicken Wings (page 334) with Really Creamy SKINNYFat Blue Cheese Dressing (or dip) (page 322) and carrot and celery sticks

DAY 17 (Tuesday)

7:30 a.m. Traditional Triple Threat Shake (page 311)

12:00 p.m. Leftover chicken wings and blue cheese dressing

3:30 p.m. Triple Threat Pudding (page 313)

7:30 p.m. Shepherd's Pie (page 351)

DAY 18 (Wednesday)

7:30 a.m. Traditional Triple Threat Shake (page 311)

12:00 p.m. Leftover Shepherd's Pie

3:30 p.m. Traditional Triple Threat Shake (page 311)

7:30 p.m. Zughetti (page 345) with grilled chicken thighs and Rich and Creamy Alfredo Sauce (page 319)

DAY 19 (Thursday)

7:30 a.m. Triple Threat Cheesecake (page 314)

12:00 p.m. Bun-less beef burger and side salad with choice of SKINNYFat dressing (pages 321–322)

3:30 p.m. Traditional Triple Threat Shake (page 311)

7:30 p.m. Thai Shrimp Noodle Soup (page 326)

DAY 20 (Friday)

7:30 a.m. Traditional Triple Threat Shake (page 311)

12:00 p.m. Leftover Thai Shrimp Noodle Soup

3:30 p.m. Traditional Triple Threat Shake (page 311)

7:30 p.m. *Rotisserie or baked whole chicken with Sweet Potato, Yam, and Apple Casserole (page 353)*

DAY 21 (Saturday)

9:00 a.m. Fried eggs served on Cauliflower Cheesy Hash Browns (page 329)

1:00 p.m. Traditional Triple Threat Shake (page 311)

5:00 p.m. Miracle Chinese Fried "Rice" (page 339)

9:00 p.m. Traditional Triple Threat Shake (page 311)

WEEK 4

DAY 22 (Sunday)

9:00 a.m. *Smoked Salmon Cream Cheese Roll-Ups (page 331) with avocado slices and berries or grapefruit*

1:00 p.m. Traditional Triple Threat Shake (page 311)

5:00 p.m. Slow-Cooked Beer-Braised Beef (page 338) and Cauliflower Mash (page 352)

9:00 p.m. Chocolate Triple Threat Ice Cream (page 314)

DAY 23 (Monday)

7:30 a.m. Triple Threat Cheesecake (page 314)

12:00 p.m. Leftover Miracle Chinese Fried "Rice"

3:30 p.m. Traditional Triple Threat Shake (page 311)

7:30 p.m. Fish and vegetables with choice of a Miracle Pesto or Miracle Butter (pages 315–318)

DAY 24 (Tuesday)

7:30 a.m. Traditional Triple Threat Shake (page 311)

12:00 p.m. Leftover Slow-Cooked Beer-Braised Beef and Cauliflower Mash

3:30 p.m. Triple Threat Pudding (page 313)

7:30 p.m. Greek Lamb Kabobs (page 341) with Tzatziki (page 320)

DAY 25 (Wednesday)

7:30 a.m. Traditional Triple Threat Shake (page 311)

12:00 p.m. Leftover Greek Lamb Kabobs on salad with choice of SKINNYFat dressing (pages 321–322)

3:30 p.m. Triple Threat Pudding (page 313)

7:30 p.m. Fabulous Fajitas (page 349) with Holy Moly Guacamole (page 324) and salsa

DAY 26 (Thursday)

7:30 a.m. Triple Threat Cheesecake (page 314)

12:00 p.m. Bun-less beef burger and Oven-Roasted Brussels Sprouts (page 352)

3:30 p.m. Traditional Triple Threat Shake (page 311)

7:30 p.m. Rustic Portobello Pizza Caps (page 344)

DAY 27 (Friday)

7:30 a.m. Traditional Triple Threat Shake (page 311)

12:00 p.m. Grilled or broiled chicken thigh on big salad with choice of SKINNYFat dressing (pages 321–322)

3:30 p.m. Triple Threat Pudding (page 313)

7:30 p.m. *Peppercorn-Crusted Beef Tenderloin (page 341) with 4-Ingredient Blender Hollandaise Sauce (page 323) and baked potato*

DAY 28 (Saturday)

9:00 a.m. Protein-Packed Morning Muffins (page 330)

1:00 p.m. Traditional Triple Threat Shake (page 311)

5:00 p.m. Grilled Tandoori Skewers (page 342) with Cooling Cucumber Raita (page 320) and Indian Garlic-Butter Cheese Non-Naan (page 354)

9:00 p.m. Chocolate Triple Threat Ice Cream (page 314)

The 28-Day Micronutrient Miracle Menu Plan Q&A

As you looked over the Signature protocol, did any questions come to mind? Here are answers to a few of the most common questions we have received from our clients.

Q: What if I don't like some of the foods in the menu plan? Can I swap foods out?

A: This 28-day menu plan is simply meant as an example of how your personalized plan might lay out. You can adjust the menu to match your taste buds and your dietary preferences. For example, if you dislike salmon, feel free to swap it out with a protein you prefer. You can also swap side dishes as you please. Just remember, you can only swap foods that fall into the same categories. You cannot swap a nonstarchy vegetable, like asparagus, with a starch, like rice. So, when swapping out asparagus, you can choose from any of the other nonstarchy vegetables—maybe broccoli or Brussels sprouts are more up your alley. If you choose to swap a nonstarchy vegetable for a starch in a particular meal, perhaps because you are dining out, then you must omit a starch from a meal in the very same week.

Q: What if my schedule doesn't allow me to eat at the times suggested?

A: Again, these are just suggestions. Remember, we explained that eating every 3 to 5 hours is key and that two of the four meals should be from shakes. We organized this 28-day menu plan to reflect many of the potential schedules you might fall into. Feel free to move the timing of the meals around to fit your "true" schedule. Also, just because a recipe is listed as dinner doesn't mean it can't make a fabulous lunch or even breakfast. Don't be afraid to alter the plan so that it is a true representation of your preferences.

Q: Should I be counting my calories?

A: We are not about counting calories. No one wants to be weighing and measuring meals. The stress caused by counting each and every morsel is unhealthy in its own right. While on the 28-day Micronutrient Miracle plan, you won't need to, either. Becoming micronutrient sufficient will alleviate your food cravings, and eating Rich Foods containing both proteins and fats and, of course, a ton of great flavors, will keep you feeling full and satisfied all day long. This doesn't mean that you should eat until your belly aches; your body doesn't need to feel stuffed to have enough energy to complete all of its metabolic functions.

The 28-Day Micronutrient Miracle Menu Plan Q&A (continued)

If, however, you are following the Weight Loss protocol, you will want to keep an eye on your portion sizes. Eat slowly and mindfully. Too much food will limit your weight loss, so many dieters find that keeping a food journal can be very helpful at the beginning. Similarly, if you find that you are working out hard and really pushing yourself using the ZMT cardiovascular training and One Set To Failure weight training, you don't want to "underfuel," or underfeed, yourself either. Your body is brilliant—trust it, not a food scale, to tell you if you require more or less food.

Q: How soon will I see results?

A: This is a tough one to answer. Many people tell us they feel more energy immediately when starting the Micronutrient Miracle plan. For others, the levels of deficiency might be far greater and the changes may take longer to occur. Everyone's body is different, so don't compare your progress with that of anyone else. Many of the complex changes occurring inside of you might not be evident right away. However, be assured that your body is experiencing something miraculous. It is receiving an incredible gift from you every single day. You are creating a micronutrient sufficient state, an environment from which health and longevity can thrive.

Remember, any health conditions you are suffering from now did not magically appear overnight. They took a while to develop. Be patient with yourself; your healing may take just as long. But feel blessed in the understanding that you are putting yourself on the path to healing—a road that you were meant to discover so that you can attain the extraordinary life that you were born to live.

Q: You said that vegans and vegetarians can follow the plan. How would you do this?

A: Following the Micronutrient Miracle plan will be harder for vegans and strict vegetarians. However, because these diets are so restrictive, focusing one's efforts on becoming micronutrient sufficient is even more important. To begin, two of your meals will still be from protein shakes; just opt for plant-based protein, preferably our IN.POWER organic plant protein. We would love for at least one of the two other meals to include poultry, eggs, or fish. If you are completely vegan, then this obviously will not be possible. So you will want to make sure you are taking in protein from beans, quinoa, chia seeds, rice, hempseed, and buckwheat. Soy is still off-limits. When you alter a recipe, simply omit the protein and add one of the previously mentioned starches in its place. This will require that you eat starches more than twice per week. However, this is necessary to fulfill your protein requirements. Also, proper food preparation is imperative for your plan. Nuts, seeds, legumes, and grains all require a bit of extra work to make their nutrients available. If eaten incorrectly, even these dense foods will leave you deficient. While micronutrient sufficiency can certainly be achieved while following a vegetarian protocol, or even a vegan lifestyle, the preparation of these problematic foods containing numerous Everyday Micronutrient Depleters makes it a bit more time-consuming. Also, remember that for you, supplementation is even more important, as some essential micronutrients are not available in plant-based foods.

Q: What if I follow a traditional whole food diet? Can I do the plan without eating protein meal replacements or taking shakes?

A: Of course, protein shakes and meal replacements are in no way mandatory. You can choose instead to simply eat three larger meals and take one snack a day, keeping the same schedule we outlined (eating every 3 to 5 hours). Make sure to eat both protein and fat in every meal so that you stay satiated. Additionally, as the Triple Threat recipes include a multivitamin, which is imperative for sufficiency, you will still need to add multivitamin supplementation into your schedule. We have clients who have been extremely successful following a whole food program. It might look something like this:

7:00 a.m. Take nutreince (or another well-formulated multivitamin) in water.

7:30 a.m. Enjoy the breakfast of your choice, such as a Greek Yogurt and Fruit Bowl (page 331) or Protein-Packed Morning Muffins (page 330).

11:30 a.m. Lunchtime. Choose from any of the entrée recipes.

3:30 p.m. Grab a snack. Make sure it contains both fat and protein (e.g., cream cheese on celery, cheese sticks, or a small piece of any of our delicious desserts).

7:30 p.m. Dinnertime. Choose from any of the entrée recipes.

9:00 p.m. Take nutreince (or another well-formulated multivitamin) in water.

The 28-Day Micronutrient Miracle Menu Plan Q&A (continued)

Q: Should I be worried that there appears to be a lot of fat in this plan? Aren't vegetables and fruits better for me than meats, fats, and eggs?

A: Carbohydrates—like fruits, grains, and vegetables—stimulate insulin, which increases the body's fat stores. Most physicians are unaware that humans have absolutely no requirement for carbohydrates. You don't even need 1 gram to survive and thrive. Individuals who eat carbohydrates all day consistently have an elevated insulin concentration in their blood. This drives the excess carbohydrates into the fat cells, which now cannot release the fat. Carbohydrates alone don't satisfy for long, and this drives you to eat more carbs and more calories throughout the day, leading to weight gain, insulin sensitivity, and possibly diabetes.

It is the combination of protein and fat that satiates and reduces hunger, and unlike carbohydrates, both of these are required by the body to maintain health. The myth of fat, especially saturated fats, being hazardous to your health is just that—a myth. This has been debunked by numerous scientific studies. It is completely untrue that eating saturated fat miraculously plugs your coronary arteries. Both sugar and wheat are much more likely to cause this to happen, which is why we eliminate both on the Micronutrient Miracle plan.

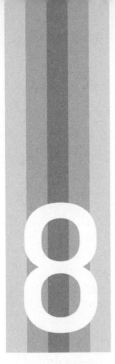

Personalizing Your Plan for Specific Health Conditions

IN THE PREVIOUS CHAPTER, you learned exactly what to do every day while following our Signature 28-day Micronutrient Miracle plan in order to set yourself on the path to micronutrient sufficiency and, ultimately, optimal health. While the Signature plan has yielded exceptional results for the vast majority of our clients, your current state of health, the conditions you might suffer from, and what miracle you aim to achieve during these first 28 days might call for a more specific protocol. That is why we have created this chapter, where you can delve a little deeper, get a bit more personalized, and focus in on what your body needs in order to achieve your desired goals. In this chapter, we identify eight different health conditions and give you specific information on how to tweak the Signature plan to create the physiological changes required to reduce, alleviate, or heal these unwanted ailments.

Don't spread yourself too thin! You can't do it all in only 28 days. You will drive yourself crazy if you try to follow more than one protocol because you currently have more than one health condition. Because they all have micronutrient sufficiency as the "core cure," you don't have to worry that you are worsening one condition while combatting another. Both will get better just because all of the plans have a state of sufficiency as their common denominator. They are tailored simply to help an individual focus deeper on a specific goal.

You can choose to follow any of the condition-specific protocols listed below.

- Fat Loss (see page 223)
- Autoimmune—Chronic Inflammation (see page 233)
- Digestive Health (see page 243)

- Blood Sugar Regulation (see page 254)
- Ketogenic (our strictest protocol; suitable for many conditions) (see page 263)

- Cardiovascular Health (see page 276)
- Bone Building (see page 287)
- Hormone Regulation (see page 298)

Personalizing Your Plan—How It Works

For each of the protocols above, we'll begin by first reviewing who might want to follow the plan and which conditions it might improve or alleviate. Next, and this part is key, we will identify the adjustments you will need to make to the Signature 28-day Micronutrient Miracle plan on page 210. This will include any alterations to the 10 Golden Rules, such as increased or decreased Zero Movement Training for cardiovascular health, or any adjustments to one's daily limitations for fruit, starches, alcohol, or caffeine. These variations from the Signature protocol are very important and will help you to achieve your goals in the most efficient and effective manner.

Next, for each protocol, we will outline the micronutrients used in the prevention and treatment of the specific health complaint. These vitamins and minerals will be the focus of your meals. To help you increase your intake of these specific essential micronutrients, we have created a go-to list of the foods richest in the micronutrients that you need the most. We want you to refer to this list of "Powerhouse Picks" whenever you are creating recipes of your own, whenever you are swapping out foods you don't enjoy from the predesigned 28-day condition-specific menu plan, or whenever you find yourself ordering at a restaurant. Remember, you can swap freely from this list, but you can only swap similar foods. For example, if you see Brussels sprouts on your menu and you don't love them, then you can choose any of the powerhouse picks listed in the same category. This means you can pick another nonstarchy vegetable as a substitute; you cannot, however, select a potato (starch) or an apple (fruit). It is pretty simple and you have a ton of delicious options to choose from. We have also listed additional supplements, both essential micronutrients as well as accessory nutrients and herbs, that you may consider adding to your protocol.

Remember, these are in no way mandatory, but they have been shown to be beneficial in studies, so you may want to add them in, at least for the first 28 days.

You will also see a 7-day menu plan that has been specially designed for your condition-specific 28-day plan. We ran out of room in this book and didn't want to leave out any vital information, so instead, we opted to provide the additional 3-week menu plans for each of the condition-specific protocols as downloads at mymiracleplan.com. These condition-specific meal plans have been altered from the Signature 28-day Micronutrient Miracle menu plan to deliver foods that are denser in the specific micronutrients your body needs. Feel free to move recipes around to fit your personal schedule and taste preferences.

Fat Loss

This plan is specifically designed for individuals who are looking to burn fat at a moderate and sustainable pace. This protocol will help you create an internal environment that is optimal for fat loss, eliminating food cravings, and achieving your genetic potential for lean muscle tissue. If you wish to lose fat at an accelerated rate, you may want to consider our Ketogenic protocol.

The Fat Loss protocol is designed for individuals who are:

- Overweight/obese
- Bingers and cravers
- Exercise enthusiasts

Adjustments you must make to the Signature 28-day Micronutrient Miracle plan for your specific condition(s):

10 GOLDEN RULES While each of the condition-specific protocols must follow all 10 of the Golden Rules, for best results with this protocol, we have identified the following rules to either be critical or require small tweaks.

#2: Ousting the obesogens is critical, as they are hormone disruptors. Make sure to be keenly aware of removing MSG, BPA, and phthalates.

#5: Stress reduction is very important for optimal fat loss, as stress increases the release of cortisol, a hormone that spikes appetite and increases fat storage in the belly region.

#6: Increase your ZMT sessions from three or four per week to six or seven. Also make an effort to get out and walk, bike, hike, row, or do any other type of physical movement as much as possible.

#7: Purchasing nontoxic household and beauty goods will ensure that they are not causing hormonal imbalances and weight gain. Try to follow our Top 10 Terrific Tricks to Reduce Household Toxins.

#8: Taking a multivitamin that contains enough calcium and magnesium is extremely important to kill cravings. Most supplements do not contain these bulky minerals. nutreince contains these and the dynamic duo of carnitine and choline, two nutrients that, when combined, have been called the "nutritional equivalent to liposuction." If you take nutreince, you will be getting what you need; however, if you opt for a different multivitamin, make sure to evaluate it using our ABCs of Optimal Supplementation Guidelines or the stack-up analysis available at MultivitaminStackUpQuiz.com.

#9: Taking your Micronutrient Miracle Triple Threat Shakes twice a day is especially important while following this protocol, as it will provide you with the amino acid L-glutamine, which has been shown to reduce sugar cravings and aid in the regulation of metabolism. Studies confirm that individuals who increased whey protein intake lost nearly twice the weight of those who skipped whey. Also, whey protein shakes reduce ghrelin (a hormone that tells your brain you're hungry).

DAILY LIMITS: The daily limits for the Fat Loss protocol are slightly stricter than for our Signature plan. For the next 28 days, adhere to the following limits.

Starches/fruits/nuts/seeds: One serving per week. You can enjoy a total of one gluten-free starch *or* one fruit *or* 1 serving of nuts/seeds a week.

Alcohol: Rather than one or two glasses a day, limit alcohol to up to three glasses per week. Eliminate gluten-free beers.

Caffeinated drinks: Two cups daily (same as the Signature plan). The chlorogenic acid found in coffee and tea has been shown to reduce insulin resistance and chronic inflammation.

SETTING YOUR SCHEDULE: Studies have verified that weight loss can be improved when undergoing an intermittent fast. To best achieve this, opt for scheduling options 4, 5, or 6 from Chapter 7 (see page 209) and make two consecutive meals Triple Threat Shakes or puddings. (In option 4, your two consecutive shakes are your last meal of the day followed by your first meal the next morning, allowing you to still achieve the fasting goal.) You don't need to do this every day, either; you can choose this option as often as you like.

Beneficial micronutrients used in the prevention and treatment of overweight/obesity:

Choline	Vitamin D	Magnesium
Vitamin A	Vitamin E	Potassium
Vitamin B$_3$	Calcium	Zinc
Vitamin B$_6$	Chromium	Omega-3 fatty acids
Vitamin B$_{12}$	Iodine	Alpha-lipoic acid
Vitamin C	Iron	CoQ10

POWERHOUSE PICKS: Choose these micronutrient powerhouses whenever possible. The Rich Foods listed below are high in the essential micronutrients shown to be beneficial for fat loss. Additionally, the spices and beverages listed below have been shown to increase metabolism or help in the prevention and treatment of overweight/obesity. We have adjusted your 28-day menu suggestions to include many of these Rich Food choices. Make an effort to choose these Rich Foods when designing personalized menus or eating out, and don't forget to properly prepare foods that contain EMDs.

PROTEINS

Beef	Mussels	Shrimp
Bone broth	Organ meats	Snapper
Chicken	Oysters	Tuna
Clams	Rainbow trout	Turkey
Cod	Salmon	Venison
Crab	Sardines	
Herring	Scallops	

DAIRY

Cheese	Milk
Cream	Yogurt

FATS

Butter	Eggs (with yolks)
Coconut oil	SKINNYFat*

*Use SKINNYFat in recipes whenever possible, as it is virtually impossible to store as body fat. Peer-reviewed published research also shows that MCT oil (the main ingredient in SKINNYFat) increases metabolism, reduces body fat, and improves insulin sensitivity and glucose tolerance, while the long-chain triglycerides in the coconut oil in SKINNYFat aid in the absorption of your essential micronutrients. In studies, individuals using MCT oil lost more total weight, total fat mass, intra-abdominal adipose tissue, and subcutaneous abdominal adipose than those eating alternative oils.

NONSTARCHY VEGETABLES

Asparagus	Dark leafy greens	Red or green chile peppers
Avocado	Garlic	Romaine lettuce
Broccoli	Jalapeño peppers	Seaweed
Brussels sprouts	Mushrooms	Snow peas
Cabbage	Onions	Tomatoes
Cauliflower	Pumpkin	Yellow bell peppers

STARCHES

Acorn Squash	Lentils	Sweet potatoes
Brown rice	Lima beans	Quinoa
Green peas	Navy beans	
Kidney beans	Potatoes	

FRUITS

Bananas	Grapefruit	Prunes
Coconut water (counts as a fruit, not as a beverage; check carefully for sugar)	Limes	Raisins
	Oranges	Strawberries
	Papaya	Watermelon

NUTS AND SEEDS

Cashews	Pine nuts	Walnuts
Chia seeds	Pumpkins seeds	
Peanuts	Sesame seeds	

BENEFICIAL SPICES

Black pepper	Cinnamon	Mustard
Cardamom	Cumin	Onion powder
Cayenne pepper	Garlic powder	Red-pepper flakes
Chile pepper (chipotle)	Ginger	Turmeric

DAILY BEVERAGES

Black tea	Green tea	Mineral water
Coffee	Oolong tea	Water

Additional essential micronutrient supplements to consider:

Iron: This mineral aids in fatty acid metabolism and is necessary for the production of carnitine, which metabolizes fat. Try to get 8 milligrams (men) or 18 milligrams (women) per day, either through your food or in supplement form.

Note: It is imperative that you take iron in supplement form at a separate time from your multivitamin (nutreince). Iron is the most competitive micronutrient, conflicting with 10 other micronutrients. Take it midday on an empty stomach.

Omega-3s: Studies show that omega-3s can both increase oxidation of fat by activating genes that break down fat and reduce the number of overall fat cells. Attempt to get the RDI of 1.6 grams (1,600 milligrams) per day from food or in supplement form.

Note: You can take omega-3s in supplement form at the same time as your multivitamin (nutreince). Opt for Origin Omega or try to find a supplement with a greater amount of EPA than DHA, if possible.

Additional beneficial supplements to consider:

Alpha-lipoic acid (ALA): This powerful antioxidant/anti-inflammatory supplement can have an "antiobesity effect," resulting in decreased appetite, increased activity levels, and decreased abdominal fat. Those deficient in ALA have been shown to have an increased likelihood of being overweight or obese.

L-carnitine/acetyl-L-carnitine: This micronutrient is critical for energy formation and an active metabolism. Alpha-lipoic acid and acetyl-L-carnitine work together to increase metabolism and lower oxidative stress more than either compound alone. A 5:1 ratio of L-carnitine to ALA may be optimal.

CoQ10: Similar to ALA and acetyl-L-carnitine, CoQ10 is a powerful antioxidant/anti-inflammatory that assists with energy production. CoQ10 has been shown to be beneficial for treating and preventing obesity, enhancing metabolism, and supporting optimal energy and endurance. In one study, individuals found to be deficient in CoQ10 were given CoQ10 supplementation (100 milligrams per day), and in only 9 weeks, they had lost an incredible average of 30 pounds.

L-glutamine: This amino acid has been shown to reduce sugar cravings and enhance metabolism. It will already be supplemented through the addition of IN.POWER whey protein. If you are omitting the protein Triple Threat meal replacement shakes, you may want to consider supplementation with 2 to 4 grams of powdered L-glutamine. You can add this to your nutreince multivitamin drink or to cold water. Take it separate from your meals.

Curcumin: According to the USDA, this active ingredient typically found in the Indian spice turmeric enhances cellular energy to speed metabolism.

Digestive enzymes: These can assist with digestion and enhance micronutrient availability and absorption. Look for a product with amylase, protease, and lipase, as well as a variety of other digestive enzymes. Bromelain, ox bile, pancreatin, papain, pepsin, and betaine HCL may all be beneficial. Betaine HCL may be especially important for this protocol, as it helps with the absorption of calcium and magnesium, two micronutrients that will assist you in eliminating food cravings.

DHEA: Levels of DHEA drop with age. Most studies on DHEA for fat or weight loss support its use for this purpose. DHEA should be taken with caution, though, because high doses may suppress the body's natural ability to make DHEA and may lead to liver damage (as shown in an animal study). Taking antioxidants—such as vitamins C and E and selenium—is recommended to prevent oxidative damage to the liver.

The Fat Loss 28-Day Menu Plan

Limited foods are *italicized* so that you can see where they fit into your plan.

Feel free to choose from any of the Miracle Pestos, Miracle Butters, SKINNYFat Salad Dressings, and SKINNYFat Infusions, as they all fit into the Fat Loss protocol.

WEEK 1

DAY 1 (Sunday)

9:00 a.m. Protein-Packed Morning Muffins (page 330)

1:00 p.m. Traditional Triple Threat Shake (page 311)

5:00 p.m. Buffalo Chicken Chili (page 340)

9:00 p.m. Triple Threat Pudding (page 313)

DAY 2 (Monday)

7:30 a.m. Traditional Triple Threat Shake (page 311)

12:00 p.m. Leftover Buffalo Chicken Chili

3:30 p.m. Traditional Triple Threat Shake (page 311)

7:30 p.m. Salmon with asparagus and choice of a Miracle Pesto or Miracle Butter (pages 315–318)

DAY 3 (Tuesday)

7:30 a.m. Triple Threat Cheesecake (page 314)

12:00 p.m. Big salad with leftover salmon and asparagus and choice of SKINNYFat dressing (pages 321–322)

3:30 p.m. Traditional Triple Threat Shake (page 311)

7:30 p.m. Greek Chicken (page 337)

DAY 4 (Wednesday)

7:30 a.m. Traditional Triple Threat Shake (page 311)

12:00 p.m. Leftover Greek Chicken

3:30 p.m. Triple Threat Pudding (page 313)

7:30 p.m. Quick Tandoori Shrimp (page 336) with Cooling Cucumber Raita (page 320) and optional Indian Garlic-Butter Cheese Non-Naan (page 354)

DAY 5 (Thursday)

7:30 a.m. Triple Threat Cheesecake (page 314)

12:00 p.m. Big salad with leftover Quick Tandoori Shrimp and choice of SKINNYFat dressing (pages 321–322)

3:30 p.m. Traditional Triple Threat Shake (page 311)

7:30 p.m. Bun-less cheeseburger and Oven-Roasted Brussels Sprouts (page 352)

DAY 6 (Friday)

7:30 a.m. Traditional Triple Threat Shake (page 311)

12:00 p.m. Broccoli Cheese Soup (page 327)

3:30 p.m. Traditional Triple Threat Shake (page 311)

7:30 p.m. Grilled steak with choice of a Miracle Pesto or Miracle Butter (pages 315–318) or 4-Ingredient Blender Hollandaise Sauce (page 323) and Cauliflower Mash (page 352)

DAY 7 (Saturday)

9:00 a.m. Speedy Salmon Cakes (page 329) and eggs any style

1:00 p.m. Traditional Triple Threat Shake (page 311)

5:00 p.m. *Fish and Chips (page 350)*

9:00 p.m. Chocolate Triple Threat Ice Cream (page 314)

WEEK 2

DAY 8 (Sunday)

9:00 a.m. French Onion Egg Tart (page 328)

1:00 p.m. Traditional Triple Threat Shake (page 311)

5:00 p.m. Zughetti (page 345) with Mom's Beef Bolognese (page 324)

9:00 p.m. Traditional Triple Threat Shake (page 311)

DAY 9 (Monday)

7:30 a.m. Traditional Triple Threat Shake (page 311)

12:00 p.m. Grilled or broiled chicken thighs, sautéed mushrooms, and choice of a Miracle Pesto or Miracle Butter (pages 315–318)

3:30 p.m. Triple Threat Cheesecake (page 314)

7:30 p.m. Moqueca (aka Brazilian Fish Stew) (page 343)

DAY 10 (Tuesday)

7:30 a.m. Traditional Triple Threat Shake (page 311)

12:00 p.m. Leftover Moqueca

3:30 p.m. Traditional Triple Threat Shake (page 311)

7:30 p.m. Coq au Vin (page 347) with Cauliflower Mash (page 352)

DAY 11 (Wednesday)

7:30 a.m. Traditional Triple Threat Shake (page 311)

12:00 p.m. Leftover Coq au Vin

3:30 p.m. Triple Threat Pudding (page 313)

7:30 p.m. Thai-Style Chopped Pork (page 347) on greens

DAY 12 (Thursday)

7:30 a.m. Traditional Triple Threat Shake (page 311)

12:00 p.m. Leftover chopped pork on a salad with choice of SKINNYFat dressing (pages 321–322)

3:30 p.m. Traditional Triple Threat Shake (page 311)

7:30 p.m. Scallops in Lemon Butter Sauce (page 334) with broccoli

DAY 13 (Friday)

7:30 a.m. Traditional Triple Threat Shake (page 311)

12:00 p.m. Mexican Chicken Wrap (page 338); use a lettuce wrap instead of the Ridiculously Simple Wrap

3:30 p.m. Triple Threat Cheesecake (page 314)

7:30 p.m. Salad and Rustic Flatbread (page 346)

DAY 14 (Saturday)

9:00 a.m. *Carrot Cake Pancakes with Cream Cheese Frosting and chopped walnuts and raisins (page 333)*

1:00 p.m. Traditional Triple Threat Shake (page 311)

5:00 p.m. Micronutrient-Packed "Offaly" Tasty Meatloaf (page 348) and steamed vegetable with choice of a Miracle Pesto or Miracle Butter (pages 315–318)

9:00 p.m. Triple Threat Pudding (page 313)

WEEK 3

DAY 15 (Sunday)

9:00 a.m. Leftover meatloaf heated in a frying pan and topped with a fried egg and covered in melted cheese

1:00 p.m. Traditional Triple Threat Shake (page 311)

5:00 p.m. *Camarão na Moranga (aka Brazilian Shrimp Stew in a Pumpkin) (page 335)*

9:00 p.m. Traditional Triple Threat Shake (page 311)

DAY 16 (Monday)

7:30 a.m. Traditional Triple Threat Shake (page 311)

12:00 p.m. Big salad with ½ can of tuna fish and choice of SKINNYFat dressing (pages 321–322)

3:30 p.m. Traditional Triple Threat Shake (page 311)

7:30 p.m. Chicken Wings (page 334) with Really Creamy SKINNYFat Blue Cheese Dressing (page 322) and carrot and celery sticks

DAY 17 (Tuesday)

7:30 a.m. Traditional Triple Threat Shake (page 311)

12:00 p.m. Leftover chicken wings and blue cheese dressing

3:30 p.m. Triple Threat Cheesecake (page 314)

7:30 p.m. Shepherd's Pie (page 351)

DAY 18 (Wednesday)

7:30 a.m. Traditional Triple Threat Shake (page 311)

12:00 p.m. Leftover Shepherd's Pie

3:30 p.m. Traditional Triple Threat Shake (page 311)

7:30 p.m. Zughetti (page 345) and grilled chicken thigh with Rich and Creamy Alfredo Sauce (page 319)

DAY 19 (Thursday)

7:30 a.m. Triple Threat Cheesecake (page 314)

12:00 p.m. Bun-less beef burger and a side salad with choice of SKINNYFat dressing (pages 321–322)

3:30 p.m. Traditional Triple Threat Shake (page 311)

7:30 p.m. Thai Shrimp Noodle Soup (page 326)

DAY 20 (Friday)

7:30 a.m. Traditional Triple Threat Shake (page 311)

12:00 p.m. Leftover Thai Shrimp Noodle Soup

3:30 p.m. Traditional Triple Threat Shake (page 311)

7:30 p.m. Rotisserie or baked whole chicken with sautéed mushrooms and onions in butter

DAY 21 (Saturday)

9:00 a.m. Fried eggs served on Cauliflower Cheesy Hash Browns (page 329)

1:00 p.m. Traditional Triple Threat Shake (page 311)

5:00 p.m. Miracle Chinese Fried "Rice" (page 339)

9:00 p.m. Traditional Triple Threat Shake (page 311)

WEEK 4

DAY 22 (Sunday)

9:00 a.m. Smoked Salmon Cream Cheese Roll-Ups (page 331) with avocado slices and an egg any style

1:00 p.m. Traditional Triple Threat Shake (page 311)

5:00 p.m. Slow-Cooked Beer-Braised Beef (page 338) and Cauliflower Mash (page 352)

9:00 p.m. Chocolate Triple Threat Ice Cream (page 314)

DAY 23 (Monday)

7:30 a.m. Traditional Triple Threat Shake (page 311)

12:00 p.m. Leftover Miracle Chinese Fried "Rice"

3:30 p.m. Traditional Triple Threat Shake (page 311)

7:30 p.m. Fish and vegetables with choice of a Miracle Pesto or Miracle Butter (pages 315–318)

DAY 24 (Tuesday)

7:30 a.m. Traditional Triple Threat Shake (page 311)

12:00 p.m. Leftover Slow-Cooked Beer-Braised Beef and Cauliflower Mash

3:30 p.m. Triple Threat Cheesecake (page 314)

7:30 p.m. Greek Lamb Kabobs (page 314) with Tzatziki (page 320)

DAY 25 (Wednesday)

7:30 a.m. Traditional Triple Threat Shake (page 311)

12:00 p.m. Leftover Greek Lamb Kabobs on a salad with Tzatziki

3:30 p.m. Triple Threat Pudding (page 313)

7:30 p.m. Fabulous Fajitas (page 349) with Holy Moly Guacamole (page 324) and salsa (omit the wraps)

DAY 26 (Thursday)

7:30 a.m. Traditional Triple Threat Shake (page 311)

12:00 p.m. Bun-less beef burger and Oven-Roasted Brussels Sprouts (page 352)

3:30 p.m. Traditional Triple Threat Shake (page 311)

7:30 p.m. Rustic Portobello Pizza Caps (page 344)

DAY 27 (Friday)

7:30 a.m. Traditional Triple Threat Shake (page 311)

12:00 p.m. Grilled or broiled chicken thigh on a big salad with choice of SKINNYFat dressing (pages 321–322)

3:30 p.m. Triple Threat Cheesecake (page 314)

7:30 p.m. *Peppercorn-Crusted Beef Tenderloin (page 341) with 4-Ingredient Blender Hollandaise Sauce (page 323) and Sweet Potato, Yam, and Apple Casserole (page 353) or baked potato*

DAY 28 (Saturday)

9:00 a.m. Protein-Packed Morning Muffins (page 330)

1:00 p.m. Traditional Triple Threat Shake (page 311)

5:00 p.m. Grilled Tandoori Skewers (page 342) with Cooling Cucumber Raita (page 320) and optional Indian Garlic-Butter Cheese Non-Naan (page 354)

9:00 p.m. Chocolate Triple Threat Ice Cream (page 314)

Autoimmune—Chronic Inflammation

This plan is specifically designed for individuals who are suffering from an autoimmune condition. This protocol will help you to create an internal environment that will reduce chronic inflammation while working toward healing the digestive system and reducing intestinal permeability (leaky gut). If you wish to focus more directly on enhanced gut health, you may want to consider our Digestive Health protocol. We have also had great success using our Ketogenic protocol with our clients with autoimmune issues.

The Autoimmune protocol is designed for individuals who have:

- Addison's disease
- Alopecia
- Alzheimer's
- Asthma
- Celiac disease
- Chronic fatigue syndrome
- Chronic inflammation

- Crohn's disease
- Eczema
- Graves' disease
- Hashimoto's thyroiditis
- Lupus
- Multiple sclerosis
- Parkinson's disease

- Pernicious anemia
- Psoriasis
- Raynaud's phenomenon
- Rheumatoid arthritis
- Scleroderma
- Type 1 diabetes
- Vitiligo

Adjustments you must make to the Signature 28-day Micronutrient Miracle plan for your specific condition(s):

10 GOLDEN RULES: While each of the condition-specific protocols must follow all 10 of the Golden Rules, for best results with this protocol, we have identified the following rules to either be critical or require small tweaks.

#5: Stress reduction is very important for the autoimmune protocol. Chronic stress has been shown to trigger and worsen autoimmune conditions by altering the effectiveness of cortisol to regulate inflammatory responses.

#7: Purchasing new nontoxic alternatives for your beauty, cleaning, and hygiene products is especially important while following this protocol.

#8: Multivitamin supplementation is key, as micronutrient sufficiency has been shown to greatly improve autoimmune conditions. Take a well-formulated multivitamin, like nutreince, or compare others at MultivitaminStackUpQuiz.com.

#9: Taking your Micronutrient Miracle Triple Threat Shakes twice a day is especially important while following this protocol, as it will provide you with the amino acid L-glutamine, which has been shown to have an anti-inflammatory effect that can aid in the healing of the intestinal lining by repelling gut irritants.

EMD ALERT: During this protocol, avoid antacids as well as aspirin, ibuprofen, or other NSAIDs, as they could irritate your gastrointestinal tract lining.

DAILY LIMITS: The daily limits for this protocol are slightly stricter than for our Signature plan. For the next 28 days, adhere to the following limits.

Starches/fruit/nuts/seeds: Two servings per week, but with restrictions. You can still enjoy a total of two gluten-free starches *or* two fruits each week (*or* one of each). However, eliminate all grains, nuts, seeds, berries, beans, and nightshades (i.e., potatoes [not sweet potatoes], eggplant, tomatoes, hot peppers, and bell peppers), as they may cause gut irritation or inflammation within the body.

Alcohol: Rather than having one or two glasses a day, eliminate alcohol altogether for the next 28 days to allow for gut healing.

Caffeinated drinks: Try to eliminate caffeinated drinks during this protocol and drink only decaffeinated beverages; however, if you *need* caffeine, limit your intake to one cup per day.

Bone broth: Add this food to your daily protocol. Try to drink a small cup of homemade bone broth each morning for the next 28 days.

Beneficial micronutrients used in the prevention and treatment of autoimmune conditions:

Vitamin A	*Vitamin B$_{12}$*	*Magnesium*
Vitamin B$_1$	*Choline*	*Manganese*
Vitamin B$_2$	*Vitamin C*	*Potassium*
Vitamin B$_3$	*Vitamin D*	*Selenium*
Vitamin B$_5$	*Vitamin E*	*Silicon*
Vitamin B$_6$	*Calcium*	*Zinc*
Vitamin B$_7$	*Iodine*	*Omega-3 fatty acids*
Vitamin B$_9$	*Iron*	

POWERHOUSE PICKS: Choose these micronutrient powerhouses whenever possible. The Rich Foods listed below are high in the essential micronutrients shown to be beneficial for autoimmune conditions. Additionally, the spices and beverages listed below have been shown to have an anti-inflammatory effect. We have adjusted your 28-day menu suggestions to include many of these Rich Food choices. Choose these Rich Foods when designing personalized menus or eating out, and don't forget to properly prepare foods that contain EMDs.

PROTEINS

Beef	*Lamb*	*Sardines*
Bone broth	*Mussels*	*Scallops*
Chicken	*Organ meats*	*Shrimp*
Clams	*Oysters*	*Snapper*
Cod	*Pork*	*Tuna*
Crab	*Rainbow trout*	*Turkey*
Herring	*Salmon*	*Venison*

DAIRY

Cheese	*Milk*
Cream	*Yogurt*

FATS

Butter	*Eggs (with yolks)*
Coconut oil	*SKINNYFat**

*Using SKINNYFat and SKINNYFat Olive in lieu of olive oil will boost brainpower and metabolism as well as reduce inflammation caused by eating too many omega-6 fatty acids from olive oil. Additionally, there is a lot of good research on MCT oil (the main ingredient in both SKINNYFat varieties) being particularly beneficial for patients with heart disease, diabetes, or Alzheimer's.

NONSTARCHY VEGETABLES

Asparagus	Dark leafy greens	Seaweed
Avocado	Garlic	Snow peas
Broccoli	Mushrooms	Spinach (cooked)
Brussels sprouts	Mustard greens	Sprouts
Cabbage	Onions	Swiss chard
Cauliflower	Pumpkin	
Celery	Romaine lettuce	

STARCHES

Acorn squash	Green peas	Sweet potatoes

FRUITS

Apples	Dates	Papaya
Bananas	Grapefruit	Pineapple
Coconut water (counts as a fruit, not as a beverage; check carefully for sugar)	Limes	Prunes
	Mango	Raisins
	Melons	Tart cherries
	Oranges	Watermelon

NUTS AND SEEDS

Eliminated

BENEFICIAL SPICES

Cinnamon	Ginger	Turmeric
Cloves	Onion powder	
Garlic powder	Sage	

SAFE SPICES (for the autoimmune protocol, omit any spices that do not appear under either Beneficial or Safe Spices)

Basil	Horseradish	Saffron
Bay leaf	Lemongrass	Spearmint
Chives	Oregano	Tarragon
Cilantro	Parsley	Thyme
Curry leaf	Peppermint	Unrefined salt
Dill	Rosemary	Vanilla extract

DAILY BEVERAGES

Coffee	Mineral water
Green tea	Water

Additional essential micronutrient supplements to consider:

Iron: This mineral aids in the prevention and treatment of several autoimmune conditions, including chronic fatigue syndrome, celiac disease, and Crohn's disease. Try to get 8 milligrams (men) or 18 milligrams (women) per day, either through your food or in supplement form.

Note: It is imperative that you take iron in supplement form at a separate time from your multivitamin (nutreince). Iron is the most competitive micronutrient, conflicting with 10 other micronutrients. Take it midday on an empty stomach.

Omega-3s: Omega-3 supplementation has demonstrated benefits (reduced pain and inflammation) for individuals suffering from autoimmune conditions, including psoriasis, Crohn's disease, lupus, rheumatoid arthritis, and multiple sclerosis. Attempt to get the RDI of 1.6 grams (1,600 milligrams) per day from food or in supplement form.

Note: You can take approximately 1,000 milligrams of omega-3s in supplement form with your AM multivitamin (nutreince) and 1,000 milligrams with your PM multivitamin. Opt for Origin Omega or try to find an omega-3 supplement with a greater amount of EPA than DHA, if possible.

Selenium and iodine: Most people with Hashimoto's are not iodine deficient, but taking a multivitamin with iodine can be helpful to support thyroid function. Caution should be exercised when taking high doses of iodine, because iodine has been implicated in triggering Hashimoto's. The doses of iodine present in nutreince are well tolerated by most people with Hashimoto's. Iodine absorption is greatly improved with the supplementation of a key synergist, selenium. While the AM dose of nutreince already contains 70 micrograms of selenium, we suggest that those with Hashimoto's take an additional 200 micrograms in the form of selenomethionine with their AM nutreince. Iodine's other synergistic micronutrients—vitamins A and E, iron, and zinc—are already supplied in ample amounts, as is vitamin D, which is likely deficient in those with this condition. nutreince is approved for individuals with Hashimoto's.

Additional beneficial supplements to consider:

Digestive enzymes: These can assist with digestion and enhance micronutrient availability and absorption. Look for a product with amylase, protease, and lipase, as well as a variety of other digestive enzymes. Betaine with pepsin may especially be beneficial for eliminating fatigue.

Curcumin: This active ingredient that gives turmeric its yellow color has an anti-inflammatory effect similar to that of cortisone, the prescription drug commonly dispensed for inflammation. In studies, it has been shown to remove amyloid plaque buildup in the brain that can cause Alzheimer's.

The Autoimmune 28-Day Menu Plan

Limited foods are *italicized* so that you can see where they fit into your plan.

Approved Miracle Pesto: Dairy-Free, Nut-Free Basil Miracle Pesto

Approved Miracle Butters: Herb Miracle Butter, Avocado Potassium-Packed Miracle Butter, Garlic-Parmesan Miracle Butter

Approved SKINNYFat Infusion: SKINNYFat Pizza in a Bottle Italian-Infused Oil (omit the hot peppers)

Approved SKINNYFat Salad Dressings: Simple SKINNYFat Italian Dressing (omit black pepper), SKINNYFat Parmesan-Peppercorn Dressing (omit peppercorn), Really Creamy SKINNYFat Blue Cheese Dressing

WEEK 1

DAY 1 (Sunday)

9:00 a.m. *Greek Yogurt and Fruit Bowl (page 331) or Baked Apple à la Micronutrient Miracle Mode (page 332)*

1:00 p.m. Traditional Triple Threat Shake (page 311)

5:00 p.m. Miracle Chinese Fried "Rice" (page 339)

9:00 p.m. Triple Threat Cheesecake (page 314)

DAY 2 (Monday)

7:30 a.m. Traditional Triple Threat Shake (page 311)

12:00 p.m. Leftover Miracle Chinese Fried "Rice"

3:30 p.m. Traditional Triple Threat Shake (page 311)

7:30 p.m. Salmon with asparagus and choice of approved Miracle Pesto or Miracle Butter (pages 315–318)

DAY 3 (Tuesday)

7:30 a.m. Triple Threat Cheesecake (page 314)

12:00 p.m. Big salad with leftover salmon and asparagus with choice of SKINNYFat dressing (pages 321–322)

3:30 p.m. Traditional Triple Threat Shake (page 311)

7:30 p.m. Greek Lamb Kabobs (page 341) and Tzatziki (page 320); omit the tomato from kabobs

DAY 4 (Wednesday)

7:30 a.m. Traditional Triple Threat Shake (page 311)

12:00 p.m. Leftover Greek Lamb Kabobs and Tzatziki

3:30 p.m. Triple Threat Pudding (page 313)

7:30 p.m. Quick Tandoori Shrimp (page 342) with Cooling Cucumber Raita (page 320); omit the cayenne pepper, paprika, and garam masala and replace with 1 tsp each of garlic powder, cinnamon, and onion powder

DAY 5 (Thursday)

7:30 a.m. Traditional Triple Threat Shake (page 311)

12:00 p.m. Big salad with leftover Quick Tandoori Shrimp and choice of SKINNYFat dressing (pages 321–322)

3:30 p.m. Triple Threat Pudding (page 313)

7:30 p.m. Bun-less beef burger and Oven-Roasted Brussels Sprouts (page 352)

DAY 6 (Friday)

7:30 a.m. Traditional Triple Threat Shake (page 311)

12:00 p.m. Broccoli Cheese Soup (page 327)

3:30 p.m. Traditional Triple Threat Shake (page 311)

7:30 p.m. Grilled steak with choice of approved Miracle Pesto or Miracle Butter (pages 315–318) and Cauliflower Mash (page 352)

DAY 7 (Saturday)

9:00 a.m. *Speedy Salmon Cakes (page 329) and eggs any style with grapefruit (or preferred fruit)*

1:00 p.m. Traditional Triple Threat Shake (page 311)

5:00 p.m. Fish with sautéed spinach, onions, and garlic

9:00 p.m. Chocolate Triple Threat Ice Cream (page 314)

WEEK 2

DAY 8 (Sunday)

9:00 a.m. French Onion Egg Tart (page 328)

1:00 p.m. Traditional Triple Threat Shake (page 311)

5:00 p.m. Zughetti (page 345) and shrimp with Rich and Creamy Alfredo Sauce (page 319)

9:00 p.m. Traditional Triple Threat Shake (page 311)

DAY 9 (Monday)

7:30 a.m. Traditional Triple Threat Shake (page 311)

12:00 p.m. *Grilled or broiled chicken thighs, choice of approved Miracle Pesto or Miracle Butter, and baked sweet potato*

3:30 p.m. Triple Threat Cheesecake (page 314)

7:30 p.m. Pork tenderloin and green beans in choice of approved Miracle Butter

DAY 10 (Tuesday)

7:30 a.m. Traditional Triple Threat Shake (page 311)

12:00 p.m. Big salad with leftover pork tenderloin and choice of SKINNYFat dressing (pages 321–322)

3:30 p.m. Traditional Triple Threat Shake (page 311)

7:30 p.m. Shepherd's Pie (page 351)

DAY 11 (Wednesday)

7:30 a.m. Traditional Triple Threat Shake (page 311)

12:00 p.m. Leftover Shepherd's Pie

3:30 p.m. Triple Threat Cheesecake (page 314)

7:30 p.m. Thai-Style Chopped Pork (page 347) on greens

DAY 12 (Thursday)

7:30 a.m. Traditional Triple Threat Shake (page 311)

12:00 p.m. Leftover chopped pork on a salad with choice of SKINNYFat dressing (pages 321–322)

3:30 p.m. Traditional Triple Threat Shake (page 311)

7:30 p.m. Scallops in Lemon Butter Sauce (page 334) with broccoli

DAY 13 (Friday)

7:30 a.m. Traditional Triple Threat Shake (page 311)

12:00 p.m. Mexican Chicken Wrap (page 338); use a lettuce wrap instead of the Ridiculously Simple Wrap, omit the salsa, and use fresh avocado instead of the guacamole

3:30 p.m. Traditional Triple Threat Shake (page 311)

7:30 p.m. Salad and Rustic Flatbread (page 346)

DAY 14 (Saturday)

9:00 a.m. *Carrot Cake Pancakes with Cream Cheese Frosting and chopped walnuts and raisins (page 333)*

1:00 p.m. Traditional Triple Threat Shake (page 311)

5:00 p.m. Micronutrient-Packed "Offaly" Tasty Meatloaf (page 348) and steamed vegetable with choice of approved Miracle Pesto or Miracle Butter

9:00 p.m. Triple Threat Cheesecake (page 314)

WEEK 3

DAY 15 (Sunday)

9:00 a.m. *Leftover meatloaf heated in a frying pan and topped with a fried egg and covered in melted cheese with a bowl of cut melon*

1:00 p.m. Traditional Triple Threat Shake (page 311)

5:00 p.m. Bun-less ground lamb burger seasoned with cinnamon, turmeric, and garlic served with Oven-Roasted Brussels Sprouts (page 352)

9:00 p.m. Traditional Triple Threat Shake (page 311)

DAY 16 (Monday)

7:30 a.m. Traditional Triple Threat Shake (page 311)

12:00 p.m. Big salad with ½ can of tuna fish and choice of SKINNYFat dressing (pages 321–322)

3:30 p.m. Traditional Triple Threat Shake (page 311)

7:30 p.m. Chicken Wings (page 334) tossed in Garlic-Parmesan Miracle Butter (page 317) with Really Creamy SKINNYFat Blue Cheese Dressing (page 322) and carrot and celery sticks

DAY 17 (Tuesday)

7:30 a.m. Traditional Triple Threat Shake (page 311)

12:00 p.m. Leftover chicken wings and blue cheese dressing

3:30 p.m. Triple Threat Cheesecake (page 314)

7:30 p.m. Steak with mushrooms and onions sautéed in garlic and butter

DAY 18 (Wednesday)

7:30 a.m. Traditional Triple Threat Shake (page 311)

12:00 p.m. Leftover steak strips on a salad with choice of SKINNYFat dressing (pages 321–322)

3:30 p.m. Traditional Triple Threat Shake (page 311)

7:30 p.m. Zughetti (page 345) and grilled chicken thigh with Rich and Creamy Alfredo Sauce (page 319)

DAY 19 (Thursday)

7:30 a.m. Triple Threat Cheesecake (page 314)

12:00 p.m. Bun-less beef burger and a side salad with choice of SKINNYFat dressing (pages 321–322)

3:30 p.m. Traditional Triple Threat Shake (page 311)

7:30 p.m. Thai Shrimp Noodle Soup (page 326)

DAY 20 (Friday)

7:30 a.m. Traditional Triple Threat Shake (page 311)

12:00 p.m. Leftover Thai Shrimp Noodle Soup

3:30 p.m. Traditional Triple Threat Shake (page 311)

7:30 p.m. *Rotisserie or baked whole chicken with Sweet Potato, Yam, and Apple Casserole (page 353)*

DAY 21 (Saturday)

9:00 a.m. Fried eggs served on Cauliflower Cheesy Hash Browns (page 329)

1:00 p.m. Traditional Triple Threat Shake (page 311)

5:00 p.m. Miracle Chinese Fried "Rice" (page 339)

9:00 p.m. Traditional Triple Threat Shake (page 311)

WEEK 4

DAY 22 (Sunday)

9:00 a.m. Smoked Salmon Cream Cheese Roll-Ups (page 331) with avocado slices and an egg

1:00 p.m. Traditional Triple Threat Shake (page 311)

5:00 p.m. Micronutrient-Packed "Offaly" Tasty Meatloaf (page 348) with vegetables and choice of approved Miracle Pesto or Miracle Butter

9:00 p.m. Chocolate Triple Threat Ice Cream (page 314)

DAY 23 (Monday)

7:30 a.m. Traditional Triple Threat Shake (page 311)

12:00 p.m. Leftover Miracle Chinese Fried "Rice"

3:30 p.m. Triple Threat Cheesecake (page 314)

7:30 p.m. Fish and vegetables with choice of approved Miracle Pesto or Miracle Butter

DAY 24 (Tuesday)

7:30 a.m. Traditional Triple Threat Shake (page 311)

12:00 p.m. Leftover meatloaf with a side salad and choice of SKINNYFat dressing

3:30 p.m. Triple Threat Pudding (page 313)

7:30 p.m. *Fish and Chips (page 350); substituting the rice flour with ⅔ cup coconut flour and ⅓ cup arrowroot powder; only use sweet potato for chips*

DAY 25 (Wednesday)

7:30 a.m. Traditional Triple Threat Shake (page 311)

12:00 p.m. Broccoli Cheese Soup (page 327)

3:30 p.m. Triple Threat Cheesecake (page 314)

7:30 p.m. Grilled Tandoori Skewers (page 342); omit the tomatoes and cayenne pepper

DAY 26 (Thursday)

7:30 a.m. Traditional Triple Threat Shake (page 311)

12:00 p.m. Bun-less beef burger and Oven-Roasted Brussels Sprouts (page 352)

3:30 p.m. Traditional Triple Threat Shake (page 311)

7:30 p.m. Chicken thigh with broccoli sautéed in lemon butter sauce (use the sauce recipe from the scallops on page 334)

DAY 27 (Friday)

7:30 a.m. Traditional Triple Threat Shake (page 311)

12:00 p.m. Leftover Grilled Tandoori Skewers on a big salad with choice of SKINNYFat dressing

3:30 p.m. Triple Threat Pudding (page 313)

7:30 p.m. *Peppercorn-Crusted Beef Tenderloin (page 341) with 4-Ingredient Blender Hollandaise (page 323) and baked potato (omit the peppercorn and rub with sage)*

DAY 28 (Saturday)

9:00 a.m. Protein-Packed Morning Muffins (page 330); omit the tomato

1:00 p.m. Traditional Triple Threat Shake (page 311)

5:00 p.m. Fabulous Fajitas (page 349) with Holy Moly Guacamole (page 324) and sour cream; replace the bell peppers with cauliflower and broccoli, and make the guacamole without tomato, jalapeño pepper, and black pepper.

9:00 p.m. Chocolate Triple Threat Ice Cream (page 314)

Digestive Health

This plan is specifically designed for individuals who are suffering from a digestive health issue. This protocol will help you to create an internal environment that will aid in healing the digestive system and reduce intestinal permeability (leaky gut).

The Digestive Health protocol is designed for individuals who have:

- Irritable bowel syndrome
- Leaky gut
- Inflammatory bowel disease
- Colitis or ulcerative colitis
- Heartburn/gastroesophageal reflux disease (the Ketogenic protocol also works well for this)

Adjustments you must make to the Signature 28-day Micronutrient Miracle plan for your specific condition(s):

10 GOLDEN RULES: While each of the condition-specific protocols must follow all 10 of the Golden Rules, for best results with this protocol, we have identified the following rules to either be critical or require small tweaks.

#7: Purchasing new nontoxic alternatives for your beauty, cleaning, and hygiene products is especially important while following this protocol.

#8: Individuals suffering from digestive issues often have difficulty absorbing the micronutrients in food, as well as in capsules and pills. Therefore, taking a well-formulated liquid multivitamin, like nutreince, is essential for sufficiency. Use the free online stack-up quiz to compare any other prospective multivitamin (MultivitaminStackUpQuiz.com).

#9: Taking your Micronutrient Miracle Triple Threat Shakes twice a day is especially important while following this protocol, as it will provide you with the amino acid L-glutamine, which has been shown to have an anti-inflammatory effect that can aid in the healing of the intestinal lining by repelling gut irritants. And researchers believe that the whey component alpha-lactalbumin may help prevent gastric injury, ulcers, and other gastrointestinal pathologies.

EMD ALERT: During this protocol, avoid antacids as well as aspirin, ibuprofen, or other NSAIDs, as they could irritate your gastrointestinal tract lining.

DAILY LIMITS: The daily limits for the Digestive Health protocol are slightly stricter than for our Signature plan. For the next 28 days, adhere to the following limits.

Starches/fruits/nuts/seeds: Two servings per week, but with restrictions. You can still enjoy a total of two gluten-free starches *or* two fruits each week (*or* one of each). However, eliminate all grains, nuts, seeds, berries, and beans, as they may cause digestive issues in some.

Alcohol: Rather than having one or two glasses a day, eliminate alcohol altogether for the next 28 days to allow for gut healing.

Caffeinated drinks: Try to eliminate caffeinated drinks during this protocol and drink only decaffeinated beverages; however, if you *need* caffeine, limit your intake to one cup per day.

Bone broth: Add this food to your daily protocol. Try to drink a small cup of homemade bone broth each morning for the next 28 days.

Beneficial micronutrients used in the prevention and treatment of digestive conditions:

Vitamin A	Vitamin B_7	Iron
Vitamin B_1	Vitamin B_9	Magnesium
Vitamin B_2	Vitamin B_{12}	Phosphorus
Vitamin B_3	Vitamin C	Zinc
Vitamin B_5	Vitamin D	Omega-3 fatty acids
Vitamin B_6	Calcium	

POWERHOUSE PICKS: Choose these micronutrient powerhouses whenever possible. The Rich Foods listed below are high in the essential micronutrients shown to be beneficial to digestive health. Additionally, the spices and beverages listed below have been shown to have an anti-inflammatory effect. We have adjusted your 28-day menu suggestions to include many of these Rich Food choices. Choose these Rich Foods when designing personalized menus or eating out, and don't forget to properly prepare foods that contain EMDs.

PROTEINS

Beef	Mussels	Shrimp
Bone broth	Organ meats	Snapper
Chicken	Oysters	Tuna
Clams	Pork	Turkey
Crab	Rainbow trout	Venison
Dungeness crab	Salmon	
Herring	Sardines	
Lamb	Scallops	

DAIRY

Cheese

Cream

Milk

Yogurt

FATS

Butter

Coconut oil

Eggs (with yolks)

SKINNYFat*

*SKINNYFat is perfect for the more than 25 million Americans with a removed or poorly functioning gall-bladder. Because MCTs (the main ingredient in SKINNYFat) do not need bile salts or pancreatic enzymes for digestion, SKINNYFat is easily digestible.

NONSTARCHY VEGETABLES

Asparagus

Avocado

Bell peppers

Broccoli

Brussels sprouts

Cabbage

Cauliflower

Chile peppers

Dark leafy greens

Garlic

Kale

Mushrooms

Onion

Romaine lettuce

Snow peas

Spinach (cooked)

Sprouts

Swiss chard

STARCHES

Green peas

Potatoes

Sweet potatoes

FRUITS

Bananas

Grapefruit

Limes

Oranges

Prunes

Raisins

Strawberries

Watermelon

NUTS AND SEEDS

Eliminated

BENEFICIAL SPICES

Cardamom

Chile spice

Cinnamon

Cloves

Dill

Garlic powder

Ginger

Onion powder

Sage

Turmeric

DAILY BEVERAGES

Coffee	*Herbal teas*	*Water*
Green tea	*Mineral water*	

Additional essential micronutrient supplements to consider:

Iron: Individuals suffering from leaky gut and other digestive health issues are prone to iron deficiency due to malabsorption. Try to get 8 milligrams (men) or 18 milligrams (women) per day, either through your food or in supplement form.

Note: It is imperative that you take iron in supplement form at a separate time from your multivitamin (nutreince). Iron is the most competitive micronutrient, conflicting with 10 other micronutrients. Take it midday on an empty stomach.

Omega-3: Omega-3s play a vital role in helping to ensure optimum digestion and healthy bowel function. In studies, supplementation has been shown to reduce the inflammation and pain associated with leaky gut and ulcerative colitis. Attempt to get the RDI of 1.6 grams (1,600 milligrams) per day from food or in supplement form.

Note: You can take approximately 1,000 milligrams of omega-3s in supplement form with your AM multivitamin (nutreince) and 1,000 milligrams with your PM multivitamin. Opt for Origin Omega or try to find an omega-3 supplement with a greater amount of EPA than DHA, if possible.

Additional beneficial supplements to consider:

Digestive enzymes: These can assist with digestion and enhance micronutrient availability and absorption. Look for a product with amylase, protease, and lipase, as well as a variety of other digestive enzymes, such as bromelain, ox bile, pancreatin, papain, pepsin, and betaine HCL. Remember, taking betaine HCL with pepsin can eleviate heartburn efficiently with medication.

Curcumin: This active ingredient found in the Indian spice turmeric can be very helpful for digestive issues. Not only can it treat pain directly, but it also has anti-inflammatory properties similar to cortisone, the prescription drug commonly dispensed for inflammation. In studies, it has been shown to prevent ulcerations, including gastritis, peptic ulcers, irritable bowel syndrome, and colitis.

Licorice root: Drink this herbal tea or chew it in wafers (look for DGL—a specific type of licorice) before meals to guard against digestive issues. Licorice root increases the production of mucin, which protects the gut lining from stomach acid.

Peppermint oil capsules: Choose capsules that are enteric coated to ensure that they make it deep into your digestive tract before dissolving. This oil relaxes the muscles of the intestinal walls, preventing dyspepsia (indigestion).

Ginger tea: Ginger soothes the gut and has been used for generations as a digestive aid.

L-glutamine: This amino acid that heals the epithelial cells lining the small intestine will already be supplemented through the addition of IN.POWER whey protein. If you are omitting the protein Triple Threat meal replacement shakes, you may want to consider supplementation with 2 to 4 grams of powdered L-glutamine. You can add this to your nutreince multivitamin drink or to cold water taken separately from your meals.

The Digestive Health 28-Day Menu Plan

Limited foods are *italicized* so that you can see where they fit into your plan.

Approved Miracle Pesto: Dairy-Free, Nut-Free Basil Miracle Pesto

Approved Miracle Butters: All Miracle Butters

Approved SKINNYFat Infusions: All SKINNYFat Infusions

Approved SKINNYFat Salad Dressings: All SKINNYFat salad dressings

WEEK 1

DAY 1 (Sunday)

9:00 a.m. *Greek Yogurt and Fruit Bowl (page 331)* or *Baked Apple à la Micronutrient Miracle Mode (page 332)*

1:00 p.m. Traditional Triple Threat Shake (page 311)

5:00 p.m. Buffalo Chicken Chili (page 340)

9:00 p.m. Triple Threat Pudding (page 313)

DAY 2 (Monday)

7:30 a.m. Traditional Triple Threat Shake (page 311)

12:00 p.m. Leftover Buffalo Chicken Chili

3:30 p.m. Traditional Triple Threat Shake (page 311)

7:30 p.m. Salmon with asparagus and choice of approved Miracle Pesto or Miracle Butter (pages 315–318)

DAY 3 (Tuesday)

7:30 a.m. Triple Threat Cheesecake (page 314)

12:00 p.m. Big salad with leftover salmon and asparagus with choice of SKINNYFat salad dressing (pages 321–322)

3:30 p.m. Traditional Triple Threat Shake (page 311)

7:30 p.m. Greek Chicken (page 337)

DAY 4 (Wednesday)

7:30 a.m. Traditional Triple Threat Shake (page 311)

12:00 p.m. Leftover Greek Chicken

3:30 p.m. Triple Threat Pudding (page 313)

7:30 p.m. Quick Tandoori Shrimp (page 336) with Cooling Cucumber Raita (page 320)

DAY 5 (Thursday)

7:30 a.m. Triple Threat Cheesecake (page 314)

12:00 p.m. Big salad with leftover Quick Tandoori Shrimp and choice of SKINNYFat dressing (pages 321–322)

3:30 p.m. Traditional Triple Threat Shake (page 311)

7:30 p.m. Bun-less beef burger and Oven-Roasted Brussels Sprouts (page 352)

DAY 6 (Friday)

7:30 a.m. Traditional Triple Threat Shake (page 311)

12:00 p.m. Broccoli Cheese Soup (page 327)

3:30 p.m. Traditional Triple Threat Shake (page 311)

7:30 p.m. Grilled steak with choice of approved Miracle Pesto or Miracle Butter (pages 315–318) and Cauliflower Mash (page 352)

DAY 7 (Saturday)

9:00 a.m. Speedy Salmon Cakes (page 319) and eggs any style

1:00 p.m. Traditional Triple Threat Shake (page 311)

5:00 p.m. *Fish and Chips (page 350); substituting the rice flour with ⅔ cup coconut flour and ⅓ cup arrowroot flour*

9:00 p.m. Chocolate Triple Threat Ice Cream (page 314)

WEEK 2

DAY 8 (Sunday)

9:00 a.m. French Onion Egg Tart (page 328)

1:00 p.m. Traditional Triple Threat Shake (page 311)

5:00 p.m. Zughetti (page 345) with Mom's Beef Bolognese (page 324)

9:00 p.m. Traditional Triple Threat Shake (page 311)

DAY 9 (Monday)

7:30 a.m. Traditional Triple Threat Shake (page 311)

12:00 p.m. *Grilled or broiled chicken thighs, choice of approved Miracle Pesto or Miracle Butter, and baked sweet potato*

3:30 p.m. Triple Threat Pudding (page 313)

7:30 p.m. Moqueca (aka Brazilian Fish Stew) (page 343)

DAY 10 (Tuesday)

7:30 a.m. Traditional Triple Threat Shake (page 311)

12:00 p.m. Leftover Moqueca

3:30 p.m. Traditional Triple Threat Shake (page 311)

7:30 p.m. Coq au Vin (page 347) served with Cauliflower Mash (page 352)

DAY 11 (Wednesday)

7:30 a.m. Traditional Triple Threat Shake (page 311)

12:00 p.m. Leftover Coq au Vin

3:30 p.m. Triple Threat Cheesecake (page 314)

7:30 p.m. Thai-Style Chopped Pork (page 347) on greens

DAY 12 (Thursday)

7:30 a.m. Traditional Triple Threat Shake (page 311)

12:00 p.m. Leftover chopped pork on a salad with choice of SKINNYFat dressing (pages 321–322)

3:30 p.m. Traditional Triple Threat Shake (page 311)

7:30 p.m. Scallops in Lemon Butter Sauce (page 334) with broccoli

DAY 13 (Friday)

7:30 a.m. Traditional Triple Threat Shake (page 311)

12:00 p.m. Mexican Chicken Wrap (page 338); use a lettuce wrap instead of the Ridiculously Simple Wrap

3:30 p.m. Traditional Triple Threat Shake (page 311)

7:30 p.m. Salad and Rustic Flatbread (page 346)

DAY 14 (Saturday)

9:00 a.m. *Carrot Cake Pancakes with Cream Cheese Frosting and chopped walnuts and raisins (page 333)*

1:00 p.m. Traditional Triple Threat Shake (page 311)

5:00 p.m. Micronutrient-Packed "Offaly" Tasty Meatloaf (page 348) and steamed vegetable with choice of approved Miracle Pesto or Miracle Butter

9:00 p.m. Triple Threat Cheesecake (page 314)

WEEK 3

DAY 15 (Sunday)

9:00 a.m. Leftover meatloaf heated in a frying pan and topped with a fried egg and covered in melted cheese

1:00 p.m. Traditional Triple Threat Shake (page 311)

5:00 p.m. *Camarão na Moranga (aka Brazilian Shrimp Stew in a Pumpkin) (page 335)*

9:00 p.m. Traditional Triple Threat Shake (page 311)

DAY 16 (Monday)

7:30 a.m. Traditional Triple Threat Shake (page 311)

12:00 p.m. Big salad with ½ can of tuna fish and choice of SKINNYFat dressing (pages 321–322)

3:30 p.m. Traditional Triple Threat Shake (page 311)

7:30 p.m. Chicken Wings (page 301) with Really Creamy SKINNYFat Blue Cheese Dressing (page 319) and carrot and celery sticks

DAY 17 (Tuesday)

7:30 a.m. Traditional Triple Threat Shake (page 311)

12:00 p.m. Leftover chicken wings and blue cheese dressing

3:30 p.m. Triple Threat Cheesecake (page 314)

7:30 p.m. Shepherd's Pie (page 352)

DAY 18 (Wednesday)

7:30 a.m. Traditional Triple Threat Shake (page 311)

12:00 p.m. Leftover Shepherd's Pie

3:30 p.m. Traditional Triple Threat Shake (page 311)

7:30 p.m. Zughetti (page 345) and grilled chicken thigh with Rich and Creamy Alfredo Sauce (page 319)

DAY 19 (Thursday)

7:30 a.m. Triple Threat Cheesecake (page 314)

12:00 p.m. Bun-less beef burger and a side salad with choice of SKINNYFat dressing (pages 321–322)

3:30 p.m. Traditional Triple Threat Shake (page 311)

7:30 p.m. Thai Shrimp Noodle Soup (page 326)

DAY 20 (Friday)

7:30 a.m. Traditional Triple Threat Shake (page 311)

12:00 p.m. Leftover Thai Shrimp Noodle Soup

3:30 p.m. Traditional Triple Threat Shake (page 311)

7:30 p.m. *Rotisserie or baked whole chicken with Sweet Potato, Yam, and Apple Casserole (page 353)*

DAY 21 (Saturday)

9:00 a.m. Fried eggs served on Cauliflower Cheesy Hash Browns (page 352)

1:00 p.m. Traditional Triple Threat Shake (page 311)

5:00 p.m. Miracle Chinese Fried "Rice" (page 339)

9:00 p.m. Traditional Triple Threat Shake (page 311)

WEEK 4

DAY 22 (Sunday)

9:00 a.m. *Smoked Salmon Cream Cheese Roll-Ups (page 331) with avocado slices and berries or grapefruit*

1:00 p.m. Traditional Triple Threat Shake (page 311)

5:00 p.m. Slow-Cooked Beer-Braised Beef (page 338) and Cauliflower Mash (page 352)

9:00 p.m. Chocolate Triple Threat Ice Cream (page 314)

DAY 23 (Monday)

7:30 a.m. Traditional Triple Threat Shake (page 311)

12:00 p.m. Leftover Miracle Chinese Fried "Rice"

3:30 p.m. Traditional Triple Threat Shake (page 311)

7:30 p.m. Fish and vegetables with choice of approved Miracle Pesto or Miracle Butter

DAY 24 (Tuesday)

7:30 a.m. Traditional Triple Threat Shake (page 311)

12:00 p.m. Leftover Slow-Cooked Beer-Braised Beef and Cauliflower Mash

3:30 p.m. Triple Threat Cheesecake (page 314)

7:30 p.m. Greek Lamb Kabobs (page 341) with Tzatziki (page 320)

DAY 25 (Wednesday)

7:30 a.m. Traditional Triple Threat Shake (page 311)

12:00 p.m. Leftover Greek Lamb Kabobs on a salad with Tzatziki

3:30 p.m. Triple Threat Pudding (page 313)

7:30 p.m. Fabulous Fajitas (page 349) with Holy Moly Guacamole (page 324) and salsa (omit the wraps)

DAY 26 (Thursday)

7:30 a.m. Traditional Triple Threat Shake (page 311)

12:00 p.m. Bun-less beef burger and Oven-Roasted Brussels Sprouts (page 352)

3:30 p.m. Traditional Triple Threat Shake (page 311)

7:30 p.m. Rustic Portobello Pizza Caps (page 344)

DAY 27 (Friday)

7:30 a.m. Triple Threat Cheesecake (page 311)

12:00 p.m. Grilled or broiled chicken thigh on a big salad with choice of SKINNYFat dressing (pages 321–322)

3:30 p.m. Traditional Triple Threat Shake (page 311)

7:30 p.m. *Peppercorn-Crusted Beef Tenderloin (page 341) with 4-Ingredient Blender Hollandaise (page 323) and baked potato*

DAY 28 (Saturday)

9:00 a.m. Protein-Packed Morning Muffins (page 330)

1:00 p.m. Traditional Triple Threat Shake (page 311)

5:00 p.m. Grilled Tandoori Skewers (page 309) with Cooling Cucumber Raita (page 287)

9:00 p.m. Chocolate Triple Threat Ice Cream (page 314)

Blood Sugar Regulation

This plan is specifically designed for individuals who are suffering from blood sugar–related health issues. This protocol will help you create an internal environment that will aid in regulating your blood sugar levels naturally. You may also want to consider our Ketogenic protocol.

The Blood Sugar Regulation protocol is designed for individuals who have:

- Dysglycemia
- Hypoglycemia
- Type 1 or 2 diabetes

Adjustments you must make to the Signature 28-day Micronutrient Miracle plan for your specific condition(s):

10 GOLDEN RULES: While each of the condition-specific protocols must follow all 10 of the Golden Rules, for best results with this protocol, we have identified the following rules to either be critical or require small tweaks.

#2: Make sure to be keenly aware of eliminating MSG, BPA, and phthalates. Research indicates that BPA triggers the release of almost double the insulin actually needed to break down food. High insulin levels can desensitize the body to the hormone over time, which in some people may then lead to weight gain and type 2 diabetes.

#6: Make sure to practice both ZMT and One Set To Failure; a 2012 study published in the *Archives of Internal Medicine* (now *JAMA Internal Medicine*) showed that men who lifted weights and added in regular cardiovascular exercise (like our ZMT training) slashed their risk of type 2 diabetes by 59 percent.

#8: Micronutrient supplementation is key for regulating blood sugar levels. Make sure that your multivitamin contains beneficial quantities of key micronutrients, such as vitamins D and K, magnesium, and all eight forms of vitamin E. nutreince contains beneficial quantities of all these, along with the safest, most-absorbable form of chromium—chromium polynicotinate, a pure niacin-bound form identified by US government researchers as the active component of true GTF (Glucose Tolerance Factor), which regulates the body's use of glucose and helps to balance blood sugar levels. Vanadium, a mineral that studies suggest may improve glucose tolerance, is also added to nutreince. Use the free online quiz to compare other prospective multivitamins at MultivitaminStackUpQuiz.com.

#9: Taking your Micronutrient Miracle Triple Threat Shakes twice a day is especially important while following this protocol, as whey protein supplementation has been shown to lower blood glucose levels by nearly 30 percent. It will also provide you with the amino acid L-glutamine, which has been shown to aid in sugar cravings. In addition to your Triple Threat Shakes, studies suggest that taking whey protein (in the equivalent of one scoop of IN.POWER) approximately 30 minutes before each solid meal significantly reduced blood glucose levels even in subjects with the most severe insulin resistance—without affecting the rate of insulin secretion.

EMD ALERT: Be extremely cautious. Read all ingredient labels to verify that products do not contain any hidden sugar. Additionally, don't forget to properly prepare foods that contain EMDs to reduce possible depletion.

DAILY LIMITS: The daily limits for the Blood Sugar Regulation protocol are slightly stricter than for our Signature plan. For the next 28 days, adhere to the following limits.

Starches/fruits/nuts/seeds: One serving per week. You can enjoy a total of one gluten-free starch or one fruit or 1 serving of nuts/seeds once a week.

Alcohol: Rather than having one or two glasses a day, limit alcohol to up to three glasses a week. Eliminate gluten-fee beers, or limit yourself to one.

Caffeinated drinks: Two cups daily (same as the Signature plan). The chlorogenic acid found in coffee and tea has been shown to reduce insulin resistance and chronic inflammation.

Bone broth: Add this food to your daily protocol. Try to drink homemade bone broth frequently; your collagen—the structural matrix of your body—can be damaged due to chronically high blood sugar levels.

Beneficial micronutrients used in the prevention and treatment of blood sugar regulation:

Choline	Vitamin C	Magnesium
Vitamin B_3	Vitamin D	Manganese
Vitamin B_5	Vitamin E	Zinc
Vitamin B_6	Vitamin K	Omega-3 fatty acids
Vitamin B_7	Chromium	

POWERHOUSE PICKS: Choose these micronutrient powerhouses whenever possible. The Rich Foods listed below are high in the essential micronutrients shown to be beneficial to blood sugar regulation. We have adjusted your 28-day menu suggestions to include many of these Rich Food choices. Make an effort to choose these Rich Foods when designing personalized menus or eating out.

PROTEINS

Beef	Lamb	Sardines
Bone broth	Mussels	Scallops
Chicken	Organ meats	Shrimp
Clams	Oysters	Snapper
Crab	Pork	Tuna
Dungeness crab	Rainbow trout	Turkey
Herring	Salmon	Venison

DAIRY

Cheese, specifically Gouda	Milk
Cream	Yogurt

FATS

Butter	Eggs (with yolks)
Coconut oil	SKINNYFat*

*Use SKINNYFat in recipes whenever possible as it is virtually impossible to store as body fat. Peer-reviewed published research also shows that MCT oil (the main ingredient in SKINNYFat) increases metabolism, reduces body fat, and improves insulin sensitivity and glucose tolerance, while the long-chain triglycerides in the coconut oil in SKINNYFat aid in the absorption of your essential micronutrients.

NONSTARCHY VEGETABLES

Avocado	Chile peppers	Onions
Bell peppers	Dark leafy greens	Romaine lettuce
Broccoli	Garlic	Snow peas
Brussels sprouts	Kale	Spinach (cooked)
Cabbage	Mushrooms	Swiss chard
Cauliflower	Mustard greens	Tomatoes

STARCHES

Green peas	Quinoa
Potatoes	Sweet potatoes

FRUITS

Bananas	Grapefruit	Pineapple
Coconut water (counts as a fruit, not as a beverage; check carefully for sugar)	Limes	Strawberries
	Oranges	Watermelon
	Papaya	

NUTS AND SEEDS

Almonds	Hazelnuts	Sesame seeds
Cashews	Peanuts	Sunflower seeds
Chia seeds	Pine nuts	Walnuts
Flaxseed	Pumpkins seeds	

BENEFICIAL SPICES

Chile spice	Marjoram	Rosemary
Cinnamon	Onion powder	Turmeric
Garlic powder	Oregano	

DAILY BEVERAGES

Coffee	Mineral water
Green tea	Water

Additional essential micronutrient supplements to consider:

Omega-3s: Studies show that people on a weight-loss diet that included fat-rich fish daily had improved glucose and insulin metabolism. Attempt to get the RDI of 1.6 grams (1,600 milligrams) per day from food or in supplement form.

Note: You can take approximately 1,000 milligrams of omega-3s in supplement form with your AM multivitamin (nutreince) and 1,000 milligrams with your PM multivitamin. Opt for Origin Omega or try to find an omega-3 supplement with a greater amount of EPA than DHA, if possible.

Additional beneficial supplements to consider:

Curcumin: In studies, curcumin, the active ingredient in the Indian spice turmeric, has been shown to switch on the liver genes that keep glucose levels in check. It improves the pancreas's ability to make insulin and helps slow down the metabolism of carbohydrates after meals.

Blood Sugar Regulation 28-Day Menu Plan

Limited foods are *italicized* so that you can see where they fit into your plan.

Feel free to choose from any of the Miracle Pestos, Miracle Butters, SKINNYFat Salad Dressings, and SKINNYFat Infusions, as they all fit into the Blood Sugar Regulation protocol.

WEEK 1

DAY 1 (Sunday)

9:00 a.m. Greek Yogurt and Fruit Bowl (page 331) and an egg any style; omit the fruit

1:00 p.m. Traditional Triple Threat Shake (page 311)

5:00 p.m. Buffalo Chicken Chili (page 340)

9:00 p.m. Triple Threat Pudding (page 313)

DAY 2 (Monday)

7:30 a.m. Triple Threat Cheesecake (page 314)

12:00 p.m. Leftover Buffalo Chicken Chili

3:30 p.m. Traditional Triple Threat Shake (page 311)

7:30 p.m. Salmon with broccoli and choice of a Miracle Pesto or Miracle Butter (pages 315–318)

DAY 3 (Tuesday)

7:30 a.m. Triple Threat Cheesecake (page 314)

12:00 p.m. Big salad with leftover salmon and broccoli with choice of SKINNYFat dressing (pages 321–322)

3:30 p.m. Traditional Triple Threat Shake (page 311)

7:30 p.m. Greek Chicken (page 337)

DAY 4 (Wednesday)

7:30 a.m. Traditional Triple Threat Shake (page 311)

12:00 p.m. Leftover Greek Chicken

3:30 p.m. Triple Threat Pudding (page 313)

7:30 p.m. Quick Tandoori Shrimp (page 336) with Cooling Cucumber Raita (page 320) and optional Indian Garlic-Butter Cheese Non-Naan (page 354)

DAY 5 (Thursday)

7:30 a.m. Traditional Triple Threat Shake (page 311)

12:00 p.m. Big salad with leftover Quick Tandoori Shrimp and choice of SKINNYFat dressing (pages 321–322)

3:30 p.m. Triple Threat Pudding (page 313)

7:30 p.m. Bun-less beef burger and Oven-Roasted Brussels Sprouts (page 352)

DAY 6 (Friday)

7:30 a.m. Traditional Triple Threat Shake (page 311)

12:00 p.m. Broccoli Cheese Soup (page 327)

3:30 p.m. Traditional Triple Threat Shake (page 311)

7:30 p.m. Grilled steak with choice of a Miracle Pesto (page 315–318) and Cauliflower Mash (page 352)

DAY 7 (Saturday)

9:00 a.m. Speedy Salmon Cakes (page 329) and eggs any style

1:00 p.m. Traditional Triple Threat Shake (page 311)

5:00 p.m. *Fish and Chips (page 350)*

9:00 p.m. Chocolate Triple Threat Ice Cream (page 314)

WEEK 2

DAY 8 (Sunday)

9:00 a.m. French Onion Egg Tart (page 328)

1:00 p.m. Traditional Triple Threat Shake (page 311)

5:00 p.m. Zughetti (page 345) with shrimp sautéed in Sun-Dried Tomato Miracle Pesto (page 316)

9:00 p.m. Traditional Triple Threat Shake (page 311)

DAY 9 (Monday)

7:30 a.m. Traditional Triple Threat Shake (page 311)

12:00 p.m. Grilled or broiled chicken thighs and spinach sautéed in choice of a Miracle Pesto or Miracle Butter (pages 315–318)

3:30 p.m. Triple Threat Cheesecake (page 311)

7:30 p.m. Moqueca (aka Brazilian Fish Stew) (page 343)

DAY 10 (Tuesday)

7:30 a.m. Triple Threat Cheesecake (page 314)

12:00 p.m. Leftover Moqueca

3:30 p.m. Traditional Triple Threat Shake (page 314)

7:30 p.m. Coq au Vin (page 347) served with Cauliflower Mash (page 352)

DAY 11 (Wednesday)

7:30 a.m. Traditional Triple Threat Shake (page 311)

12:00 p.m. Leftover Coq au Vin

3:30 p.m. Triple Threat Pudding (page 313)

7:30 p.m. Thai-Style Chopped Pork (page 347) on greens

DAY 12 (Thursday)

7:30 a.m. Traditional Triple Threat Shake (page 311)

12:00 p.m. Leftover chopped pork on a salad with choice of SKINNYFat dressing (pages 321–322)

3:30 p.m. Traditional Triple Threat Shake (page 311)

7:30 p.m. Scallops in Lemon Butter Sauce (page 334) with broccoli

DAY 13 (Friday)

7:30 a.m. Traditional Triple Threat Shake (page 311)

12:00 p.m. Mexican Chicken Wrap (page 338); choice of using Ridiculously Simple Wrap or lettuce wrap

3:30 p.m. Traditional Triple Threat Shake (page 311)

7:30 p.m. Salad and Rustic Flatbread (page 346)

DAY 14 (Saturday)

9:00 a.m. *Carrot Cake Pancakes with Cream Cheese Frosting and chopped walnuts and raisins (page 333)*

1:00 p.m. Traditional Triple Threat Shake (page 311)

5:00 p.m. Micronutrient-Packed "Offaly" Tasty Meatloaf (page 348) and steamed vegetable with choice of a Miracle Pesto or Miracle Butter (pages 315–318)

9:00 p.m. Triple Threat Pudding (page 313)

WEEK 3

DAY 15 (Sunday)

9:00 a.m. Leftover meatloaf heated in a frying pan topped with a slice of cream cheese, a fried egg, and melted cheese

1:00 p.m. Traditional Triple Threat Shake (page 311)

5:00 p.m. *Camarão na Moranga (aka Brazilian Shrimp Stew in a Pumpkin) (page 335)*

9:00 p.m. Traditional Triple Threat Shake (page 311)

DAY 16 (Monday)

7:30 a.m. Traditional Triple Threat Shake (page 311)

12:00 p.m. Big salad with ½ can of tuna fish and choice of SKINNYFat dressing (pages 321–322)

3:30 p.m. Traditional Triple Threat Shake (page 311)

7:30 p.m. Chicken Wings (page 334) with Really Creamy SKINNYFat Blue Cheese Dressing (page 322) and carrot and celery sticks

DAY 17 (Tuesday)

7:30 a.m. Traditional Triple Threat Shake (page 311)

12:00 p.m. Leftover chicken wings and blue cheese dressing

3:30 p.m. Triple Threat Cheesecake (page 314)

7:30 p.m. Shepherd's Pie (page 351)

DAY 18 (Wednesday)

7:30 a.m. Traditional Triple Threat Shake (page 311)

12:00 p.m. Leftover Shepherd's Pie

3:30 p.m. Traditional Triple Threat Shake (page 311)

7:30 p.m. Zughetti (page 345) and grilled chicken thigh with Rich and Creamy Alfredo Sauce (page 319)

DAY 19 (Thursday)

7:30 a.m. Triple Threat Cheesecake (page 311)

12:00 p.m. Bun-less beef burger and a side salad with choice of SKINNYFat dressing (pages 321–322)

3:30 p.m. Traditional Triple Threat Shake (page 311)

7:30 p.m. Thai Shrimp Noodle Soup (page 326)

DAY 20 (Friday)

7:30 a.m. Traditional Triple Threat Shake (page 311)

12:00 p.m. Leftover Thai Shrimp Noodle Soup

3:30 p.m. Traditional Triple Threat Shake (page 311)

7:30 p.m. Rotisserie or baked whole chicken with sautéed mushrooms and onions

DAY 21 (Saturday)

9:00 a.m. Fried eggs served on Cauliflower Cheesy Hash Browns (page 329)

1:00 p.m. Traditional Triple Threat Shake (page 311)

5:00 p.m. Miracle Chinese Fried "Rice" (page 339)

9:00 p.m. Traditional Triple Threat Shake (page 311)

WEEK 4

DAY 22 (Sunday)

9:00 a.m. Smoked Salmon Cream Cheese Roll-Ups (page 331) with avocado slices and an egg any style

1:00 p.m. Traditional Triple Threat Shake (page 311)

5:00 p.m. Slow-Cooked Beer-Braised Beef (page 338) and Cauliflower Mash (page 352)

9:00 p.m. Chocolate Triple Threat Ice Cream (page 314)

DAY 23 (Monday)

7:30 a.m. Traditional Triple Threat Shake (page 311)

12:00 p.m. Leftover Miracle Chinese Fried "Rice"

3:30 p.m. Traditional Triple Threat Shake (page 311)

7:30 p.m. Fish and vegetables with choice of a Miracle Pesto or Miracle Butter (pages 315–318)

DAY 24 (Tuesday)

7:30 a.m. Traditional Triple Threat Shake (page 311)

12:00 p.m. Leftover Slow-Cooked Beer-Braised Beef and Cauliflower Mash

3:30 p.m. Triple Threat Cheesecake (page 314)

7:30 p.m. Greek Lamb Kabobs (page 341) with Tzatziki (page 320)

DAY 25 (Wednesday)

7:30 a.m. Traditional Triple Threat Shake (page 311)

12:00 p.m. Leftover Greek Lamb Kabobs on a salad with Tzatziki

3:30 p.m. Triple Threat Pudding (page 313)

7:30 p.m. Fabulous Fajitas (page 349) with Holy Moly Guacamole (page 324), salsa, and sour cream

DAY 26 (Thursday)

7:30 a.m. Traditional Triple Threat Shake (page 311)

12:00 p.m. Bun-less beef burger and Oven-Roasted Brussels Sprouts (page 352)

3:30 p.m. Traditional Triple Threat Shake (page 311)

7:30 p.m. Rustic Portobello Pizza Caps (page 344)

DAY 27 (Friday)

7:30 a.m. Traditional Triple Threat Shake (page 311)

12:00 p.m. Grilled or broiled chicken thigh on a big salad with choice of SKINNYFat dressing (pages 321–322)

3:30 p.m. Triple Threat Cheesecake (page 314)

7:30 p.m. *Peppercorn-Crusted Beef Tenderloin (page 341) with 4-Ingredient Blender Hollandaise (page 323) and Sweet Potato, Yam, and Apple Casserole (page 353) or baked potato*

DAY 28 (Saturday)

9:00 a.m. Protein-Packed Morning Muffins (page 330)

1:00 p.m. Traditional Triple Threat Shake (page 311)

5:00 p.m. Grilled Tandoori Skewers (page 342) with Cooling Cucumber Raita (page 320) and Indian Garlic-Butter Cheese Non-Naan (page 354)

9:00 p.m. Chocolate Triple Threat Ice Cream (page 314)

Ketogenic

This advanced plan is specifically designed for individuals who are looking to burn fat at an accelerated pace or who are suffering from chronic health conditions. It will help you to create an internal environment that is optimal for healing and rebalancing the body, as well as accelerated fat loss. When deciding between the Fat Loss and Ketogenic protocols, it is important to consider your level of commitment, as the Ketogenic plan will require far greater limitations. *Note:* If you plan on following the Ketogenic protocol and you have a condition for which we have offered a separate condition-specific plan, please make sure to read that condition-specific protocol and incorporate the tips and tweaks into your Ketogenic plan.

The Ketogenic protocol is designed for individuals who are/have:

- Overweight/obese
- Neurological problems (multiple sclerosis, Parkinson's, Alzheimer's)
- Epilepsy
- Type 2 diabetes
- Cancer
- Osteoporosis/osteopenia
- High cholesterol/triglycerides
- ADHD (attention deficit hyperactivity disorder)
- AIDS
- Digestive conditions

Adjustments you must make to the Signature 28-day Micronutrient Miracle plan for your specific condition(s):

10 GOLDEN RULES: While each of the condition-specific protocols must follow all 10 of the Golden Rules, for best results with this protocol, we have identified the following rules to either be critical or require small tweaks.

#2: Research indicates that BPA triggers the release of almost double the insulin actually needed to break down food. High insulin levels can desensitize the body to the hormone over time, which in some people may lead to weight gain and type 2 diabetes. Make sure to be keenly aware of eliminating MSG, BPA, and phthalates.

#5: Stress reduction is very important for optimal fat loss, as stress increases the release of cortisol, a hormone that spikes appetite and increases fat storage in the belly region.

#6: If accelerated fat loss is your goal, increase your ZMT sessions from three or four per week to six or seven. Also, make an effort to get out and walk, bike, hike, row, or do any other type of physical movement at a moderate pace for 45 minutes per day.

#7: Purchasing nontoxic household and beauty goods will ensure that they are not causing a hormonal imbalance, resulting in weight gain. Try to follow our Top 10 Terrific Tricks to Reduce Household Toxins.

#8: As diets become more restrictive, the micronutrients supplied in the allowed foods are often limited. For this reason, taking nutreince, or another well-formulated multivitamin, is imperative on a ketogenic plan.

#9: Taking your Micronutrient Miracle Triple Threat Shakes twice a day is especially important while following this protocol, as it will provide you with the amino acids L-glutamine and L-tryptophan, which have been shown to reduce sugar cravings, aid in the regulation of metabolism, and promote healthy cholesterol levels. Additionally, the SKINNYFat in each shake will keep you in a ketogenic state and satiate you throughout the day. Make sure to prepare all puddings and ice creams with heavy cream instead of coconut milk. This will reduce your overall carbohydrate count.

DAILY LIMITS: The daily limits for the Ketogenic protocol are much stricter than for our Signature plan. For the next 28 days, adhere to the following limits.

Starches/fruits/nuts/seeds: You will eliminate all starches and fruits, but you can enjoy 1 serving of nuts or seeds per week.

Fat and protein: While other protocols do not require a specific ratio of fat to protein intake, the Ketogenic protocol does. We do not restrict calories in this protocol, but maintaining a ratio of at least 70 percent fat and 30 percent protein is imperative. To accomplish this ratio, you must eat an equal number of grams for both fat and protein. For example, if you eat 25 grams of fat and 25 grams of protein, you would be at this beneficial 70/30 ratio. However, a ratio of 80 percent fat and 20 percent protein is optimal. To accomplish this, you must eat *more* grams of fat than protein at each meal. This would mean that if you eat 25 grams of protein, you would need to eat 45 grams of fat. To determine a meal's ratio, make sure to look at its calories. While each gram of fat has 9 calories, each gram of protein has only 4. Let's look at an example to determine a meal's percentage of both fat and protein.

25 grams of fat x 9 calories = 225 calories of fat

25 grams of protein x 4 calories = 100 calories of protein

225 calories of fat ÷ 325 total calories (225 + 100 = 325) = 70% fat

This means that 70 percent of the caloric value of the meal is from fat, leaving 30 percent of the calories from protein. While on this protocol, make sure the number of grams of fat in each meal never drops below the grams of protein. When in doubt, always err on the side of more fat. Additionally, you will be ingesting a minimal amount of carbohydrates on this protocol (which contain 4 calories per gram). Keep these to below 10 percent of your total caloric intake.

Nonstarchy vegetables: Keep approved vegetables to a minimum. Either choose half servings or eliminate them entirely from either one or both meals in order to best achieve ketosis.

Alcohol: Rather than having one or two glasses a day, limit alcohol to up to three glasses a week. Gluten-free beer is off-limits. Spirits are the preferable source of alcohol on the Ketogenic protocol, followed by red wine, then white wine.

Caffeinated drinks: Two cups daily (same as the Signature plan). The chlorogenic acid in coffee and tea has been shown to reduce insulin resistance and chronic inflammation.

SETTING YOUR SCHEDULE: When following the Ketogenic protocol, it is very important to keep the body primed with fat, and therefore it is imperative to eat every 3 to 5 hours. Also, studies have verified that weight loss can be improved when undergoing an intermittent fast. To best achieve this, opt for scheduling options 4, 5, or 6 from Chapter 7 (see page 209) and make two consecutive meals Triple Threat Shakes or puddings. (In option 4, your two consecutive shakes are your last meal of the day followed by your first meal the next morning, allowing you to still achieve the fasting goal.) You don't need to do this every day, either; you can choose this option as often as you like.

Beneficial micronutrients while on a Ketogenic protocol for accelerated fat loss or healing:

Vitamin A	Vitamin D	Phosphorus
Vitamin B_1	Vitamin E	Potassium
Vitamin B_2	Vitamin K	Selenium
Vitamin B_3	Calcium	Silicon
Vitamin B_5	Chromium	Zinc
Vitamin B_6	Copper	Omega-3 fatty acids
Vitamin B_7	Iodine	Omega-6 fatty acids
Vitamin B_9	Iron	(GLA)
Vitamin B_{12}	Magnesium	Alpha-lipoic acid
Choline	Manganese	CoQ10
Vitamin C	Molybdenum	

POWERHOUSE PICKS: Choose these micronutrient powerhouses whenever possible. The Rich Foods listed below are high in the essential micronutrients shown to be beneficial to fat loss, healing, and rebalancing. We have adjusted your 28-day menu suggestions to include these Rich Food choices in the optimal fat/protein ratio. Choose these Rich Foods when designing personalized menus or eating out, and don't forget to properly prepare foods that contain EMDs.

PROTEINS

Beef	Lamb	Scallops
Bone broth	Mussels	Shrimp
Chicken (dark meat)	Organ meats	Snapper
Clams	Oysters	Tuna
Cod	Pork	Turkey (dark meat)
Crab	Rainbow trout	Venison
Dungeness crab	Salmon	
Herring	Sardines	

DAIRY

Cream	High-fat cheese, specifically Gouda

FATS

Butter

Cocoa butter

Coconut oil

Eggs (with yolks)

SKINNYFat*

*Use SKINNYFat in recipes whenever possible, as it is virtually impossible to store as body fat. Peer-reviewed published research also shows that MCT oil (the main ingredient in SKINNYFat) increases ketone production, which then boosts metabolism, reduces body fat, and improves insulin sensitivity and glucose tolerance. Meanwhile, the long-chain triglycerides in the coconut oil in SKINNYFat aid in the absorption of essential micronutrients.

NONSTARCHY VEGETABLES

Avocado

Asparagus

Cabbage

Celery

Dark leafy greens

Garlic

Mushrooms

Onions

Red or green chile peppers

Romaine lettuce

Sauerkraut

Seaweed

Sprouts

STARCHES

Eliminated

FRUITS

Eliminated

NUTS AND SEEDS

Brazil nuts

Macadamia nuts

Pecans

Walnuts

BENEFICIAL SPICES

Black pepper

Cardamom

Cayenne pepper

Chile pepper (chipotle)

Cinnamon

Cumin

Garlic powder

Ginger

Jalapeño pepper

Mustard

Onion powder

Red-pepper flakes

Turmeric

DAILY BEVERAGES

Black tea

Coffee

Green tea

Mineral water

Oolong tea

Water

Additional essential micronutrient supplements to consider:

Iron: This mineral aids in fatty acid metabolism and is necessary for the production of carnitine, which metabolizes fat. Try to get 8 milligrams (men) or 18 milligrams (women) per day, either through your food or in supplement form.

Note: It is imperative that you take iron in supplement form at a separate time from your multivitamin (nutreince). Iron is the most competitive micronutrient, conflicting with 10 other micronutrients. Take it midday on an empty stomach.

Omega-3s: Studies show that omega-3s can both increase oxidation of fat by activating genes that break down fat and reduce the number of overall fat cells. Additionally, studies show that people on a weight-loss diet that included fat-rich fish daily had improved glucose and insulin metabolism. Omega-3 supplementation has demonstrated benefits (reduced pain and inflammation) for individuals suffering from multiple sclerosis, Parkinson's, and Alzheimer's. Individuals with heart disease should also supplement with omega-3s; in a large study of more than 11,000 people with heart disease, the daily consumption of about 1 gram of fish oil reduced cardiovascular mortality by 30 percent and sudden cardiac death by 45 percent. And for those following the Ketogenic plan to treat osteoporosis, EPA and DHA from animal-derived omega-3s help to maintain or increase bone mass; enhance calcium absorption, retention, and bone deposits; and improve bone strength. Attempt to get the RDI of 1.6 grams (1,600 milligrams) per day from food or in supplement form.

Note: You can take omega-3s in supplement form at the same time as your multivitamin (nutreince). Opt for Origin Omega or try to find a supplement with a greater amount of EPA than DHA, if possible.

Omega-6 (GLA): While we strive to keep omega-6 levels low and in balance with omega-3s on the Micronutrient Miracle plan, gamma-linolenic acid (GLA) is an omega-6 fatty acid that has anti-inflammatory properties similar to omega-3s, unlike other omega-6s, which are considered inflammatory. Studies show that supplementing with GLA can help prevent heart disease, osteoporosis, and hypertension.

Note: You can take GLA in supplement form at the same time as your multivitamin.

Additional beneficial supplements to consider:

Alpha-lipoic acid (ALA): This is a powerful antioxidant/anti-inflammatory supplement that can have an "antiobesity effect," resulting in decreased appetite, increased activity levels, and decreased abdominal fat. Individuals deficient in ALA have been shown to have an increased likelihood of being overweight or obese. (If using nutreince, take with PM dose.)

L-carnitine/acetyl-L-carnitine: This micronutrient is critical for energy formation and an active metabolism. Alpha-lipoic acid, along with acetyl-L-carnitine, work together to increase metabolism and lower oxidative stress more than either compound alone. A 5:1 ratio of L-carnitine to ALA may be optimal.

CoQ10: Similar to ALA and acetyl-L-carnitine, CoQ10 is a powerful antioxidant/anti-inflammatory that assists with energy production. CoQ10 has been shown to be beneficial for treating and preventing obesity, enhancing metabolism, and supporting optimal energy and endurance. In one study, individuals found to be deficient in CoQ10 were given CoQ10 supplementation (100 milligrams/day) and in only 9 weeks they had lost an incredible average of 30 pounds. If you are currently taking a statin, we highly suggest supplementing with CoQ10.

L-glutamine: This amino acid has been shown to reduce sugar cravings and enhance metabolism. It will already be supplemented through the addition of IN.POWER whey protein. If you are omitting the protein Triple Threat meal replacement shakes, you may want to consider supplementation with 2 to 4 grams of powdered L-glutamine. You can add this to your nutreince multivitamin drink or into cold water taken separately from your meals.

Curcumin: This active ingredient found in the Indian spice turmeric can be very helpful both as an anti-inflammatory and as a blood sugar regulator. In studies, it has been shown to switch on the liver genes that keep glucose levels in check. It improves the pancreas's ability to make insulin and helps slow down the metabolism of carbohydrates after meals. Additionally, curcumin can be very helpful in maintaining heart health by reducing cholesterol oxidation, plaque buildup and clot formation, bad cholesterol (LDL), and the proinflammatory response. Finally, it benefits those with Alzheimer's, as well, because it has been shown to reduce plaque buildup in the brain.

Digestive enzymes: Look for a product with amylase, protease, and lipase, as well as a variety of other digestive enzymes such as bromelain, ox bile, pancreatin, papain, pepsin, and betaine HCL. Betaine HCL may be especially important for this protocol, as it helps with the absorption of calcium and magnesium, two micronutrients that are critical for both building bone and eliminating cravings.

DHEA: Levels of DHEA drop with age. Most studies on the use of DHEA for fat or weight loss support its use for this purpose. This supplement has also been shown to be beneficial for stimulating bone growth and helping to prevent osteoporosis. DHEA should be taken with caution, though, because high doses may suppress the body's natural ability to make DHEA and may lead to liver damage (as shown in an animal study). Taking antioxidants—such as vitamins C and E and selenium—is recommended to prevent oxidative damage to the liver.

The Ketogenic 28-Day Menu Plan

Limited foods are *italicized* so that you can see where they fit into your plan. Feel free to choose from any of the Miracle Pestos, Miracle Butters, SKINNYFat Salad Dressings, and SKINNYFat Infusions, as they all fit into the Ketogenic protocol. You should also remember that with this protocol *more* fat is preferred, so don't be shy about adding 2 to 4 frozen butter or pesto cubes to any recipe you like!

WEEK 1

DAY 1 (Sunday)

9:00 a.m. Scrambled eggs (2 or 3) with cream cheese, Cheddar cheese, bacon or sausage, and ½ cup of mushrooms (jalapeño pepper optional)

1:00 p.m. Traditional Triple Threat Shake (page 311)

5:00 p.m. Bun-less bacon cheeseburger with Really Creamy SKINNYFat Blue Cheese Dressing (or Dip) (page 322)

9:00 p.m. Triple Threat Pudding (page 313) made with heavy cream instead of coconut milk

DAY 2 (Monday)

7:30 a.m. Traditional Triple Threat Shake (page 311)

12:00 p.m. Egg salad made with 5-Minute SKINNYFat Mayonnaise (page 321) on a small bed of lettuce or in lettuce wraps

3:30 p.m. Traditional Triple Threat Shake (page 311)

7:30 p.m. Salmon sautéed in choice of a Miracle Pesto or Miracle Butter (pages 315–318) and a small side salad with SKINNYFat salad dressing (pages 321–322)

DAY 3 (Tuesday)

7:30 a.m. Triple Threat Cheesecake (page 314)

12:00 p.m. Big salad with leftover salmon and choice of SKINNYFat dressing (pages 321–322)

3:30 p.m. Traditional Triple Threat Shake (page 311)

7:30 p.m. Fabulous Fajitas (page 349); omit the bell peppers and wraps and load up on all the toppings; add 1 Tbsp of SKINNYFat into the sour cream to make super-keto sour cream

DAY 4 (Wednesday)

7:30 a.m. Traditional Triple Threat Shake (page 311)

12:00 p.m. Leftover Fabulous Fajitas and all the toppings, including super-keto sour cream

3:30 p.m. Triple Threat Cheesecake (page 314)

7:30 p.m. *Quick Tandoori Shrimp (page 336) with Cooling Cucumber Raita (page 320) and Indian Garlic-Butter Cheese Non-Naan (page 354);* add 1 Tbsp of SKINNYFat to raita recipe, and swap the Greek yogurt out for full-fat sour cream

DAY 5 (Thursday)

7:30 a.m. Traditional Triple Threat Shake (page 311)

12:00 p.m. Big salad with leftover Quick Tandoori Shrimp and special keto-adapted Cooling Cucumber Raita

3:30 p.m. Triple Threat Pudding (page 313) made with heavy cream instead of coconut milk

7:30 p.m. Bacon and cheese baked onto two chicken thighs and served with Buffalo Wing Sauce (aka Jayson's Red Hot) (page 323) and celery sticks dipped in Really Creamy SKINNYFat Blue Cheese Dressing (page 322)

DAY 6 (Friday)

7:30 a.m. Traditional Triple Threat Shake (page 311)

12:00 p.m. Broccoli Cheese Soup (page 327); lower broccoli content to 2 cups chopped

3:30 p.m. Traditional Triple Threat Shake (page 311)

7:30 p.m. Rib eye (or another higher-fat protein) and 1 cup sautéed mushrooms with choice of 4-Ingredient Blender Hollandaise Sauce (page 323) or a Miracle Pesto or Miracle Butter (pages 315–318)

DAY 7 (Saturday)

9:00 a.m. Speedy Salmon Cakes (page 329) with 4-Ingredient Blender Hollandaise Sauce (page 323) and eggs any style

1:00 p.m. Traditional Triple Threat Shake (page 311)

5:00 p.m. Rotisserie or baked whole chicken with Buffalo Wing Sauce (aka Jayson's Red Hot) (page 323) and Really Creamy SKINNYFat Blue Cheese Dressing (page 322)

9:00 p.m. Chocolate Triple Threat Ice Cream (page 314) made with heavy cream instead of coconut milk

WEEK 2

DAY 8 (Sunday)

9:00 a.m. French Onion Egg Tart (page 328); only use ½ of the onions, adding an additional 2 Tbsp of cream cheese to the egg mixture

1:00 p.m. Triple Threat Cheesecake (page 314)

5:00 p.m. Chicken salad made with chopped celery, leftover rotisserie chicken, and lots of 5-Minute SKINNYFat Mayonnaise (page 321) or Really Creamy SKINNYFat Blue Cheese Dressing (page 322) and served in lettuce wraps

9:00 p.m. Traditional Triple Threat Shake (page 311)

DAY 9 (Monday)

7:30 a.m. Traditional Triple Threat Shake (page 311)

12:00 p.m. Grilled or broiled chicken thighs, asparagus, and choice of a Miracle Pesto or Miracle Butter (pages 315–318)

3:30 p.m. Triple Threat Pudding (page 313) made with heavy cream instead of coconut milk

7:30 p.m. Greek Lamb Kabobs (page 341) served with Tzatziki (page 320); for the skewer vegetables, use 1 onion and 6 large portobello mushrooms; swap the Greek yogurt for full-fat sour cream and add 1 Tbsp SKINNYFat to make the tzatziki

DAY 10 (Tuesday)

7:30 a.m. Traditional Triple Threat Shake (page 311)

12:00 p.m. Leftover Greek Lamb Kabobs over lettuce with keto-adapted tzatziki

3:30 p.m. Traditional Triple Threat Shake (page 311)

7:30 p.m. Chicken Wings (page 334) with Really Creamy SKINNYFat Blue Cheese Dressing (page 322) and celery sticks

DAY 11 (Wednesday)

7:30 a.m. Traditional Triple Threat Shake (page 311)

12:00 p.m. Leftover chicken wings and dressing

3:30 p.m. Triple Threat Pudding (page 313) made with heavy cream instead of coconut milk

7:30 p.m. Pork chops with sautéed mushroom and 4-Ingredient Blender Hollandaise (page 323)

DAY 12 (Thursday)

7:30 a.m. Traditional Triple Threat Shake (page 311)

12:00 p.m. Leftover pork on a salad with choice of SKINNYFat dressing (pages 321–322)

3:30 p.m. Traditional Triple Threat Shake (page 311)

7:30 p.m. Scallops in Lemon Butter Sauce (page 334) with ½ cup mushrooms sautéed in butter

DAY 13 (Friday)

7:30 a.m. Triple Threat Cheesecake (page 314)

12:00 p.m. *Mexican Chicken Wrap (page 338); limit to 2 Tbsp of salsa*

3:30 p.m. Traditional Triple Threat Shake (page 311)

7:30 p.m. Chicken thigh and mushrooms sautéed in Rich and Creamy Alfredo Sauce (page 319)

DAY 14 (Saturday)

9:00 a.m. Smoked Salmon Cream Cheese Roll-Ups (page 331) with fried eggs

1:00 p.m. Traditional Triple Threat Shake (page 311)

5:00 p.m. Micronutrient-Packed "Offaly" Tasty Meatloaf (page 348) dipped in Really Creamy SKINNYFat Blue Cheese Dressing (page 322)

9:00 p.m. Triple Threat Pudding (page 313) made with heavy cream instead of coconut milk

WEEK 3

DAY 15 (Sunday)

9:00 a.m. Leftover meatloaf heated in a frying pan topped with a slice of cream cheese, a fried egg, and melted cheese

1:00 p.m. Traditional Triple Threat Shake (page 311)

5:00 p.m. Asparagus cheese soup (start with Broccoli Cheese Soup recipe on page 327, but replace broccoli with 2 cups of asparagus)

9:00 p.m. Traditional Triple Threat Shake (page 311)

DAY 16 (Monday)

7:30 a.m. Traditional Triple Threat Shake (page 311)

12:00 p.m. *Tuna salad wrap made from ½ can of tuna fish and 5-Minute SKINNYFat Mayonnaise served with lettuce and choice of SKINNYFat dressing in a Ridiculously Simple Wrap (page 353)*

3:30 p.m. Traditional Triple Threat Shake (page 311)

7:30 p.m. Chili con keto—in a pot, combine 1.5 pounds of cooked ground chuck, ½ cup Buffalo Wing Sauce (aka Jayson's Red Hot) (page 323) with the butter added in, and an 8-ounce package of cream cheese and top with shredded Cheddar cheese and sour cream (makes 4 servings)

DAY 17 (Tuesday)

7:30 a.m. Triple Threat Cheesecake (page 314)

12:00 p.m. Leftover chili con keto

3:30 p.m. Traditional Triple Threat Shake (page 311)

7:30 p.m. Salmon or another omega-3-rich fish sautéed with choice of a Miracle Pesto or Miracle Butter (pages 315–318)

DAY 18 (Wednesday)

7:30 a.m. Traditional Triple Threat Shake (page 311)

12:00 p.m. Bun-less cheeseburger with Really Creamy SKINNYFat Blue Cheese Dressing (page 322) and sauerkraut

3:30 p.m. Traditional Triple Threat Shake (page 311)

7:30 p.m. Rotisserie or baked whole chicken with Buffalo Wing Sauce (aka Jayson's Red Hot) (page 323) and Really Creamy SKINNYFat Blue Cheese Dressing (page 322)

DAY 19 (Thursday)

7:30 a.m. Triple Threat Cheesecake (page 314)

12:00 p.m. Chicken salad made with chopped celery, leftover rotisserie chicken, and 5-Minute SKINNYFat Mayonnaise (page 321) served in lettuce wraps with choice of SKINNYFat dressing (pages 321–322)

3:30 p.m. Traditional Triple Threat Shake (page 311)

7:30 p.m. Thai Shrimp Noodle Soup (page 326); omit the carrots and green beans

DAY 20 (Friday)

7:30 a.m. Traditional Triple Threat Shake (page 311)

12:00 p.m. Leftover Thai Shrimp Noodle Soup

3:30 p.m. Traditional Triple Threat Shake (page 311)

7:30 p.m. Chicken thigh and mushrooms sautéed in Rich and Creamy Alfredo Sauce (page 319)

DAY 21 (Saturday)

9:00 a.m. Burger bites—mini bun-less beef burgers (approximately ⅙ pound each) cooked in a frying pan and then topped with a slice of cream cheese and a fried egg; eat 2

1:00 p.m. Traditional Triple Threat Shake (page 311)

5:00 p.m. Lamb chops with asparagus and choice of a Miracle Pesto or Miracle Butter (pages 315–318)

9:00 p.m. Traditional Triple Threat Shake (page 311)

WEEK 4

DAY 22 (Sunday)

9:00 a.m. Smoked Salmon Cream Cheese Roll-Ups (page 331) with fried eggs

1:00 p.m. Traditional Triple Threat Shake (page 311)

5:00 p.m. Crab legs dripping in butter

9:00 p.m. Chocolate Triple Threat Ice Cream (page 314) made with heavy cream instead of coconut milk

DAY 23 (Monday)

7:30 a.m. Traditional Triple Threat Shake (page 311)

12:00 p.m. Rustic Portobello Pizza Caps (page 344)

3:30 p.m. Traditional Triple Threat Shake (page 311)

7:30 p.m. Salmon and ½ cup mushrooms sautéed in choice of a Miracle Pesto or Miracle Butter (pages 315–318)

DAY 24 (Tuesday)

7:30 a.m. Traditional Triple Threat Shake (page 311)

12:00 p.m. Bun-less Cheddar bacon burger served with Really Creamy SKINNYFat Blue Cheese Dressing (page 322) and sauerkraut

3:30 p.m. Triple Threat Pudding (page 313) made with heavy cream instead of coconut milk

7:30 p.m. Greek Lamb Kabobs (page 341) served with Tzatziki (page 320); for the skewer vegetables, use 1 onion and 4 large portobello mushrooms; swap the Greek yogurt for full-fat sour cream and add 1 Tbsp SKINNYFat to make the tzatziki

DAY 25 (Wednesday)

7:30 a.m. Traditional Triple Threat Shake (page 311)

12:00 p.m. Leftover Greek Lamb Kabobs on a salad with keto-adapted tzatziki

3:30 p.m. Triple Threat Cheesecake (page 314)

7:30 p.m. Chicken Wings (page 334) with Really Creamy SKINNYFat Blue Cheese Dressing (page 322) and celery sticks

DAY 26 (Thursday)

7:30 a.m. Traditional Triple Threat Shake (page 311)

12:00 p.m. Leftover chicken wings and blue cheese dressing

3:30 p.m. Traditional Triple Threat Shake (page 311)

7:30 p.m. Chicken thigh personal pizzas—take 2 chicken thighs (grilled or broiled), top with 2 Tbsp of your favorite tomato sauce, make sure to put pepperoni and extra cheese on top, drizzle with SKINNYFat Pizza in a Bottle Italian-Infused Oil, and bake in the oven until melted

DAY 27 (Friday)

7:30 a.m. Traditional Triple Threat Shake (page 311)

12:00 p.m. Grilled or broiled chicken thigh on a big salad with choice of SKINNYFat dressing (pages 321–322)

3:30 p.m. Triple Threat Cheesecake (page 314)

7:30 p.m. Peppercorn-Crusted Beef Tenderloin (page 341) with 4-Ingredient Blender Hollandaise (page 323) and sautéed mushrooms

DAY 28 (Saturday)

9:00 a.m. Scrambled eggs (2 or 3) with cream cheese, Cheddar cheese, bacon or sausage, and ½ cup of spinach chopped

1:00 p.m. Traditional Triple Threat Shake (page 311)

5:00 p.m. *Grilled Tandoori Skewers (page 342) with Cooling Cucumber Raita (page 320) and Indian Garlic-*

Butter Cheese Non-Naan (page 354); for the skewer vegetables, omit the broccoli, cauliflower, and tomatoes and use 6 portobello mushrooms instead; for the raita, use sour cream and an additional Tbsp of SKINNYFat in place of the Greek yogurt

9:00 p.m. Chocolate Triple Threat Ice Cream (page 314) made with heavy cream instead of coconut milk

Cardiovascular Health

This plan is specifically designed for individuals who are suffering from cardiovascular health issues related to hypertension. This protocol will help you create an internal environment that will reduce inflammation while working toward healthy blood pressure. If you are looking to reduce your cholesterol/triglycerides levels, you may want to consider using our Ketogenic protocol.

The Cardiovascular Health protocol is designed for individuals who have:

- Hypertension/high blood pressure
- Heart disease

Adjustments you must make to the Signature 28-day Micronutrient Miracle plan for your specific condition(s):

10 GOLDEN RULES: While each of the condition-specific protocols must follow all 10 of the Golden Rules, for best results with this protocol, we have identified the following rules to either be critical or require small tweaks.

#2: New studies reveal that blood pressure rises significantly immediately after ingesting foods from containers made with BPA. For this reason, it is important to avoid all the obesogenic toxins (MSG, BPA, phthalates).

#5: Stress reduction is very important for cardiovascular health, as stress increases the release of cortisol, a hormone that spikes appetite and increases visceral fat storage in the belly region, which has been shown to increase the risk of heart disease.

#6: Check with your doctor to make sure your heart is healthy enough for three or four ZMT sessions per week. If not, get out and walk, bike, hike, row, or do any other type of physical movement at a moderate pace for 45 minutes 3 or 4 days per week. Make sure to include the One Set To Failure weight-training plan, as studies have shown that lifting weights can reduce blood pressure as well as antihypertensive drugs.

#8: Taking a well-formulated multivitamin, like nutreince, that contains both forms of niacin (one to control blood sugar and the other to help regulate cholesterol levels) is important for your condition. Additionally, vitamin K_2 has been shown to be extremely beneficial in fighting arterial plaque and directing calcium out of the blood and into the bone. nutreince is also formulated to contain statin-safe levels of vitamins C and E. If opting for another supplement, make sure to evaluate the product using the quiz at MultivitaminStackUpQuiz.com. While many cardiovascular doctors prefer the use of products that don't contain vitamin K for patients on warfarin (Coumadin), we ask that you work with your doctor to find and regulate your prescription levels rather than omit this essential micronutrient with so many heart-healthy benefits.

#9: Taking your Micronutrient Miracle Triple Threat Shakes twice a day is especially important while following this heart-healthy protocol. There are two conditions that greatly contribute to cardiovascular disease being the leading cause of death in the United States—high blood pressure and elevated LDL. Research indicates that the peptides found in whey protein improve both of these factors. Blood pressure is modulated due to the opioid-like activity of several whey peptides—including alpha-lactalbumin and beta-lactoglobulin. And whey protein has a cholesterol-lowering effect, reducing LDL cholesterol through a decrease of VLDL (very low-density lipoprotein)—the type of cholesterol that modern science is now linking to cardiovascular disease.

DAILY LIMITS: The daily limits for the Cardiovascular Health protocol are the same as for our Signature plan. However, for the next 28 days, pay particular attention to the following micronutrients.

Potassium: Insufficient levels of potassium, calcium, and magnesium have been shown to cause high blood pressure. While the Cardiovascular Health protocol is designed to deliver sufficient amounts of calcium and magnesium through your food and a properly formulated multivitamin, such as nutreince, special attention is needed to accomplish this for potassium. Make an effort to consume potassium-rich foods when available. Foods that are high in potassium include avocado, coconut water, salmon, flounder, tuna, poultry, beef, pumpkin, cauliflower, dairy products (milk, cream, cheese, yogurt), artichokes, bananas, green peas, citrus fruits, dried apricots, prunes, raisins, acorn squash, mushrooms, green leafy vegetables, legumes, melons, potatoes (with skin), and tomatoes. Some clients have had great success reducing blood pressure by adding one 16-ounce coconut water per day. For this protocol, coconut water is treated as a beverage, and one serving per day is allowed. Adding this beverage to your AM nutreince (not PM) is a great way to remember to drink it.

CoQ10: We have listed CoQ10 as an additional beneficial supplement below; however, we also want you to include foods high in CoQ10 as often as you can. These foods include beef, chicken, rainbow trout, herring, sesame seeds, pistachios, broccoli, cauliflower, eggs, and 100 percent chocolate (pure cocoa—no sugar).

Beneficial micronutrients while on the Cardiovascular Health protocol for hypertension:

Vitamin B$_1$	*Vitamin E*	*Selenium*
Vitamin B$_2$	*Vitamin K*	*Silicon*
Vitamin B$_3$	*Calcium*	*Omega-3 fatty acids*
Vitamin B$_6$	*Choline*	*Omega-6 fatty acids*
Vitamin B$_9$	*Chromium*	*(GLA)*
Vitamin B$_{12}$	*Copper*	*CoQ10*
Vitamin C	*Magnesium*	
Vitamin D	*Potassium*	

POWERHOUSE PICKS: In addition to the foods listed above, choose these micronutrient powerhouses whenever possible. The Rich Foods listed below are high in the essential micronutrients shown to be beneficial for reducing blood pressure and achieving cardiovascular health. We have adjusted your 28-day menu suggestions to include these Rich Food choices. Choose these Rich Foods when designing personalized menus or eating out, and don't forget to properly prepare foods that contain EMDs.

PROTEINS

Beef	*Lamb*	*Scallops*
Bone broth	*Mussels*	*Shrimp*
Chicken	*Organ meats*	*Snapper*
Clams	*Oysters*	*Tuna*
Cod	*Pork*	*Turkey*
Crab	*Rainbow trout*	*Venison*
Dungeness crab	*Salmon*	
Herring	*Sardines*	

DAIRY

Cheese, especially Gouda   Milk

Cream   Yogurt

FATS

Butter   Cocoa butter   Eggs (with yolks)

Chocolate (100 percent   Coconut oil   SKINNYFat*
pure)

*Using SKINNYFat can help you maintain healthy cholesterol levels by controlling LDL (bad) levels and increasing HDL (good) levels. The ketone bodies produced by SKINNYFat may actually be the preferred source of energy for both your heart and brain. This can be particularly beneficial for patients suffering from heart disease and diabetes. Use SKINNYFat in recipes whenever possible, as it is virtually impossible to store as body fat and can aid in the absorption of essential micronutrients.

NONSTARCHY VEGETABLES

Asparagus   Garlic   Romaine lettuce

Avocado   Green beans   Sauerkraut

Bell peppers   Kale   Snow peas

Broccoli   Mushrooms (crimini/   Spinach

Brussels sprouts   shiitake)   Sprouts

Cabbage   Mustard greens   Swiss chard

Cauliflower   Onions   Tomatoes

Celery   Pumpkin

Dark leafy greens   Red or green chile peppers

STARCHES

Acorn squash   Lentils   Quinoa

Brown rice   Lima beans   Sweet potatoes

Garbanzo beans   Oats

Green peas   Potatoes (with skin)

FRUITS

Apples   Mango   Raisins

Bananas   Melons   Strawberries

Dates   Oranges   Watermelon

Grapefruit   Papaya

Limes   Prunes

NUTS AND SEEDS

Almonds	Flaxseed	Pecans
Brazil nuts	Hazelnuts	Pine nuts
Cashews	Hemp seeds	Sunflower seeds
Chia seeds	Peanuts	Walnuts

BENEFICIAL SPICES

Basil	Cloves	Onion powder
Black pepper	Cumin	Oregano
Cardamom	Garlic powder	Red-pepper flakes
Cayenne pepper	Ginger	Thyme
Chile pepper (chipotle)	Jalapeño pepper	Turmeric
Cinnamon	Mustard	

DAILY BEVERAGES

Black tea	Coffee	Oolong tea
Coconut water (1 serving per day; check carefully for sugar)	Green tea	Water
	Mineral water	

Additional essential micronutrient supplements to consider:

Omega-3s: In a large study of more than 11,000 people with heart disease, the daily consumption of about 1 gram of fish oil reduced cardiovascular mortality by 30 percent and sudden cardiac death by 45 percent. Attempt to get the RDI of 1.6 grams (1,600 milligrams) per day from food or in supplement form.

Note: You can take omega-3s in supplement form at the same time as your multivitamin (nutreince). Opt for Origin Omega or try to find a supplement with a greater amount of EPA than DHA, if possible.

Omega-6s (GLA): While we strive to keep omega-6 levels low and in balance with omega-3s on the Micronutrient Miracle plan, gamma-linolenic acid (GLA) is an omega-6 fatty acid that has anti-inflammatory properties similar to those of omega-3s, unlike other omega-6s, which are considered inflammatory. Studies show that supplementing with GLA can help prevent cardiovascular disease and hypertension.

Note: You can take GLA in supplement form with your multivitamin.

Vitamin C: Studies have found that supplementing with vitamin C (1,500 to 3,000 milligrams per day) dramatically lowers the risk of vascular diseases, including heart disease and stroke. However, if you are on a statin, make sure to speak to your physician about increasing your vitamin C levels, as a dose over 200 milligrams may interfere with your medication.

Additional beneficial supplements to consider:

Alpha-lipoic acid (ALA): This is a powerful antioxidant/anti-inflammatory supplement that has been shown to strongly inhibit the production of adhesion molecules, which may aid in the prevention and treatment of atherosclerosis. Plus, individuals deficient in ALA have been shown to have an increased likelihood of being overweight or obese. (If using nutreince, take with PM dose.)

Curcumin: This active ingredient that gives turmeric its yellow color can be very helpful in maintaining heart health by reducing cholesterol oxidation, plaque buildup and clot formation, bad cholesterol (LDL), and the proinflammatory response.

CoQ10: Supplementation with this powerful antioxidant/anti-inflammatory that assists with energy production is highly recommended for individuals taking a statin. CoQ10 (100–200 milligrams/day) has been shown to be beneficial for treating and preventing obesity, enhancing metabolism, and supporting optimal energy, endurance, and cardiovascular function.

Digestive enzymes: These can assist with digestion and enhance micronutrient availability and absorption. Look for a product with amylase, protease, and lipase, as well as a variety of other digestive enzymes. Bromelain, ox bile, pancreatin, papain, pepsin, and betaine HCL may all be beneficial. Betaine HCL may be especially important for this protocol, as it helps with the absorption of calcium and magnesium—two of the three key nutrients for blood pressure regulation.

The Cardiovascular Health 28-Day Menu Plan

Limited foods are *italicized* so that you can see where they fit into your plan. Feel free to choose from any of the Miracle Pestos, Miracle Butters, SKINNYFat Salad Dressings, and SKINNYFat Infusions, as they all fit into the Cardio-vascular Health protocol.

WEEK 1

DAY 1 (Sunday)

9:00 a.m. *Yogurt and banana or Baked Apple à la Micronutrient Miracle Mode (page 332)*

1:00 p.m. Traditional Triple Threat Shake (page 311) made with coconut water instead of water

5:00 p.m. Buffalo Chicken Chili (page 340)

9:00 p.m. Triple Threat Pudding (page 313)

DAY 2 (Monday)

7:30 a.m. Traditional Triple Threat Shake (page 311) made with coconut water instead of water

12:00 p.m. Leftover Buffalo Chicken Chili

3:30 p.m. Traditional Triple Threat Shake (page 311)

7:30 p.m. Salmon with green beans and Avocado Potassium-Packed Miracle Butter (page 317)

DAY 3 (Tuesday)

7:30 a.m. Triple Threat Cheesecake (page 314) and coconut water

12:00 p.m. Big salad with leftover salmon and green beans with choice of SKINNYFat dressing (pages 321–322)

3:30 p.m. Traditional Triple Threat Shake (page 311)

7:30 p.m. Greek Chicken (page 337)

DAY 4 (Wednesday)

7:30 a.m. Traditional Triple Threat Shake (page 311) made with coconut water instead of water

12:00 p.m. Leftover Greek Chicken

3:30 p.m. Triple Threat Cheesecake (page 314)

7:30 p.m. Quick Tandoori Shrimp (page 336) with Cooling Cucumber Raita (page 320)

DAY 5 (Thursday)

7:30 a.m. Traditional Triple Threat Shake (page 311) made with coconut water instead of water

12:00 p.m. Big salad with leftover Quick Tandoori Shrimp and choice of SKINNYFat dressing (pages 321–322)

3:30 p.m. Triple Threat Cheesecake (page 314)

7:30 p.m. Bun-less beef burger with avocado wedges and Oven-Roasted Brussels Sprouts (page 352)

DAY 6 (Friday)

7:30 a.m. Traditional Triple Threat Shake (page 311) made with coconut water instead of water

12:00 p.m. Broccoli Cheese Soup (page 327)

3:30 p.m. Traditional Triple Threat Shake (page 311)

7:30 p.m. Grilled steak with choice of a Miracle Pesto (pages 315–316) and Cauliflower Mash (page 352)

DAY 7 (Saturday)

9:00 a.m. Speedy Salmon Cakes (page 329) and eggs any style

1:00 p.m. Traditional Triple Threat Shake (page 311) made with coconut water instead of water

5:00 p.m. *Fish and Chips (page 350)*

9:00 p.m. Chocolate Triple Threat Ice Cream (page 314)

WEEK 2

DAY 8 (Sunday)

9:00 a.m. French Onion Egg Tart (page 328)

1:00 p.m. Traditional Triple Threat Shake (page 311) made with coconut water

5:00 p.m. Zughetti (page 345) with Mom's Beef Bolognese (page 324)

9:00 p.m. Traditional Triple Threat Shake (page 311)

DAY 9 (Monday)

7:30 a.m. Traditional Triple Threat Shake (page 311) made with coconut water

12:00 p.m. *Grilled or broiled chicken thighs, choice of a Miracle Pesto or Miracle Butter (pages 315–318), and baked potato with skin on*

3:30 p.m. Triple Threat Cheesecake (page 314)

7:30 p.m. Moqueca (aka Brazilian Fish Stew) (page 343)

DAY 10 (Tuesday)

7:30 a.m. Traditional Triple Threat Shake (page 311) made with coconut water

12:00 p.m. Leftover Moqueca

3:30 p.m. Traditional Triple Threat Shake (page 311)

7:30 p.m. Coq au Vin (page 347) served with Cauliflower Mash (page 352)

DAY 11 (Wednesday)

7:30 a.m. Traditional Triple Threat Shake (page 311) made with coconut water

12:00 p.m. Leftover Coq au Vin

3:30 p.m. Triple Threat Pudding (page 311)

7:30 p.m. Thai-Style Chopped Pork (page 347) on greens

DAY 12 (Thursday)

7:30 a.m. Traditional Triple Threat Shake (page 311) made with coconut water

12:00 p.m. Leftover chopped pork on a salad with avocado slices and choice of SKINNYFat dressing (pages 321–322)

3:30 p.m. Traditional Triple Threat Shake (page 311)

7:30 p.m. Scallops in Lemon Butter Sauce (page 334) with broccoli

DAY 13 (Friday)

7:30 a.m. Traditional Triple Threat Shake (page 311) made with coconut water

12:00 p.m. Mexican Chicken Wrap (page 338)

3:30 p.m. Traditional Triple Threat Shake (page 311)

7:30 p.m. Salad and Rustic Flatbread (page 346); use mushroom caps on either the salad or flatbread

DAY 14 (Saturday)

9:00 a.m. *Carrot Cake Pancakes with Cream Cheese Frosting and chopped walnuts and raisins (page 333)*

1:00 p.m. Traditional Triple Threat Shake (page 311) made with coconut water

5:00 p.m. Micronutrient-Packed "Offaly" Tasty Meatloaf (page 348) and steamed vegetable with choice of a Miracle Pesto or Miracle Butter (pages 315–318)

9:00 p.m. Triple Threat Cheesecake (page 314)

WEEK 3

DAY 15 (Sunday)

9:00 a.m. Leftover meatloaf heated in a frying pan and topped with a fried egg and covered in melted cheese

1:00 p.m. Traditional Triple Threat Shake (page 311) made with coconut water

5:00 p.m. *Camarão na Moranga (aka Brazilian Shrimp Stew in a Pumpkin) (page 335)*

9:00 p.m. Traditional Triple Threat Shake (page 311)

DAY 16 (Monday)

7:30 a.m. Traditional Triple Threat Shake (page 311) made with coconut water

12:00 p.m. Big salad with ½ can of tuna fish and choice of SKINNYFat dressing (pages 321–322)

3:30 p.m. Traditional Triple Threat Shake (page 311)

7:30 p.m. Chicken Wings (page 334) with Really Creamy SKINNYFat Blue Cheese Dressing (page 322) and carrot and celery sticks

DAY 17 (Tuesday)

7:30 a.m. Traditional Triple Threat Shake (page 311) made with coconut water

12:00 p.m. Leftover chicken wings and blue cheese dressing

3:30 p.m. Triple Threat Pudding (page 313)

7:30 p.m. Shepherd's Pie (page 351)

DAY 18 (Wednesday)

7:30 a.m. Triple Threat Cheesecake (page 314) and coconut water

12:00 p.m. Leftover Shepherd's Pie

3:30 p.m. Traditional Triple Threat Shake (page 311)

7:30 p.m. Zughetti (page 345) and grilled chicken thigh with Rich and Creamy Alfredo Sauce (page 319)

DAY 19 (Thursday)

7:30 a.m. Triple Threat Cheesecake (page 314) and coconut water

12:00 p.m. Bun-less beef burger and a side salad with choice of SKINNYFat dressing (pages 321–322)

3:30 p.m. Traditional Triple Threat Shake (page 311)

7:30 p.m. Thai Shrimp Noodle Soup (page 326)

DAY 20 (Friday)

7:30 a.m. Traditional Triple Threat Shake (page 311) made with coconut water

12:00 p.m. Leftover Thai Shrimp Noodle Soup

3:30 p.m. Traditional Triple Threat Shake (page 311)

7:30 p.m. *Rotisserie or baked whole chicken with Sweet Potato, Yam, and Apple Casserole (page 353)*

DAY 21 (Saturday)

9:00 a.m. Fried eggs served on Cauliflower Cheesy Hash Browns (page 329)

1:00 p.m. Traditional Triple Threat Shake (page 311) made with coconut water

5:00 p.m. Miracle Chinese Fried "Rice" (page 339)

9:00 p.m. Traditional Triple Threat Shake (page 311)

WEEK 4

DAY 22 (Sunday)

9:00 a.m. *Smoked Salmon Cream Cheese Roll-Ups (page 331) with avocado slices and berries or grapefruit*

1:00 p.m. Traditional Triple Threat Shake (page 311) made with coconut water

5:00 p.m. Slow-Cooked Beer-Braised Beef (page 338) and Cauliflower Mash (page 352)

9:00 p.m. Chocolate Triple Threat Ice Cream (page 314)

DAY 23 (Monday)

7:30 a.m. Traditional Triple Threat Shake (page 311) made with coconut water

12:00 p.m. Leftover Miracle Chinese Fried "Rice"

3:30 p.m. Traditional Triple Threat Shake (page 311)

7:30 p.m. Rainbow trout and vegetables with Avocado Potassium-Packed Miracle Butter (page 317)

DAY 24 (Tuesday)

7:30 a.m. Traditional Triple Threat Shake (page 311) made with coconut water

12:00 p.m. Leftover Slow-Cooked Beer-Braised Beef and Cauliflower Mash

3:30 p.m. Triple Threat Cheesecake (page 314)

7:30 p.m. Greek Lamb Kabobs (page 341); swap out chicken for the lamb to increase potassium intake

DAY 25 (Wednesday)

7:30 a.m. Traditional Triple Threat Shake (page 311) made with coconut water

12:00 p.m. Leftover Greek chicken kabobs on a salad with choice of SKINNYFat dressing (pages 321–322)

3:30 p.m. Triple Threat Pudding (page 313)

7:30 p.m. Fabulous Fajitas (page 349) with Holy Moly Guacamole (page 324) and salsa

DAY 26 (Thursday)

7:30 a.m. Triple Threat Cheesecake (page 314) and coconut water

12:00 p.m. Speedy Salmon Cakes (page 329) with SKINNYFat Tartar Sauce (page 322) and Oven-Roasted Brussels Sprouts (page 352)

3:30 p.m. Traditional Triple Threat Shake (page 311)

7:30 p.m. Rustic Portobello Pizza Caps (page 344)

DAY 27 (Friday)

7:30 a.m. Traditional Triple Threat Shake (page 311) made with coconut water

12:00 p.m. Grilled or broiled chicken thigh on a big salad with choice of SKINNYFat dressing (pages 321–322)

3:30 p.m. Triple Threat Pudding (page 313)

7:30 p.m. *Peppercorn-Crusted Beef Tenderloin (page 339) with 4-Ingredient Blender Hollandaise (page 323) and baked potato*

DAY 28 (Saturday)

9:00 a.m. Protein-Packed Morning Muffins (page 330)

1:00 p.m. Traditional Triple Threat Shake (page 311) made with coconut water

5:00 p.m. Grilled Tandoori Skewers (page 342) with Cooling Cucumber Raita (page 320) and Indian Garlic-Butter Cheese Non-Naan (page 354)

9:00 p.m. Chocolate Triple Threat Ice Cream (page 314)

Bone Building

This plan is specifically designed for individuals who are suffering from osteoporosis or osteopenia. This protocol will help you to create an internal environment that is conducive to strengthening bone and preventing fractures. The Ketogenic protocol can also be used by those who are looking for an advanced bone-building plan. Mira used the Ketogenic protocol to reverse her advanced osteoporosis and then used this Bone Building protocol to help her maintain bone health. If the Ketogenic protocol interests you and you have osteoporosis, make sure to read this protocol, as well, in order to understand the detailed condition-specific information below.

The Bone Building protocol is designed for individuals who have:

- Osteoporosis
- Osteopenia
- Other joint/bone issues
- Looking to avoid bone issues as they age (especially those with small frames)

Adjustments you must make to the Signature 28-day Micronutrient Miracle plan for your specific condition(s):

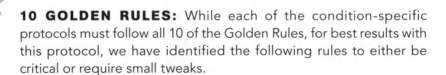

10 GOLDEN RULES: While each of the condition-specific protocols must follow all 10 of the Golden Rules, for best results with this protocol, we have identified the following rules to either be critical or require small tweaks.

#1: Pay particular attention to eliminating all sugar from your diet.

#2: Studies reveal that women with high levels of phthalates are likely to go through menopause earlier, and have estrogen disruption, which can then have an unhealthy effect on bone formation. Make sure to be keenly aware of eliminating all endocrine disruptors including phthalates, BPA, fragrances and pesticides.

#6: Adjust exercise as follows:

- Keep cardio to a minimum during this protocol; do not increase your ZMT training past the recommended 3 or 4 days per week.

- Make sure to include the One Set To Failure weight-training program. It is essential for the stimulation of bone growth.

- To reduce calcium loss from your bones during exercise, make sure to take your calcium-containing multivitamin (the AM nutreince contains all 600 milligrams of calcium) 30 minutes before your workout. This may mean changing your preferred workout time to the AM or switching your AM and PM doses so that you are taking the AM dose before your evening workout, or taking your additional calcium supplement 30 minutes prior.

- Individuals with advanced osteoporosis may find using a whole body vibration platform (Power Plate or similar) beneficial for building bone either in lieu of or in addition to the One Set To Failure weight-training program. This can be especially useful for those who are too frail to lift weights.

#8: Take a well-formulated multivitamin, like nutreince, each and every day. Our multivitamin was designed to treat Mira's advanced osteoporosis. It includes all three forms of vitamin K and beneficial quantities of calcium, magnesium, and vitamin D. Additionally, nutreince contains all eight forms of vitamin E, which is very important because new research suggests that delta-tocotrienol can completely prevent the erosion of the bone surface and was also effective in increasing bone formation and preventing bone reabsorption.

#9: Taking your Micronutrient Miracle Triple Threat Shakes twice a day is especially important. Studies have shown that supplementing elderly patients and postmenopausal women with protein causes increases in bone density, improved clinical symptoms in patients, and reduced bone loss. Additionally, each scoop of IN.POWER whey protein contains 1,000 milligrams of L-lysine, an essential amino acid that aids in calcium absorption and improves connective tissue strength. It is also critical for optimal growth and bone formation and may be particularly helpful at preventing osteoporosis in at-risk menopausal women. Taking two Triple Threat Shakes daily will also aid in lean muscle tissue growth, which is critical for balance and bone support in those with weakened bones. Try to take one Triple Threat daily as a pudding, as the extra collagen from the gelatin supports bone health.

EMD ALERT:

Oxalic acid and phytic acid: During this protocol, you should be especially mindful of reducing your consumption of foods with high levels of oxalic acid and phytic acid. If you are eating foods with these EMDs, make sure they are properly prepared to reduce their micronutrient-depleting effects.

Caffeine: Because caffeine depletes specific bone-building nutrients—including vitamins A, B_9, and D, as well as calcium—you may want to eliminate caffeinated drinks or make sure you are getting sufficient amounts of these micronutrients through diet and supplementation.

DAILY LIMITS: The daily limits for the Bone Building protocol are the same as for our Signature plan. However, for the next 28 days, pay particular attention to the following micronutrients.

Calcium and vitamins D and K_2: While our multivitamin nutreince contains 600 milligrams of calcium in the AM dose, most people need around 1,200 milligrams of calcium per day to slow down or reverse bone loss. During this protocol, you will need to make an effort to consume calcium-rich foods each day to meet this level. Foods that are high in calcium include dairy products (milk, cheese, cream, yogurt), sardines, canned salmon with the bones in, shrimp, eggs, green leafy vegetables, hazelnuts, bok choy, broccoli, almonds, and legumes. If you do not feel you are reaching beneficial levels of calcium through your diet, we recommend taking an additional 500 to 600 milligrams of calcium in supplement form. If you are taking nutreince, do not take the additional calcium with either the AM or PM doses. Take it midday, away from meals. Some people like to take additional vitamin D and vitamin K_2 at the same time. Foods that are high in vitamin D include egg yolks, liver, salmon, herring, sardines, shiitake mushrooms, and oysters. Foods that are high in vitamin K_2 are goose liver, Gouda cheese, sauerkraut, egg yolks, butter, ground beef, and liver.

Potassium: Insufficient levels of potassium have been associated with osteoporosis. Make an effort to consume potassium-rich foods when available. Foods that are high in potassium include avocado, coconut water, salmon, flounder, tuna, poultry, beef, pumpkin, cauliflower, dairy products (milk, cream, cheese, yogurt), artichokes, bananas, green peas, citrus fruit, dried apricots, prunes, raisins, acorn squash, mushrooms, green leafy vegetables, legumes, melons, potatoes (with skin), and tomatoes.

Bone broth: Add this food to your daily protocol, not for its high levels of calcium, but rather for the collagen (see page 139). Try to drink a small cup of homemade bone broth each day for the next 28 days.

Beneficial micronutrients used in the prevention and treatment of osteoporosis and osteopenia:

Vitamin A	Calcium	Silicon
Vitamin B_9	Chromium	Zinc
Vitamin B_{12}	Copper	Omega-3 fatty acids
Vitamin D	Magnesium	Omega-6 fatty acids
Vitamin E	Manganese	(GLA)
Vitamin K	Phosphorus	
Boron	Potassium	

POWERHOUSE PICKS: Choose these micronutrient powerhouses whenever possible. The Rich Foods listed below are high in the essential micronutrients shown to be beneficial for bone building. We have adjusted your 28-day menu suggestions to include these Rich Food choices. Choose these Rich Foods when designing personalized menus or eating out, and don't forget to properly prepare foods that contain EMDs.

PROTEINS

Beef	Lamb	Sardines
Bone broth	Mussels	Scallops
Chicken	Organ meats	Shrimp
Clams	Oysters	Snapper
Crab	Pork	Tuna
Dungeness crab	Rainbow trout	Turkey
Herring	Salmon	Venison

DAIRY

Cheese, especially Gouda	Yogurt
Cream	Milk

FATS

Butter	Chocolate (100 percent cocoa)	Coconut oil
Eggs (with yolks)		SKINNYFat*

*Although the majority of the fat in SKINNYFat comes from MCTs, which bypass the normal process of diges-tion and help with fat metabolism, this combination of oils was specially formulated to contain just the right amount of long-chain triglycerides to stimulate the release of the bile acids needed for the proper absorption and utilization of the fat-soluble vitamins A, D, E, and K, as well as other essential micronutrients, including carotenoids, calcium, and magnesium—many of which are essential for bone growth.

NONSTARCHY VEGETABLES

Asparagus	Garlic	Sauerkraut
Avocado	Green beans	Snow peas
Bok choy	Kale	Spinach (cooked; use infrequently)
Broccoli	Mushrooms	
Brussels sprouts	Mustard greens	Sprouts
Cabbage	Onions	Swiss chard
Cauliflower	Pumpkin	Tomatoes
Dark leafy greens	Romaine lettuce	

STARCHES

Acorn squash
Brown rice
Garbanzo beans
Green peas

Lentils
Lima beans
Oats
Potatoes (with skin)

Quinoa
Sweet potatoes

FRUITS

Apples
Bananas
Berries
Coconut water (counts as a
    fruit, not as a beverage;
    check carefully for sugar)

Dates
Mango
Melons
Papaya
Pineapple

Prunes
Raisins

NUTS AND SEEDS

Almonds
Brazil nuts
Cashews
Chia seeds
Flaxseed

Hazelnuts
Hemp seeds
Peanuts
Pecans
Pine nuts

Sesame seeds
Sunflower seeds
Walnuts

BENEFICIAL SPICES

Black pepper
Cilantro
Cinnamon
Cloves

Five-spice blend
Garlic powder
Ginger

Onion powder
Parsley
Turmeric

DAILY BEVERAGES

Coffee
Green tea

Mineral water
Water

Additional essential micronutrient supplements to consider:

Calcium: Individuals with osteoporosis and osteopenia should attempt to get the RDI of between 1,000 and 1,200 milligrams per day of this mineral from food or in supplement form.

Note: Do not combine calcium supplements with the AM or PM doses of nutreince; take the extra calcium at midday. If you are taking extra vitamin D or vitamin K, you can take them together at midday.

Vitamin D: This is important for the maintenance of bones and teeth. nutreince contains 2,000 milligrams of vitamin D_3; however, some individuals may want to supplement further.

Note: Do not take vitamin D supplements with the PM nutreince dose; take extra vitamin D either with the AM nutreince dose or at midday.

Vitamin K_2: This is necessary for the synthesis of osteocalcin, a unique protein in the bone, which attracts calcium to the bone tissue and is directly linked to bone mineral density. Vitamin K_2 is also required for the carboxylation of MPG (matrix gla protein), which directly blocks the formation of calcium crystals inside the blood vessels and arteries. nutreince contains 80 micrograms of vitamin K (27 micrograms of K_1 and 54 of K_2); however, some individuals may want to supplement further.

Note: Do not take vitamin K_2 supplements with the PM nutreince dose; take extra vitamin K_2 either with the AM nutreince dose or at midday.

Omega-3s: EPA and DHA from animal-derived omega-3s help to maintain or increase bone mass; enhance calcium absorption, retention, and bone deposits; and improve bone strength. Additionally, a deficiency in omega-3s can lead to severe bone loss and osteoporosis. Attempt to get the RDI of 1.6 grams (1,600 milligrams) per day from food or in supplement form.

Note: You can take approximately 1,000 milligrams of omega-3s in supplement form with your AM multivitamin (nutreince) and 1,000 milligrams with your PM multivitamin. Opt for Origin Omega or try to find an omega-3 supplement with a greater amount of EPA than DHA, if possible.

Omega-6s (GLA): Some studies suggest that people who don't get enough of some essential fatty acids (particularly EPA and GLA) are more likely to have bone loss than those with normal levels of these fatty acids. In a study of women over 65 with osteoporosis, those who took EPA and GLA supplements had less bone loss over 3 years than those who took a placebo. Many of these women also experienced an increase in bone density. Unlike other forms of omega-6s, which are considered inflammatory, GLA has anti-inflammatory properties similar to those of omega-3s.

Note: You can take GLA in supplement form with your multivitamin.

Additional beneficial supplements to consider:

Digestive enzymes: These can assist with digestion and enhance micronutrient availability and absorption. Look for a product with amylase, protease, and lipase, as well as a variety of other digestive enzymes. Bromelain, ox bile, pancreatin, papain, pepsin, and betaine HCL may all be beneficial. Betaine HCL may be especially important for this protocol, as it helps with the absorption of calcium and magnesium—two key micronutrients for bone health.

DHEA: This supplement has been shown to stimulate bone growth and help prevent osteoporosis. DHEA should be taken with caution, though, because high doses may suppress the body's natural ability to make DHEA and may lead to liver damage (as shown in an animal study). Taking antioxidants—such as vitamins C and E and selenium—is recommended to prevent oxidative damage to the liver.

Strontium: We do not recommend strontium, as it uses the same carrier protein as calcium for transport, thus causing micronutrient competition. It is also not an essential micronutrient, and it may cause false readings of improvement on your DEXA scan because it is denser than calcium.

The Bone Building 28-Day Menu Plan

Limited foods are *italicized* so that you can see where they fit into your plan. Feel free to choose from any of the Miracle Pestos, Miracle Butters, SKINNYFat Salad Dressings, and SKINNYFat Infusions as they all fit into the Bone Building protocol.

WEEK 1

DAY 1 (Sunday)

9:00 a.m. *Greek Yogurt and Fruit Bowl (page 331) or Baked Apple à la Micronutrient Miracle Mode (page 332)*

1:00 p.m. Traditional Triple Threat Shake (page 311)

5:00 p.m. Buffalo Chicken Chili (page 340)

9:00 p.m. Triple Threat Pudding (page 313)

DAY 2 (Monday)

7:30 a.m. Traditional Triple Threat Shake (page 311)

12:00 p.m. Leftover Buffalo Chicken Chili

3:30 p.m. Traditional Triple Threat Shake (page 311)

7:30 p.m. Salmon with green beans and choice of a Miracle Pesto or Miracle Butter (pages 315–318)

DAY 3 (Tuesday)

7:30 a.m. Triple Threat Cheesecake (page 314)

12:00 p.m. Big salad with leftover salmon and green beans with choice of SKINNYFat dressing (pages 321–322)

3:30 p.m. Traditional Triple Threat Shake (page 311)

7:30 p.m. Greek Chicken (page 337)

DAY 4 (Wednesday)

7:30 a.m. Traditional Triple Threat Shake (page 311)

12:00 p.m. Leftover Greek Chicken

3:30 p.m. Triple Threat Pudding (page 313)

7:30 p.m. Quick Tandoori Shrimp (page 336) with Cooling Cucumber Raita (page 320)

DAY 5 (Thursday)

7:30 a.m. Traditional Triple Threat Shake (page 311)

12:00 p.m. Big salad with leftover Quick Tandoori Shrimp and choice of SKINNYFat dressing (pages 321–322)

3:30 p.m. Triple Threat Pudding (page 313)

7:30 p.m. Speedy Salmon Cakes (page 329) with SKINNYFat Tartar Sauce (page 322) and Oven-Roasted Brussels Sprouts (page 352)

DAY 6 (Friday)

7:30 a.m. Triple Threat Cheesecake (page 314)

12:00 p.m. Broccoli Cheese Soup (page 327); use Gouda cheese in the recipe

3:30 p.m. Traditional Triple Threat Shake (page 311)

7:30 p.m. Grilled steak with choice of a Miracle Pesto (pages 315–316) and Cauliflower Mash (page 352)

DAY 7 (Saturday)

9:00 a.m. Speedy Salmon Cakes (page 329) and eggs any style

1:00 p.m. Traditional Triple Threat Shake (page 311)

5:00 p.m. *Fish and Chips (page 350)*

9:00 p.m. Chocolate Triple Threat Ice Cream (page 314)

WEEK 2

DAY 8 (Sunday)

9:00 a.m. French Onion Egg Tart (page 328); make sure to use Gouda cheese

1:00 p.m. Traditional Triple Threat Shake (page 311)

5:00 p.m. Rustic Portobello Pizza Caps (page 344)

9:00 p.m. Triple Threat Pudding (page 311)

DAY 9 (Monday)

7:30 a.m. Traditional Triple Threat Shake (page 311)

12:00 p.m. *Grilled or broiled chicken thighs, choice of a Miracle Pesto or Miracle Butter (pages 321–322), and baked sweet potato*

3:30 p.m. Triple Threat Pudding (page 313)

7:30 p.m. Moqueca (aka Brazilian Fish Stew) (page 343)

DAY 10 (Tuesday)

7:30 a.m. Traditional Triple Threat Shake (page 311)

12:00 p.m. Leftover Moqueca

3:30 p.m. Traditional Triple Threat Shake (page 311)

7:30 p.m. Shepherd's Pie (page 351)

DAY 11 (Wednesday)

7:30 a.m. Traditional Triple Threat Shake (page 311)

12:00 p.m. Leftover Shepherd's Pie

3:30 p.m. Triple Threat Pudding (page 313)

7:30 p.m. Thai-Style Chopped Pork (page 347) on greens

DAY 12 (Thursday)

7:30 a.m. Triple Threat Cheesecake (page 314)

12:00 p.m. Leftover chopped pork on a salad with choice of SKINNYFat dressing (pages 321–322)

3:30 p.m. Traditional Triple Threat Shake (page 314)

7:30 p.m. Scallops in Lemon Butter Sauce (page 334) with broccoli

DAY 13 (Friday)

7:30 a.m. Triple Threat Cheesecake (page 314)

12:00 p.m. Mexican Chicken Wrap (page 338)

3:30 p.m. Traditional Triple Threat Shake (page 311)

7:30 p.m. Salad and Rustic Flatbread (page 346)

DAY 14 (Saturday)

9:00 a.m. *Carrot Cake Pancakes with Cream Cheese Frosting and chopped walnuts and raisins (page 333)*

1:00 p.m. Traditional Triple Threat Shake (page 311)

5:00 p.m. Micronutrient-Packed "Offaly" Tasty Meatloaf (page 348) and steamed vegetable with choice of Miracle Pesto or Miracle Butter (pages 315–318)

9:00 p.m. Triple Threat Pudding (page 313)

WEEK 3

DAY 15 (Sunday)

9:00 a.m. Leftover meatloaf heated in a frying pan topped with a fried egg and covered with Gouda cheese

1:00 p.m. Traditional Triple Threat Shake (page 311)

5:00 p.m. *Camarão na Moranga (aka Brazilian Shrimp Stew in a Pumpkin) (page 335)*

9:00 p.m. Triple Threat Pudding (page 313)

DAY 16 (Monday)

7:30 a.m. Traditional Triple Threat Shake (page 311)

12:00 p.m. Big salad with ½ can of tuna fish, Gouda cheese, and choice of SKINNYFat dressing (pages 321–322)

3:30 p.m. Traditional Triple Threat Shake (page 311)

7:30 p.m. Chicken Wings (page 334) with Really Creamy SKINNYFat Blue Cheese Dressing (page 322) and carrot and celery sticks

DAY 17 (Tuesday)

7:30 a.m. Traditional Triple Threat Shake (page 311)

12:00 p.m. Leftover chicken wings and blue cheese dressing

3:30 p.m. Triple Threat Pudding (page 313)

7:30 p.m. Coq au Vin (page 347) served with Cauliflower Mash (page 352)

DAY 18 (Wednesday)

7:30 a.m. Traditional Triple Threat Shake (page 311)

12:00 p.m. Leftover Coq au Vin

3:30 p.m. Triple Threat Pudding (page 313)

7:30 p.m. Zughetti (page 345) and grilled chicken thigh with Rich and Creamy Alfredo Sauce (page 319)

DAY 19 (Thursday)

7:30 a.m. Triple Threat Cheesecake (page 314)

12:00 p.m. Bun-less beef burger covered with melted Gouda cheese and a side salad with choice of SKINNYFat dressing (pages 321–322)

3:30 p.m. Traditional Triple Threat Shake (page 311)

7:30 p.m. Thai Shrimp Noodle Soup (page 326)

DAY 20 (Friday)

7:30 a.m. Traditional Triple Threat Shake (page 311)

12:00 p.m. Leftover Thai Shrimp Noodle Soup

3:30 p.m. Triple Threat Pudding (page 313)

7:30 p.m. *Rotisserie or baked whole chicken with Sweet Potato, Yam, and Apple Casserole (page 353)*

DAY 21 (Saturday)

9:00 a.m. Fried eggs served on Cauliflower Cheesy Hash Browns (page 329); use Gouda cheese in the hash browns

1:00 p.m. Triple Threat Cheesecake (page 314)

5:00 p.m. Miracle Chinese Fried "Rice" (page 339)

9:00 p.m. Traditional Triple Threat Shake (page 311)

WEEK 4

DAY 22 (Sunday)

9:00 a.m. *Smoked Salmon Cream Cheese Roll-Ups (page 331) with avocado slices and berries or grapefruit*

1:00 p.m. Traditional Triple Threat Shake (page 311)

5:00 p.m. Slow-Cooked Beer-Braised Beef (page 338) and Cauliflower Mash (page 352)

9:00 p.m. Chocolate Triple Threat Ice Cream (page 314)

DAY 23 (Monday)

7:30 a.m. Triple Threat Cheesecake (page 314)

12:00 p.m. Leftover Miracle Chinese Fried "Rice"

3:30 p.m. Traditional Triple Threat Shake (page 311)

7:30 p.m. Fish and vegetables with choice of a Miracle Pesto or Miracle Butter (pages 315–318)

DAY 24 (Tuesday)

7:30 a.m. Traditional Triple Threat Shake (page 311)

12:00 p.m. Leftover Slow-Cooked Beer-Braised Beef and Cauliflower Mash

3:30 p.m. Triple Threat Pudding (page 313)

7:30 p.m. Greek Lamb Kabobs (page 341)

DAY 25 (Wednesday)

7:30 a.m. Traditional Triple Threat Shake (page 311)

12:00 p.m. Leftover Greek Lamb Kabobs on a salad with choice of SKINNYFat dressing (pages 321–322)

3:30 p.m. Triple Threat Pudding (page 313)

7:30 p.m. Fabulous Fajitas (page 349) with Holy Moly Guacamole (page 324) and salsa; use Gouda cheese.

DAY 26 (Thursday)

7:30 a.m. Triple Threat Cheesecake (page 314)

12:00 p.m. Bun-less beef burger and Oven-Roasted Brussels Sprouts (page 352)

3:30 p.m. Traditional Triple Threat Shake (page 311)

7:30 p.m. Zughetti (page 345) with Mom's Beef Bolognese (page 324)

DAY 27 (Friday)

7:30 a.m. Traditional Triple Threat Shake (page 311)

12:00 p.m. Grilled or broiled chicken thigh on a big salad with choice of SKINNYFat dressing (pages 321–322)

3:30 p.m. Triple Threat Pudding (page 313)

7:30 p.m. *Peppercorn-Crusted Beef Tenderloin (page 341) with 4-Ingredient Blender Hollandaise (page 323) and baked potato with skin on*

DAY 28 (Saturday)

9:00 a.m. Protein-Packed Morning Muffins (page 330)

1:00 p.m. Traditional Triple Threat Shake (page 311)

5:00 p.m. Grilled Tandoori Skewers (page 342) with Cooling Cucumber Raita (page 320) and Indian Garlic-Butter Cheese Non-Naan (page 354)

9:00 p.m. Chocolate Triple Threat Ice Cream (page 314)

Hormone Regulation

This plan is specifically designed for individuals who are suffering from hormone imbalances. This protocol will help you to create an internal environment that will help to regulate and rebalance your hormones naturally. **The Hormone Regulation protocol is designed for individuals who have:**

- Excess or low levels of cortisol, progesterone, estrogen, androgens, testosterone, or thyroid hormone
- Hypothyroidism

Adjustments you must make to the Signature 28-day Micronutrient Miracle plan for your specific condition(s):

10 GOLDEN RULES: While each of the condition-specific protocols must follow all 10 of the Golden Rules, for best results with this protocol, we have identified the following rules to either be critical or require small tweaks.

#2: Ousting the obesogens is critical, as they are hormone disruptors. Make sure to be keenly aware of eliminating MSG, BPA, and phthalates.

#5: Stress reduction is very important for hormonal balance, as stress increases the release of cortisol, the hormone that spikes appetite and increases visceral fat storage in the belly region. Even if you're doing everything else right, high levels of cortisol will throw all your hormones off-balance. Make sure to practice stress-reducing techniques.

#6: While long, extended cardio sessions can cause further hormonal and adrenal fatigue, both our ZMT cardiovascular workout and our One Set To Failure weight training can be beneficial. These types of workouts stimulate a flurry of beneficial hormonal reactions within the body.

#7: Purchasing nontoxic household and beauty goods will ensure they are not causing hormonal imbalances. Try to follow our Top 10 Terrific Tricks to Reduce Household Toxins.

#8: Using nutreince as your multivitamin during this protocol can be extremely helpful because it is the only multivitamin that we know of on the market that contains adequate amounts of many of the essential micronutrients shown to be beneficial in preventing and treating hormone imbalances, including all eight forms of natural vitamin E, 400 milligrams of ionic magnesium citrate, 600 milligrams of ionic calcium citrate, 425 milligrams of choline, and 2,000 IU of vitamin D_3. If you choose to use an alternative multivitamin, make sure to review the ABCs of Optimal Supplementation Guidelines and use the stack-up quiz to evaluate your choice (MultivitaminStackUpQuiz.com).

#9: Taking your Micronutrient Miracle Triple Threat Shakes twice a day is especially important while following this protocol, as the hormone leptin is key to managing all of the other hormones. Think of it as the master hormone that helps to control hunger and feelings of satiety. Taking your Triple Threat for breakfast, first thing in the morning, will start your day off right with the proper amount of protein and fat, which is key to keeping your leptin levels in check for the rest of the day.

DAILY LIMITS: The daily limits for the Hormone Regulation protocol are the same as for our Signature plan. However, for the next 28 days, pay particular attention to the following recommendation.

Saturated fat: Make sure to take in enough fat for optimal results with this protocol. This is the best way to boost testosterone and other hormones. Cholesterol is needed for the formation of healthy cell membranes and is a precursor to all steroid hormones (progesterone, estrogen, follicle-stimulating hormone, etc.). One cannot have proper hormonal balance without adequate amounts of saturated fats. Focus on consuming SKINNYFat, egg yolks, coconut oil, avocados, and other healthy sources of saturated fat.

Beneficial micronutrients while on the Hormone Regulation protocol for hormone rebalancing:

Vitamin A	Vitamin E	Magnesium
Vitamin B$_1$	Calcium	Selenium
Vitamin B$_5$	Choline	Zinc
Vitamin B$_6$	Chromium	Omega-3 fatty acids
Vitamin C	Copper	Omega-6 fatty acids
Vitamin D	Iron	(GLA)

POWERHOUSE PICKS: Choose these micronutrient powerhouses whenever possible. The Rich Foods listed below are high in the essential micronutrients shown to be beneficial to hormone regulation. We have adjusted your 28-day menu suggestions to include these Rich Food choices. Choose these Rich Foods when designing personalized menus or eating out, and don't forget to properly prepare foods that contain EMDs.

PROTEINS

Beef	Lamb	Sardines
Bone broth	Mussels	Scallops
Chicken	Organ meats	Shrimp
Clams	Oysters	Snapper
Cod	Pork	Tuna
Crab	Rainbow trout	Turkey
Herring	Salmon	Venison

DAIRY

Cheese	Milk
Cream	Yogurt

FATS

Butter	Cocoa butter	SKINNYFat*
Chocolate (100 percent pure)	Eggs (with yolks)	

*Use SKINNYFat in recipes whenever possible, as it is virtually impossible to store as body fat. Peer-reviewed published research also shows that MCT oil (the main ingredient in SKINNYFat) increases metabolism, reduces body fat, and improves insulin sensitivity and glucose tolerance. Additionally, the ingredients in SKINNYFat have been shown to optimize the production of thyroid hormones and help with the absorption and utilization of key micronutrients beneficial to hormone regulation, including vitamins A, D, and E, and the minerals calcium and magnesium.

NONSTARCHY VEGETABLES

Asparagus	Celery	Onions
Avocado	Dark leafy greens	Romaine lettuce
Bell peppers	Garlic	Sauerkraut
Broccoli	Kale	Snow peas
Brussels sprouts	Mushrooms (crimini/ shiitake)	Spinach
Cabbage		Swiss chard
Cauliflower	Mustard greens	Tomatoes

STARCHES

Brown rice	Lentils	Sweet potatoes
Green peas	Potatoes (with skin)	
Kidney beans	Quinoa	

FRUITS

Bananas	Oranges	Raisins
Grapefruit	Papaya	Strawberries
Limes	Prunes	Watermelon

NUTS AND SEEDS

Almonds	Hazelnuts	Pumpkin seeds
Brazil nuts	Hemp seeds	Sesame seeds
Cashews	Peanuts	Sunflower seeds
Chia seeds	Pecans	Walnuts
Flaxseed	Pine nuts	

BENEFICIAL SPICES

Anise	Garlic powder	Saffron
Black pepper	Mustard	Turmeric
Cinnamon	Onion powder	

DAILY BEVERAGES

Black tea	Green tea	Oolong tea
Coffee	Mineral water	Water

Additional essential micronutrient supplements to consider:

Vitamin C: Studies have found that supplementing with vitamin C can help to increase progesterone and balance cortisol levels. However, if you are on a statin, make sure to speak to your physician about increasing your vitamin C levels, as a dose over 100 milligrams may interfere with your medication.

Vitamin D: If you are using a multivitamin other than nutreince (which contains 2,000 IU of vitamin D_3), you may want to supplement with 2,000 IU of vitamin D if you suffer from excess androgens or low thyroid.

Omega-3s: It is important to achieve a balance of omega-3s and omega-6s to properly regulate hormone levels. Omega-3s can also help control high cortisol levels. Attempt to get the RDI of 1.6 grams (1,600 milligrams) per day from food or in supplement form.

Note: You can take omega-3s in supplement form at the same time as your multivitamin (nutreince). Opt for Origin Omega or try to find a supplement with a greater amount of EPA than DHA, if possible.

Omega-6s (GLA): While we strive to keep omega-6 levels low and in balance with omega-3s on the Micronutrient Miracle plan, gamma-linolenic acid (GLA) is an omega-6 fatty acid that has anti-inflammatory properties similar to those of omega-3s, unlike other omega-6s, which are considered inflammatory. Studies show that supplementing with GLA can help support healthy progesterone levels.

Note: You can take GLA in supplement form with your AM multivitamin (nutreince) or your PM multivitamin.

Selenium and iodine: Taking a multivitamin with iodine can be helpful to support thyroid function. Caution should be exercised when taking high doses of iodine; however, the doses of iodine present in nutreince are well tolerated by most people with hypothyroidism. Iodine absorption is greatly improved with the supplementation of a key synergist, selenium. While the AM dose of nutreince already contains 70 micrograms of selenium, we suggest that those with hypothyroidism take an additional 200 micrograms in the form of selenomethionine with their morning nutreince. Iodine's other synergistic micronutrients—vitamins A and E, iron, and zinc—are already supplied in ample amounts, as is vitamin D, which is likely deficient in those with this condition.

Additional beneficial supplements to consider:

Digestive enzymes: These can assist with digestion and enhance micronutrient availability and absorption. Look for a product with amylase, protease, and lipase, as well as a variety of other digestive enzymes, such as bromelain, ox bile, pancreatin, papain, pepsin, and betaine HCL. Digestive enzymes are key to protein/amino acid absorption, and many amino acids can restore the endocrine glands' ability to produce normal levels of hormones.

Phosphatidylserine: This is often used for reducing cortisol levels.

L-theanine: This amino acid, found in green tea, has been shown to lower stress hormones, including cortisol. It also improves sleep and reduces anxiety.

L-lysine and L-arginine: Together these amino acids can help to lower cortisol levels and feelings of anxiety.

Ashwagandha: This herbal supplement can reduce anxiety and lower cortisol levels.

Rhodiola: This is used for reducing stress, improving mental focus, and decreasing cortisol levels and feelings of depression.

Chasteberry: This supplement is safe and effective for increasing progesterone.

St. John's wort: Used for those with low progesterone or estrogen levels, this herbal supplement has been shown to relieve behavioral and physical PMS symptoms.

Saw palmetto: This supplement acts to lower androgens in those suffering with excess androgens.

Maca root: This is a tuber in the radish family that has a history of boosting hormone production and libido. Many women report fewer PMS symptoms, improved skin, and increased fertility, while men notice increased libido, increased sperm production, and better sleep.

The Hormone Regulation 28-Day Menu Plan

Limited foods are *italicized* so that you can see where they fit into your plan. Feel free to choose from any of the Miracle Pestos, Miracle Butters, SKINNYFat Salad Dressings, and SKINNYFat Infusions, as they all fit into the Hormone Regulation protocol.

WEEK 1

DAY 1 (Sunday)

9:00 a.m. *Greek Yogurt and Fruit Bowl (page 331)* or Baked Apple à la Micronutrient Miracle Mode (page 332)

1:00 p.m. Traditional Triple Threat Shake (page 311)

5:00 p.m. Buffalo Chicken Chili (page 340) with optional Ridiculously Simple Wrap (page 353) for dipping

9:00 p.m. Triple Threat Pudding (page 313)

DAY 2 (Monday)

7:30 a.m. Traditional Triple Threat Shake (page 311)

12:00 p.m. Leftover Buffalo Chicken Chili

3:30 p.m. Traditional Triple Threat Shake (page 311)

7:30 p.m. Salmon with snow peas and choice of a Miracle Pesto or Miracle Butter (pages 315–318)

DAY 3 (Tuesday)

7:30 a.m. Triple Threat Cheesecake (page 314)

12:00 p.m. Big salad with leftover salmon and snow peas with choice of SKINNYFat dressing (pages 321–322)

3:30 p.m. Traditional Triple Threat Shake (page 311)

7:30 p.m. Greek Chicken (page 337)

DAY 4 (Wednesday)

7:30 a.m. Traditional Triple Threat Shake (page 311)

12:00 p.m. Leftover Greek Chicken

3:30 p.m. Triple Threat Cheesecake (page 314)

7:30 p.m. Quick Tandoori Shrimp (page 336) with Cooling Cucumber Raita (page 320)

DAY 5 (Thursday)

7:30 a.m. Traditional Triple Threat Shake (page 311)

12:00 p.m. Big salad with leftover Quick Tandoori Shrimp and choice of SKINNYFat dressing (pages 321–322)

3:30 p.m. Triple Threat Pudding (page 313)

7:30 p.m. Mexican Chicken Wrap (page 338)

DAY 6 (Friday)

7:30 a.m. Traditional Triple Threat Shake (page 311)

12:00 p.m. Broccoli Cheese Soup (page 327)

3:30 p.m. Traditional Triple Threat Shake (page 311)

7:30 p.m. Grilled steak with choice of a Miracle Pesto (pages 315–318) and Cauliflower Mash (page 352)

DAY 7 (Saturday)

9:00 a.m. French Onion Egg Tart (page 328)

1:00 p.m. Traditional Triple Threat Shake (page 311)

5:00 p.m. *Fish and Chips (page 350)*

9:00 p.m. Chocolate Triple Threat Ice Cream (page 314)

WEEK 2

DAY 8 (Sunday)

9:00 a.m. Speedy Salmon Cakes (page 329) and eggs any style

1:00 p.m. Traditional Triple Threat Shake (page 311)

5:00 p.m. Rustic Portobello Pizza Caps (page 344)

9:00 p.m. Traditional Triple Threat Shake (page 311)

DAY 9 (Monday)

7:30 a.m. Traditional Triple Threat Shake (page 311)

12:00 p.m. *Grilled or broiled chicken thighs, choice of a Miracle Pesto or Miracle Butter (pages 315–318), and baked sweet potato*

3:30 p.m. Triple Threat Cheesecake (page 314)

7:30 p.m. Moqueca (aka Brazilian Fish Stew) (page 343)

DAY 10 (Tuesday)

7:30 a.m. Traditional Triple Threat Shake (page 311)

12:00 p.m. Leftover Moqueca

3:30 p.m. Traditional Triple Threat Shake (page 311)

7:30 p.m. Coq au Vin (page 347) served with Cauliflower Mash (page 352)

DAY 11 (Wednesday)

7:30 a.m. Traditional Triple Threat Shake (page 311)

12:00 p.m. Leftover Coq au Vin

3:30 p.m. Triple Threat Pudding (page 313)

7:30 p.m. Thai-Style Chopped Pork (page 347) on greens

DAY 12 (Thursday)

7:30 a.m. Traditional Triple Threat Shake (page 311)

12:00 p.m. Leftover chopped pork on a salad with choice of SKINNYFat dressing (pages 321–322)

3:30 p.m. Traditional Triple Threat Shake (page 311)

7:30 p.m. Scallops in Lemon Butter Sauce (page 334) with broccoli

DAY 13 (Friday)

7:30 a.m. Traditional Triple Threat Shake (page 311)

12:00 p.m. Mexican Chicken Wrap (page 338)

3:30 p.m. Traditional Triple Threat Shake (page 311)

7:30 p.m. Salad and Rustic Flatbread (page 346)

DAY 14 (Saturday)

9:00 a.m. *Carrot Cake Pancakes with Cream Cheese Frosting and chopped walnuts and raisins (page 333)*

1:00 p.m. Traditional Triple Threat Shake (page 311)

5:00 p.m. Micronutrient-Packed "Offaly" Tasty Meatloaf (page 348) and steamed vegetable with choice of a Miracle Pesto or Miracle Butter (pages 315–318)

9:00 p.m. Triple Threat Cheesecake (page 314)

WEEK 3

DAY 15 (Sunday)

9:00 a.m. Leftover meatloaf heated in a frying pan and topped with a fried egg and covered in melted cheese

1:00 p.m. Traditional Triple Threat Shake (page 311)

5:00 p.m. *Camarão na Moranga (aka Brazilian Shrimp Stew in a Pumpkin) (page 335)*

9:00 p.m. Traditional Triple Threat Shake (page 311)

DAY 16 (Monday)

7:30 a.m. Traditional Triple Threat Shake (page 311)

12:00 p.m. Big salad with ½ can of tuna fish and choice of SKINNYFat dressing (pages 321–322)

3:30 p.m. Traditional Triple Threat Shake (page 311)

7:30 p.m. Chicken Wings (page 334) with Really Creamy SKINNYFat Blue Cheese Dressing (page 322) and carrot and celery sticks

DAY 17 (Tuesday)

7:30 a.m. Traditional Triple Threat Shake (page 311)

12:00 p.m. Leftover chicken wings and blue cheese dressing

3:30 p.m. Triple Threat Cheesecake (page 314)

7:30 p.m. Shepherd's Pie (page 351)

DAY 18 (Wednesday)

7:30 a.m. Traditional Triple Threat Shake (page 311)

12:00 p.m. Leftover Shepherd's Pie

3:30 p.m. Traditional Triple Threat Shake (page 311)

7:30 p.m. Zughetti (page 345) and grilled chicken thigh with Rich and Creamy Alfredo Sauce (page 319)

DAY 19 (Thursday)

7:30 a.m. Triple Threat Cheesecake (page 314)

12:00 p.m. Bun-less beef or turkey burger and a side salad with choice of SKINNYFat dressing (pages 321–322)

3:30 p.m. Traditional Triple Threat Shake (page 311)

7:30 p.m. Thai Shrimp Noodle Soup (page 326)

DAY 20 (Friday)

7:30 a.m. Traditional Triple Threat Shake (page 311)

12:00 p.m. Leftover Thai Shrimp Noodle Soup

3:30 p.m. Traditional Triple Threat Shake (page 311)

7:30 p.m. *Rotisserie or baked whole chicken with Sweet Potato, Yam, and Apple Casserole (page 353)*

DAY 21 (Saturday)

9:00 a.m. Fried eggs served on Cauliflower Cheesy Hash Browns (page 329)

1:00 p.m. Traditional Triple Threat Shake (page 311)

5:00 p.m. Miracle Chinese Fried "Rice" (page 339)

9:00 p.m. Traditional Triple Threat Shake (page 311)

WEEK 4

DAY 22 (Sunday)

9:00 a.m. *Smoked Salmon Cream Cheese Roll-Ups (page 331) with avocado slices and berries or grapefruit*

1:00 p.m. Traditional Triple Threat Shake (page 311)

5:00 p.m. Slow-Cooked Beer-Braised Beef (page 338) and Cauliflower Mash (page 352)

9:00 p.m. Chocolate Triple Threat Ice Cream (page 314)

DAY 23 (Monday)

7:30 a.m. Traditional Triple Threat Shake (page 311)

12:00 p.m. Leftover Miracle Chinese Fried "Rice"

3:30 p.m. Traditional Triple Threat Shake (page 311)

7:30 p.m. Fish and vegetables with choice of a Miracle Pesto or Miracle Butter (pages 315–318)

DAY 24 (Tuesday)

7:30 a.m. Traditional Triple Threat Shake (page 311)

12:00 p.m. Leftover Slow-Cooked Beer-Braised Beef and Cauliflower Mash

3:30 p.m. Triple Threat Pudding (page 313)

7:30 p.m. Greek Lamb Kabobs (page 341)

DAY 25 (Wednesday)

7:30 a.m. Traditional Triple Threat Shake (page 311)

12:00 p.m. Leftover Greek Lamb Kabobs on a salad with choice of SKINNYFat dressing (pages 321–322)

3:30 p.m. Triple Threat Cheesecake (page 314)

7:30 p.m. Fabulous Fajitas (page 349) with Holy Moly Guacamole (page 324) and salsa

DAY 26 (Thursday)

7:30 a.m. Traditional Triple Threat Shake (page 311)

12:00 p.m. Bun-less beef burger and Oven-Roasted Brussels Sprouts (page 352)

3:30 p.m. Traditional Triple Threat Shake (page 311)

7:30 p.m. Zughetti (page 345) with Mom's Beef Bolognese (page 324)

DAY 27 (Friday)

7:30 a.m. Traditional Triple Threat Shake (page 311)

12:00 p.m. Grilled or broiled chicken thigh on a big salad with choice of SKINNYFat dressing (pages 321–322)

3:30 p.m. Triple Threat Cheesecake (page 314)

7:30 p.m. *Peppercorn-Crusted Beef Tenderloin (page 341) with 4-Ingredient Blender Hollandaise (page 323) and baked potato*

DAY 28 (Saturday)

9:00 a.m. Protein-Packed Morning Muffins (page 330)

1:00 p.m. Traditional Triple Threat Shake (page 311)

5:00 p.m. Grilled Tandoori Skewers (page 342) with Cooling Cucumber Raita (page 320) and Indian Garlic-Butter Cheese Non-Naan (page 354)

9:00 p.m. Chocolate Triple Threat Ice Cream (page 314)

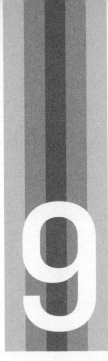

Extraordinarily Delicious Recipes

GET READY TO ENJOY some of the most delicious food you have ever eaten! We mean it! Some of these dishes will have you literally humming through the meal. We collected many of these incredible recipes during our travels around the world during the Calton Project. While we tweaked some a bit here and there to fit into our Micronutrient Miracle protocol, these recipes still include a wide variety of enticing and deeply satisfying flavors for you to enjoy.

Remember to put all the information we covered in Chapter 5 into practice when purchasing ingredients for the recipes in this chapter. Do your best over the next 28 days to locate and purchase the highest-quality local, organic, pasture-raised, grass-fed, non-GMO food you can. Don't forget that to accommodate availability and your budget, you can use our Good, Better, Best system when purchasing proteins and pantry staples and the Fab 14 and Terrible 20 lists when choosing produce. To help you find some of the more unique ingredients in the recipes, and to make shopping a little easier and less expensive, make sure to visit us at mymiracleplan.com. Not only will you find money saving coupons, but we will also have links to some of our favorite kitchen gadgets and gizmos. We are also linking you up to some of our favorite online purveyors who we know offer great high quality foods and home products at savings you can't find in the traditional grocery stores.

As you make your way through the recipes, feel free to change things up a bit to fit your personal taste preferences. For example, if the recipe calls for fish but you prefer shrimp, or if you would rather have broccoli than asparagus, swap it out. Or if you can't stand one of the spices, simply leave it out or reduce the suggested amount. Additionally, you will notice that our Triple Threat recipes always include nutreince for the micronutrients, SKINNYFat for the medium- and long-chain fats, and IN.POWER for the protein. Here, too, feel free to swap items to fit your dietary preferences. For example, if you use another multivitamin or prefer a plant-based protein, you can switch out nutreince or IN.POWER for your brand (if you are using a multivitamin pill, simply take it at the same time; do not put it into the recipe as a pill), or if you would like to use a different fat source in place of SKINNYFat, that's fine too. While your alterations will likely reduce the overall benefits slightly and will change the micronutrient profile or flavor a bit, the most important thing is that you are able to create a delicious option that will satisfy your dietary preferences.

Oh, and one last thing: Each of the recipes clearly state the serving size, but we find that many people following the Micronutrient Miracle plan enjoy doubling the recipes and either eating that meal several times over the week or freezing a portion for later use. This makes things really easy when you find yourself in a time crunch, so you may want to consider this time-saving tactic as well.

You can also watch us cook some of our favorite recipes in our free Cooking with the Caltons videos located in the Micronutrient Miracle Motivation and Resource Center at mymiracleplan.com.

TRIPLE THREAT RECIPES

If you are new to SKINNYFat, when making shakes or coffees begin by adding only 1 teaspoon and slowly increase to the required amount. It may take about a week for your stomach to become accustomed to this oil.

Traditional Triple Threat Shake

Those of smaller stature, whose goal weight is under 150 pounds, should use the small–medium recipe, while those whose goal weights are higher, above 150, may opt for the medium–large recipe, which will supply a greater amount of protein per shake.

Serves 1

SMALL–MEDIUM

- 8 oz water
- Small scoop of ice
- 1 packet either AM or PM nutreince
- 1 Tbsp SKINNYFat Original
- 1 scoop IN.POWER protein

MEDIUM–LARGE

- 8 oz water
- Small scoop of ice
- 1 packet either AM or PM nutreince
- 2 Tbsp SKINNYFat Original
- 2 scoops IN.POWER protein

1. Place the water in a blender with the ice and blend until smooth.

2. On low, add the nutreince while blending. Add the SKINNYFat while continuing to blend. Finally, add the IN.POWER while blending.

3. Increase the speed from low to medium for 20 to 30 seconds simply to fluff the delicious shake.

Optional: *Swap the water for prechilled coffee. If you only have hot coffee, use ½ cup hot coffee and 1 cup ice in lieu of the 8 ounces of water. It is delicious with the vanilla AM.*

Double Chocolate Mocha Triple Threat

Serves 1

8 oz chilled organic fair trade coffee

1 scoop IN.POWER protein

1 packet nutreince chocolate PM

1 tsp Stevita Delight chocolate drink mix

1 Tbsp SKINNYFat Original

Combine all of the ingredients in a blender and pour over ice, or blend in the ice for a frozen beverage.

Optional: *Want a Double Chocolate Mocha Triple Threat in the morning? No problem. Simply make this recipe with a nutreince vanilla or unflavored AM packet and add in more chocolate Stevita Delight to taste.*

Cinnamon Spice Triple Threat Shake

A holiday favorite!

Serves 1

8 oz cold flat or sparkling water

1 scoop IN.POWER protein

1 Tbsp SKINNYFat Original

1 packet nutreince vanilla AM

½ tsp organic cinnamon

Combine all of the ingredients in a blender and enjoy!

Gingerbread Triple Threat Coffee

Who needs a gingerbread cookie when you have this Triple Threat around?

Serves 1

8 oz warm organic fair trade coffee

1 scoop IN.POWER protein

1 packet nutreince vanilla

5–10 drops toffee-flavored Stevita drops

1 Tbsp SKINNYFat Original

½ tsp organic vanilla extract

½ tsp organic cinnamon

⅛ tsp organic ground ginger

Combine all of the ingredients in a blender and enjoy! If you are an iced coffee fan, you can certainly use chilled coffee and pour it over ice for the same delicious treat—but cold!

Triple Threat Pudding

This pudding is great for a quick and easy breakfast or for a midafternoon snack!

Makes 4 puddings to be used as meal replacements!

¾ Tbsp grass-fed gelatin (we like the Great Lakes brand in the red-orange can)

1 cup water

1 cup full-fat coconut milk (BPA-free can) or organic, grass-fed heavy cream

½ Tbsp organic vanilla extract

½ Tbsp organic cinnamon

1 Tbsp Stevita Delight chocolate drink mix (if making nutreince chocolate PM)

1 Tbsp organic, grass-fed, salted butter (the salt helps to bring out sweetness in desserts)

1 Tbsp SKINNYFat Original

4 packets nutreince chocolate PM (That's right, the multivitamin is in the pudding!)

4 scoops IN.POWER protein

1. On low heat, dissolve the gelatin into the water.

2. Place the milk or cream in the blender with the vanilla, cinnamon, Stevita Delight (if making chocolate pudding), butter, and SKINNYFat and blend.

3. Once the gelatin is dissolved, add the gelatin mixture into blender while blending on low.

4. Add in the nutreince and IN.POWER while blending.

5. Blend thoroughly then pour into 4 ramekins. Cover and put in the refrigerator.

Note: If you are trying to gain a lot of muscle, you may want to add in an additional 4 scoops IN.POWER so that you will have a total of 2 in each of the 4 puddings.

Triple Threat Cheesecake

Makes 4 cheesecakes to be used as meal replacements!

¾ Tbsp gelatin (great lakes or similar)

1 cup water

1 block (16 Tbsp) organic cream cheese

½ Tbsp cinnamon

½ Tbsp vanilla

½ Tbsp Stevita delight chocolate drink mix (if making nutreince chocolate PM)

4 packets nutreince (AM or PM)

4 scoops IN.POWER protein

1 Tbsp. SKINNYfat Original

1. Melt the gelatin into the water over medium heat.

2. Place all of the remaining ingredients into a blender or food processor and blend or process with the gelatinized water.

3. Separate into 4 ramekins and chill.

4. Eat as one meal! Enjoy!

Triple Threat Ice Cream—Chocolate or Vanilla

Makes 4 servings of ice cream to be used as meal replacements!

1. Start with the recipe for the Triple Threat Pudding.

2. Create Triple Threat pudding (either chocolate or vanilla), but do not place in ramekins.

3. Place in an ice cream maker and follow the machine's instructions.

MIRACLE PESTOS, MIRACLE BUTTERS, AND SKINNYFAT INFUSIONS

Why do we call these specialty butters and oils miraculous? Not only are they great for you because of the nutrients contained in the herbs, spices, and other ingredients, but they also give you more time in every single day. That's right! You save precious time by making these fabulous fats ahead of time, freezing them in ice cube trays or silicon molds, and then popping them out when you need them for recipes. They add a punch of flavor to any recipe. Serve dishes made with them at dinner parties and you will impress your friends.

Traditional Miracle Pesto

Makes 1 batch

2 cups packed fresh organic basil leaves

½ cup freshly grated organic Parmesan or Romano cheese

¼ cup organic pine nuts

2 large cloves garlic, quartered

Unrefined sea salt to taste

¼–½ cup SKINNYFat Olive

1. Combine the basil, cheese, pine nuts, garlic, and salt in a food processor and blend until evenly and finely chopped.

2. On a low setting, slowly add the SKINNYFat until the sauce has a thick, even texture.

3. Refrigerate or freeze in ice cube trays to use later in recipes.

Dairy-Free, Nut-Free Basil Miracle Pesto

Makes 1 batch

4 cups packed fresh organic basil leaves

Juice of ½ lemon

2 large cloves garlic, quartered

Unrefined sea salt to taste

¼ cup SKINNYFat Olive

1. Combine all of the ingredients in a blender or food processor and blend or process until smooth.

2. Refrigerate or freeze in ice cube trays to use later in recipes.

Sun-Dried Tomato Miracle Pesto (Dairy-Free)

Makes 1 batch

1 cup organic dry-packed sun-dried tomatoes

Handful of organic macadamia nuts

2 cloves garlic

Unrefined sea salt and organic pepper to taste

¼ cup SKINNYFat Olive

1. Reconstitute the dried tomatoes by soaking them in warm water for 30 minutes.

2. Combine all of the ingredients in a blender or food processor until smooth. Add extra SKINNYFat if necessary.

3. Refrigerate or freeze in ice cube trays to use later in recipes.

Herb Miracle Butter

Choose fresh organic herbs if available. If not, then use dried organic herbs.

Makes 1 batch

½ Tbsp organic thyme

½ Tbsp organic sage

½ Tbsp organic rosemary

½ Tbsp organic parsley

2 Tbsp SKINNYFat Olive

8 Tbsp (1 stick) organic, grass-fed, salted butter, softened at room temperature

1. Combine the seasonings with the SKINNYFat in a blender or food processor until smooth.

2. Add in the butter and blend or process until smooth.

3. Refrigerate or freeze in ice cube trays to use later in recipes.

Can't Get Enough Curry Miracle Butter

Makes 1 batch

2 tsp organic curry powder

2 tsp organic turmeric

2 tsp freshly grated ginger

2 Tbsp SKINNYFat Original

8 Tbsp (1 stick) organic, grass-fed, salted butter, softened at room temperature

1. In a skillet, toast the curry and turmeric for about 2 minutes.

2. Combine all of the ingredients in a blender or food processor and blend or process until smooth.

3. Refrigerate or freeze in ice cube trays to use later in recipes.

Garlic-Parmesan Miracle Butter

Makes 1 batch

8 Tbsp (1 stick) organic, grass-fed, salted butter, softened at room temperature

2 Tbsp SKINNYFat Olive

½ cup freshly grated organic Parmesan cheese

1 tsp organic garlic powder

½ tsp organic onion salt

¼ tsp organic pepper

1. Combine all of the ingredients in a blender or food processor until smooth.

2. Refrigerate or freeze in ice cube trays to use later in recipes.

Avocado Potassium-Packed Miracle Butter

Makes 1 batch

2 small avocados, halved, pitted, and peeled

2 Tbsp SKINNYFat Olive

Juice of 1 lemon

4 Tbsp (½ stick) organic, grass-fed, salted butter, softened at room temperature

1 clove garlic, minced

2 tsp organic ground cumin

Unrefined sea salt and organic pepper to taste

1. Combine all of the ingredients in a blender or food processor until smooth.

2. Refrigerate or freeze in ice cube trays to use later in recipes.

Spicy Fat-Loss Miracle Butter

Makes 1 batch

½ tsp organic chili powder

½ tsp organic paprika

½ Tbsp organic garlic powder

¼ tsp organic onion powder

¼ tsp organic ground red cayenne pepper

2 Tbsp SKINNYFat Olive

8 Tbsp (1 stick) organic, grass-fed, salted butter, softened at room temperature

1. Combine the seasonings with the SKINNYFat in a blender or food processor until smooth.

2. Add in the butter and blend or process until smooth.

3. Refrigerate or freeze in ice cube trays to use later in recipes.

SKINNYFat Pizza in a Bottle Italian-Infused Oil

Makes 1 batch

1 oz fresh organic basil, whole

1 oz fresh organic oregano

3 cloves garlic, chopped

1–2 hot peppers, halved (optional)

1 bottle SKINNYFat Olive

1. Preheat the oven to 300°F.

2. Clean the basil and oregano and place all of the ingredients in an oven-safe bowl or baking dish. Cover with the SKINNYFat.

3. Bake for 40 minutes.

4. Let cool, then strain the oil before pouring it back into the glass SKINNYFat bottle.

Note: Make sure to label the bottle. You don't want to accidently use this for your Triple Threat shake!

SKINNYFat Hot Pepper-Infused Oil

Makes 1 batch

5–15 organic hot peppers, halved (try a variety and mix it up)

1 bottle SKINNYFat Olive

1. Preheat the oven to 300°F.

2. Place the peppers in an oven-safe bowl or baking dish and cover with the SKINNYFat.

3. Bake for 40 minutes.

4. Let cool, strain, and pour the oil back into the glass SKINNYFat bottle.

Note: Omit seeds or choose peppers lower on the heat index if you want to reduce the spiciness of the oil. And make sure to label the bottle. You don't want to accidently use this for your Triple Threat shake!

SAUCES, DIPS, DRESSINGS, AND CONDIMENTS

Rich and Creamy Alfredo Sauce

Makes 1 batch

4 Tbsp (½ stick) organic, grass-fed, unsalted butter

1 large organic, pasture-raised egg, beaten

½ cup organic, grass-fed heavy cream

1 clove garlic, minced

⅔ cup freshly grated organic Parmesan cheese

Organic pepper to taste

1. Melt the butter in a skillet over low heat.

2. Add in the egg and cream and combine, raising the heat to medium.

3. Add in the garlic and slowly add in the cheese while stirring, to avoid forming clumps.

4. When fully combined, season with the pepper.

5. Refrigerate or freeze in ice cube trays to use later in recipes.

Optional: Add in sliced portobello mushrooms for an earthy, meatlike quality.

Tzatziki (Greek Cucumber Sauce)

Serves 4

2 cups organic plain Greek yogurt (try and find one that has some fat in it)

2 Tbsp SKINNYFat Olive

2 large organic cucumbers, seeded, grated, and drained to remove excess water (leave the skin on for color)

4 cloves garlic, finely minced

2 tsp lemon zest

2 Tbsp fresh lemon juice

4 Tbsp chopped fresh organic dill

Unrefined sea salt to taste

Combine all of the ingredients in a mixing bowl and let sit for at least 30 minutes prior to eating.

Cooling Cucumber Raita

This cooling, traditionally Indian salad is perfect as an accompaniment to Quick Tandoori Shrimp (page 336), Grilled Tandoori Skewers (page 342), or Indian Garlic-Butter Cheese Non-Naan (page 354).

Serves 4

2 cups organic plain Greek yogurt (try and find one that has some fat in it)

2 Tbsp SKINNYFat Olive

2 large organic seedless cucumbers, 1 chopped and 1 shredded with vegetable peeler and drained to remove excess water (leave the skin on for color)

¼ tsp organic ground coriander

¼ tsp organic ground cumin

¼ cup fresh organic cilantro, chopped

Unrefined sea salt to taste

Combine all of the ingredients in a mixing bowl and let sit for at least 30 minutes prior to eating.

5-Minute SKINNYFat Mayonnaise

You'll never buy bottled or jarred again after tasting this marvelous 5-minute mayonnaise. By using the healthiest ingredients, you'll be the talk of the town with the best spread around.

Makes 1 batch

2 large organic, pasture-raised egg yolks	¼ tsp unrefined sea salt
	¼ tsp organic pepper
1 large organic, pasture-raised whole egg	1 Tbsp fresh lemon juice or organic white vinegar (or apple cider vinegar)
1 Tbsp organic mustard	1 cup SKINNYFat Original

1. Combine the eggs, mustard, salt, pepper, and lemon juice or vinegar in a blender or food processor at low to medium speed until smooth.

2. Slowly pour the SKINNYFat into the blender while mixing.

3. Once all of the SKINNYFat has been mixed in, you will have a creamy, smooth, homemade mayonnaise.

4. Keep refrigerated.

Note: Remove the eggs from the refrigerator and bring them to room temperature. Never attempt to make mayonnaise using chilled eggs.

Optional

· *Curry mayo: Add organic curry powder and organic ground red cayenne pepper to taste. Great in chicken salad.*

· *Cajun mayo: Add organic Cajun spice and organic ground red cayenne pepper to taste. Tasty on Speedy Salmon Cakes (page 329).*

Simple SKINNYFat Italian Dressing

Makes 1 batch

⅔ cup SKINNYFat Olive	1 Tbsp minced garlic
4 Tbsp organic red wine vinegar	Unrefined sea salt and organic pepper to taste

Combine all of the ingredients in a glass jar with a lid that seals tightly. Shake before using. Enjoy!

SKINNYFat Parmesan-Peppercorn Dressing

Makes 1 batch

½ cup Simple SKINNYFat Italian Dressing (page 321)

4 heaping tsp shredded organic Parmesan cheese (buy whole and shred it yourself to avoid added cellulose powder)

¼ cup organic full-fat sour cream or organic plain Greek yogurt

Freshly cracked organic peppercorn to taste

Use an immersion blender to combine the dressing, cheese, and sour cream or yogurt in a mixing bowl. Add the peppercorn and enjoy!

SKINNYFat Tartar Sauce

Makes 1 batch

½ cup 5-Minute SKINNYFat Mayonnaise (page 321)

2 Tbsp diced pickles (we love Bubbies)

1 Tbsp organic white vinegar or white wine vinegar

1 tsp favorite organic mustard

Juice of ¼ lemon

Pinch of unrefined sea salt

Pinch of organic pepper

Combine all of the ingredients in a small bowl and let sit for at least 30 minutes before serving.

Really Creamy SKINNYFat Blue Cheese Dressing (or Dip)

This is one of Jayson's favorites. He uses it on wings, in lettuce wraps, and pretty much anytime he has some handy. Remember: This fat burns fat! You no longer need to dip lightly!

Makes 1 batch

½ of 5-Minute SKINNYFat Mayonnaise recipe (page 321)

4 oz organic blue cheese (gluten-free!)

⅓ cup organic sour cream

4 oz organic cream cheese

Combine all of the ingredients in a blender until smooth. If you prefer chunky blue cheese, mix the mayonnaise with the sour cream and cream cheese and then hand-crumble the blue cheese into the recipe.

Buffalo Wing Sauce (aka Jayson's Red Hot)

This stores really well and gives any meal a kick!

Makes ½ cup

⅔ cup organic white vinegar (apple cider, rice, and white wine vinegar work, as well)

2 tsp SKINNYFat Original

2 tsp organic chili powder

¼ tsp organic smoked paprika

½ tsp organic sweet paprika

1 Tbsp organic garlic powder

½ tsp organic onion powder

½ tsp organic ground red cayenne pepper

¼ tsp unrefined sea salt

Stevia to taste (Jayson uses ½–1 scoop of stevia using the tiny scooper in the bottle; start with just a little and add to taste)

1 tsp grass-fed gelatin

2 Tbsp organic, grass-fed salted butter, melted

1. In a small pot, stir together all of the ingredients except for the gelatin and the butter.

2. Place over medium-high heat. Once warm, slowly stir in the gelatin, to avoid clumping. Keep over the heat until the sauce starts to bubble and thicken.

3. Remove from the heat and allow to cool.

4. Store in an airtight glass bottle and keep refrigerated.

5. When you are ready to serve (likely tossing over your chicken wings; see recipe on page 334), warm the finished sauce and combine with the butter. Do not add the butter until you are ready to coat the wings or any other protein; the sauce will not keep well after you add the butter.

4-Ingredient Blender Hollandaise Sauce

Serves 4

3 organic, pasture-raised egg yolks

¼ tsp organic Dijon mustard

1 Tbsp fresh lemon juice

½ cup organic, grass-fed, unsalted butter, melted

1. Combine the egg yolks, mustard, and lemon juice in a blender or food processor. Blend or process for 10 seconds.

2. Set the blender or food processor on high speed and pour a thin stream of the butter into the egg mixture. It should thicken almost immediately.

3. Keep the sauce warm by placing it in a water bath on the stove. (Place the finished sauce in a bowl resting in a pot of hot water that reaches only about halfway up the sides of the bowl.)

Holy Moly Guacamole

Serves 1 batch

2 ripe avocados	1 organic jalapeño pepper
1 small organic onion	Juice of 1 lime
1 clove garlic	Unrefined sea salt to taste
1 ripe organic tomato	Organic pepper to taste

1. Slice open the avocados, remove the pits, and scoop out the flesh into a bowl.

2. Mince the onion and garlic.

3. Chop the tomato and jalapeño.

4. Mash the avocado in the bowl and stir in the onion, garlic, tomato, and jalapeño to taste.

5. Season with the lime juice, salt, and pepper.

6. Chill for 30 minutes before serving.

Optional: In a hurry? Mash the avocado and simply add 2 Tbsp of organic salsa. It might not be homemade, but it will be a home run!

Mom's Beef Bolognese

Okay, so it isn't Mira's Italian mom's sauce recipe at all. But it is a simple way to take a high-quality sugar-free sauce (like Mom's Organic brand, which is our favorite) and beef it up with grass-fed beef goodness to create a superfast dinnertime solution.

Serves 4

1 Tbsp SKINNYFat Olive	¼ cup freshly grated organic hard Italian cheese, like Parmesan, Asiago, or Pecorino Romano (leave out if your diet is dairy-free)
1½ lb organic, grass-fed ground beef	
1½ jars favorite tomato sauce (we use the 24 oz size Mom's Organic; make sure to choose a sauce that is organic, sugar-free, soy-free, and free of GMO oils)	

1. In a deep, heavy-bottom pot over medium heat, heat the SKINNYFat and brown the beef.

2. When the beef is cooked through, add the tomato sauce and cheese.

3. Allow to simmer for at least 30 minutes to blend the flavors.

4. Serve over Zughetti (page 345) or your favorite gluten-free pasta for a starch option that week.

Killer Ketchup That Won't Kill You!

Makes 1 batch

This is a *ketchup* recipe that has *caught up* to the times. It is sugar-free, organic, and stores well in the refrigerator.

1 can (12 oz) organic tomato paste (BPA-free can)

½ cup water

2 Tbsp organic white vinegar

1 tsp organic onion powder

1 tsp organic allspice

½ tsp organic garlic powder

Organic ground red cayenne pepper to taste

Unrefined sea salt and organic pepper to taste

Stevia extract to taste

1. If possible, pressure-cook the tomato paste first to eliminate lectins.

2. In a saucepan over medium heat, combine all of the ingredients and stir until smooth.

3. Cool and store in a canning jar, preferably opaque, in the fridge.

SOUPS

Bone Broth

Makes 1 batch

Bones (You can use raw or cooked chicken carcasses, marrow bones from the butcher, ribs, etc. Try and use bones from high-quality grass-fed/ pasture-raised proteins.)

2–3 Tbsp organic apple cider vinegar

Garlic to taste (chopped at least 15 minutes before heating)

Unrefined sea salt to taste

1. Place all of the ingredients in a slow cooker. Add enough water to cover the bones. Do not forget to add the vinegar. This is the ingredient that pulls the minerals from the bones.

2. Set to high heat to bring to a boil, and then reduce the heat to low.

3. Remember, patience is a virtue. The longer you let your broth brew, the better it will be. Leave chicken broth in the slow cooker for 24 hours and beef broth for up to 48 hours.

4. Turn it off and cool.

5. Strain the cooled broth using cheesecloth or a fine-mesh metal strainer, and only keep the liquid.

6. Refrigerate. Once cooled, the broth may form a thick, waxy layer of fat (tallow) on the surface. Skim it off and either toss it or save it for cooking.

Thai Shrimp Noodle Soup

Serves 4

2 cups coconut milk

1 cup chicken broth (homemade or an organic, sugar-free, store-bought version)

⅔ cup coconut aminos

1 cup fresh organic cilantro, chopped

¼ cup fresh lime juice (or the juice of 1 lime)

2 cloves garlic, minced

4 Tbsp freshly grated ginger

1½ lb wild-caught shrimp, peeled and deveined

1 Tbsp SKINNYFat Original

2 cups organic green beans

2 organic carrots, chopped into long strips

Organic red-pepper flakes to taste

1 pack Miracle Noodles (optional)

1. Combine the coconut milk, broth, coconut aminos, cilantro, lime, garlic, ginger, and red pepper flakes in a mixing bowl.

2. Add in the shrimp and toss to coat well.

3. In a large pot over medium heat, warm the SKINNYFat. Add the shrimp mixture and cook for about 15 minutes.

4. Add in the green beans and carrots and cook for 5 minutes.

5. Optional: Stir in the Miracle Noodles* for a heartier soup.

*Coupon is available at mymiracleplan.com.

Broccoli Cheese Soup

Serves 4

3 cups chicken broth (homemade or an organic, sugar-free, store-bought version)

1 head organic broccoli, chopped into pieces (you can use the stems, too)

8 oz organic cream cheese

2 Tbsp organic, grass-fed salted butter

1 cup organic, grass-fed heavy cream

2 cups shredded organic Cheddar cheese (buy it in a block and shred it yourself to avoid added cellulose powder)

Unrefined sea salt to taste

Organic pepper to taste

1. By cooking the broccoli in the broth, you will preserve the nutrients that broccoli loses during boiling.

2. When the broccoli is cooked through (fork-soft), move about half of the florets to a small bowl and set aside.

3. Place the broth and the remainder of the broccoli in a blender or food processor and combine until smooth.

4. In a large pot, combine the cream cheese, butter, heavy cream, and Cheddar cheese. Keep the heat low and stir frequently to avoid burning.

5. When the cheese mixture is completely melted, pour in the pureed broccoli and broth and combine over low heat.

6. Add the reserved broccoli florets for texture.

7. Add the salt and pepper.

BREAKFASTS: TO BE ENJOYED ANY TIME OF THE DAY

French Onion Egg Tart

This recipe was inspired by our time in France. We fell in love with onion tarts in Nice and brought that taste back home in this recipe.

Serves 2 as a stand-alone dish or 4 with a side

1 Tbsp organic, grass-fed salted butter, plus more to cook eggs

2 medium organic yellow onions, cut into 1–2 inch pieces

1 large clove garlic (or 2 small cloves), minced

3 sprigs fresh organic thyme

½ tsp organic red-pepper flakes, or to taste (we use 1 tsp because we like it spicy)

¼ tsp unrefined sea salt

¼ tsp organic pepper

4 organic, pasture-raised eggs

2 Tbsp freshly grated organic Parmesan cheese (or a similar cheese)

1 cooked, leftover, organic boneless chicken thigh, diced (if you don't have one in the fridge, you can substitute another leftover meat or quickly dice and brown a thigh in an additional skillet)

3 oz freshly grated organic Gruyère cheese (organic Gouda is a great option for the Bone Building and Cardiovascular Health protocols)

1. Melt the butter in a 10½-inch ceramic skillet or similar.

2. Add the onions, garlic, thyme, red-pepper flakes, salt, and black pepper.

3. Cook over medium to high heat until the onions are caramelized. Remove the thyme stems.

4. Remove the onions from the heat and set them aside in a small bowl.

5. Crack the eggs into a bowl and scramble. Add the Parmesan.

6. Place the skillet over medium heat and add a little butter.

7. Pour the egg and Parmesan mixture into the skillet so that it covers the bottom.

8. Cover and cook until the egg solidifies like a pancake (about 2 to 3 minutes).

9. Distribute the cooked chicken evenly over the egg and cover everything with the caramelized onions.

10. Place the shredded Gruyère over the whole tart.

11. Cover and cook for approximately 5 minutes, or until the cheese is melted.

12. Cut into 4 pieces and enjoy!

Cauliflower Cheesy Hash Browns

Serve under eggs or as a delicious side dish with meat.

Serves 4

1 head organic cauliflower

1 organic, pasture-raised egg, beaten

1 scoop IN.POWER protein

½ cup shredded organic Cheddar cheese (buy a block and shred it yourself to avoid added cellulose powder)

¼ cup freshly grated organic Parmesan cheese

½ tsp unrefined sea salt

1 tsp organic pepper

1 tsp organic onion powder

1 tsp organic garlic powder

1 tsp organic Cajun spice

Organic, grass-fed salted butter

1. Steam the cauliflower until soft.

2. Mash with a potato masher but leave a bit chunky.

3. Stir in the remaining ingredients, except the butter

4. Melt the butter in a skillet, add in the cauliflower, and cook over medium high heat until crispy.

Speedy Salmon Cakes

Serves 4

2 cans wild-caught salmon (we love the Wild Red sockeye salmon from Vital Choice)

2 organic, pasture-raised eggs

1 scoop IN.POWER protein

½ organic onion, finely diced

2 tsp seafood seasoning (we like Simply Organic Seafood Seasoning)

2 tsp organic Cajun spice

Unrefined sea salt to taste

Organic pepper to taste

Organic, grass-fed salted butter

1. Combine all the ingredients in a bowl. Create either 4 large or 8 small salmon cakes.

2. In a large nonstick skillet, melt some butter. Brown the salmon cakes on one side, then flip to cook the other side.

3. Remove from the heat.

Optional

· *For egg sandwiches: Place cooked salmon cakes on a baking sheet with ½ oz of organic cream cheese on each. Broil until the cheese is melted. Fry up 1 egg per salmon cake. Place the fried eggs on top of the cakes to serve.*

· *For a salad: Place the cooked salmon cakes on top of salad greens. Add colorful vegetables and your favorite SKINNYFat dressing.*

Protein-Packed Morning Muffins

You can use up any of your leftovers in these muffins to create delicious and freezable portable morning treats.

Makes 6 muffins

6 slices organic, pasture-raised bacon

⅓ organic onion, finely diced

1 clove garlic, chopped

5 large organic, pasture-raised eggs

¼ cup organic sour cream (you choose the fat content)

⅔ cup freshly chopped or grated organic cheese or cheese combo of your choice

Unrefined sea salt to taste

Organic pepper to taste

Organic ground red cayenne pepper to taste

Organic seasonings, as desired

⅓ organic tomato, chopped

⅓ cup cooked organic spinach or asparagus

1. Preheat the oven to 325°F.

2. Grease a muffin tin with ghee, coconut oil, SKINNYFat, butter, or retained and collected fat, or use a nonstick tin. You will use only 6 of the muffin molds (perhaps 7, depending on the bulk of the vegetables and bacon).

3. Brown the bacon and chop. Use the remaining bacon fat to cook the onion and garlic until the onion is translucent.

4. Beat the eggs in a small bowl and blend with the sour cream, cheese, and seasonings.

5. Pour the egg mixture into the muffin molds until two-thirds full, keeping enough room on top for the bacon and vegetables.

6. Combine the cooked onion and garlic, tomato, and spinach or asparagus with the bacon in the now-empty egg bowl. Distribute the mixture evenly into the egg mixture.

7. Bake for approximately 25 minutes, or until cooked through. Allow to completely cool before removing from the muffin tin.

Smoked Salmon Cream Cheese Roll-Ups

Serve these roll-ups for a Norwegian omega-3–filled breakfast. Jayson loves to eat an egg alongside, as they are a delicious way to soak up the nutrient-dense yolk. They are also great premade for when you have to run out of the house quickly in the morning. And these roll-ups also make for a great appetizer at a dinner party.

Serves 2

8 oz sliced wild-caught smoked salmon

8 oz organic cream cheese, softened at room temperature

1 Tbsp fresh lemon juice

¼ tsp unrefined sea salt

⅛ tsp organic pepper

Minced organic dill, jalapeños, or arugula (optional)

1. Place the salmon on a baking sheet. Line up the salmon slices side by side, slightly overlapping them to form a rectangle of flattened salmon.

2. Combine all of the other ingredients (and any other seasonings you love) in a bowl until smooth.

3. Spread the mixture evenly across the salmon.

4. Slowly roll the salmon up tightly. You should be left with a cylindrical salmon tube.

5. Cut the salmon roll-ups in 1-inch pieces. (Cut on a diagonal, if you want to get fancy!)

Greek Yogurt and Fruit Bowl

Serves 1

¾ cup organic full-fat plain Greek yogurt

1 tsp organic cinnamon

Stevia to taste

1 serving favorite fruit

Combine all of the ingredients in a bowl and enjoy.

Yogurt Conversions

▪ If you can only find nonfat Greek yogurt, add 2 Tbsp SKINNYFat and stir well to incorporate into the sweetened yogurt mixture.

▪ If you can only find regular (not Greek) full-fat plain yogurt, add 1 scoop IN.POWER protein to sweetened yogurt mixture.

▪ If you can only find regular (not Greek) nonfat plain yogurt, add both 1 Tbsp SKINNYFat and 1 scoop IN.POWER protein to sweetened yogurt mixture.

Baked Apple à la Micronutrient Miracle Mode

Serves 1

1 organic apple

1 Tbsp organic, grass-fed salted butter

1 tsp organic cinnamon

Stevia powder or drops to taste

½ cup organic plain Greek yogurt (try and find one with a higher fat content, for creaminess)

10 vanilla stevia drops (or organic vanilla extract and stevia to taste)

1. Preheat the oven to 350°F.

2. To make an "apple cup," core the apple, removing all the seeds and creating a hole approximately 1 inch around. Do not pierce through the bottom.

3. Place the butter, cinnamon, and stevia inside the apple cup.

4. Place the apple in a baking dish and fill the dish with water halfway up the apple.

5. Cook for 30 to 45 minutes, or until soft.

6. In a small bowl, combine the yogurt and vanilla stevia or sweetened extract.

7. Remove the apple from the oven and place in a bowl to serve. Top with the sweetened Greek yogurt. If full-fat Greek yogurt is unavailable, refer to the Yogurt Conversions in the Greek Yogurt and Fruit Bowl recipe on page 331.

Carrot Cake Pancakes with Cream Cheese Frosting

What's up, Doc? Who doesn't want dessert for breakfast? These delicious glazed pancakes are bound to please the crowd, regardless of age.

Serves 2

PANCAKES

- 1 organic carrot, grated
- ⅓ cup IN.POWER protein
- ⅓ cup coconut flour
- ¾ tsp aluminum-free baking powder
- ¾ tsp organic cinnamon
- ¾ tsp organic pumpkin pie spice
- 2 carrots chopped (about 1 cup)
- Pinch unrefined sea salt
- ¼ cup organic plain Greek yogurt
- 4 whole organic, pastured-raised eggs
- ½ cup water
- ½ cup full-fat coconut milk (BPA-free can)

- Stevia to taste
- ¼ tsp organic vanilla extract
- Chopped walnuts, raisins, or unsweetened coconut (optional)
- Organic, grass-fed salted butter

FROSTING

- 2 Tbsp organic cream cheese, softened at room temperature
- 2 Tbsp organic heavy cream or coconut cream
- Stevia or 4 Tbsp Lakanto sweetener

1. Set aside the grated carrot.

2. In a medium bowl, combine IN.POWER, coconut flour, baking powder, cinnamon, pumpkin pie spice, chopped carrots, and salt.

3. Combine the yogurt, eggs, water, coconut milk, stevia, and vanilla extract in a blender or food processor on low.

4. Add the dry ingredients and blend until well combined. Set the blender bowl aside to let batter stand for 10 minutes.

5. Heat a small amount (about 1 teaspoon) of butter in a skillet or griddle on medium.

6. Stir the grated carrots into the blender to finish the batter.

7. Drop the batter by ¼ cupfuls on hot griddle. Cook one side, and then flip to cook the other.

8. While the pancakes are cooking, prepare the cream cheese frosting by whipping up all the ingredients in a bowl.

9. Glaze the pancakes with the frosting and enjoy!

MAIN COURSES

Chicken Wings

Serves 4

SKINNYFat Original

2 lb organic, pasture-raised chicken wings

Buffalo Wing Sauce (aka Jayson's Red Hot) with melted butter added (page 323) or melted Garlic-Parmesan Miracle Butter (page 317)

8 medium organic carrots, cut into sticks

8 stalks organic celery, cut into sticks

1. Fill a deep fryer to the fill line with the SKINNYFat and heat 325°F, or use a deep skillet and thermometer, if you don't have a fryer.

2. Fry the chicken wings until crispy.

3. In a large pot, warm the sauce of your choice.

4. Remove the finished wings and place them on a plate covered with paper towels to absorb the excess oil.

5. Place the wings in a bowl with the desired sauce and toss quickly to coat.

Serve these wings with celery and carrot sticks and a healthy side of Really Creamy SKINNYFat Blue Cheese Dressing (page 322) for dipping.

Scallops in Lemon Butter Sauce

Serves 4

¾ cup organic, grass-fed salted butter

3 Tbsp minced garlic

2 lb large sea scallops (about 20)

2 Tbsp freshly grated organic Parmesan cheese

1 tsp unrefined sea salt

⅛ tsp organic pepper

Juice of 1 lemon

1. In a large skillet, melt the butter.

2. Stir in the garlic and cook for about 30 seconds.

3. Add in the scallops and cook for several minutes on one side. Flip over and cook until opaque.

4. Remove the scallops. Whisk the remaining ingredients into the butter.

5. Pour the sauce over the scallops to serve.

Camarão na Moranga
(aka Brazilian Shrimp Stew in a Pumpkin)

Each time we visit Rio de Janeiro, we make a reservation at our favorite restaurant on Ipanema beach. From the first time we had this dish, we were in love. There is nothing more exciting than when it arrives at the table—this big, orange pumpkin turned into a serving bowl with shrimp just pouring out of the top. Now we make this for guests when they visit us at home. The creamy flavors are just as satisfying to the palette as the incredible presentation is to the eye.

Serves 4

1 medium organic pumpkin

2 lb large wild-caught shrimp, peeled and deveined, shells saved

3 cups coconut milk

2 organic bay leaves

½ tsp freshly ground nutmeg

½ tsp unrefined sea salt

½ tsp organic pepper

2 medium organic onions, finely diced (divided)

4 large cloves garlic, chopped (divided)

2 Tbsp SKINNYFat Original

3 sprigs fresh organic rosemary, chopped

2 Tbsp organic curry powder

10 large organic Roma tomatoes, chopped (you can also use a can of organic diced tomatoes)

1 organic serrano pepper

1 cup fresh organic cilantro, roughly chopped

8 oz organic cream cheese, softened at room temperature

1. Preheat the oven to 400°F.

2. Cut a circular opening in the top of the pumpkin. Using a spoon and your hands, remove all the seeds and strings from inside the pumpkin. Wash the pumpkin thoroughly inside and out, and then dry the inside with a paper towel (like you might if you were carving a jack-o'-lantern).

3. Wrap the pumpkin in foil and place it on a baking sheet with the opening facing down. Cook in the oven for about 1 hour, or until soft.

4. Meanwhile, in a small pot over medium heat, simmer the shells from the deveined shrimp, coconut milk, bay leaves, nutmeg, salt, pepper, ½ of the onions, and ½ of the garlic for 20 minutes.

5. Strain the liquid from the small pot. Throw away everything left in the strainer. Put aside this creamy, fragrant sauce.

6. In a large skillet over medium-high heat, heat the SKINNYFat. Add the remaining onion. Cook until softened.

7. Add the rosemary, curry powder, tomatoes, pepper, and the remaining garlic, and cover and cook for 25 minutes.

8. Remove the lid and add in the shrimp and the sauce. Cook until the shrimp turns pink and opaque.

9. Remove from the heat. Add in the cilantro and set aside.

10. When the pumpkin is finished and soft, remove it from the oven and turn it right side up.

11. Spread the cream cheese over the warm, softened "meat" on the inside of the pumpkin. Make a thin layer all the way around.

12. Pour in the shrimp stew mixture.

13. Place the whole pumpkin, still in its foil, back on the baking sheet and cook for 20 minutes.

14. Remove from the oven and allow to cool. Place on a large presentation plate. When serving, make sure to put some of the flesh of the pumpkin coated with cream cheese in every bowl along with the stew. Enjoy!

Quick Tandoori Shrimp
Serves 4

1 tsp organic chili powder

¾ tsp organic curry powder

½ tsp organic ground cumin

¼ tsp organic cinnamon

¼ tsp unrefined sea salt

½–1 tsp organic ground red cayenne pepper (optional)

1½ lb medium to large wild-caught shrimp, peeled and deveined (you can also do a tandoori mixed grill by cutting other protein into bite-size pieces for broiling)

1 medium organic onion, thinly sliced into rings

10 sprigs fresh organic cilantro, chopped

Juice of 1 lime

1. Raise the oven rack to just 6 inches from the broiler.

2. Preheat the broiler.

3. Combine all the dry spices in a bowl.

4. Toss the shrimp and onion rings in the bowl to coat them.

5. Arrange the coated shrimp and onions on a baking sheet.

6. Cook the shrimp and onions until pink and opaque (approximately 7 minutes).

7. Remove the shrimp from the oven and sprinkle them with the cilantro and lime juice.

8. Serve with the Cooling Cucumber Raita (page 320).

Greek Chicken

Serves 4

SPINACH LAYER

SKINNYFat Original

10 oz organic spinach

4 oz organic feta cheese

2 large organic, pasture-raised eggs

1 medium organic onion, diced

CHICKEN MIXTURE

2 Tbsp SKINNYFat Original

1½ lb organic, pasture-raised chicken thighs, cut into 1-inch pieces

2 tsp organic garlic powder

2 tsp organic dried oregano

TOPPING

3 oz organic feta cheese to sprinkle

½–1 cup organic tomato sauce

1. Preheat the oven to 325°F.

2. Coat a baking dish with a thin layer of SKINNYFat.

3. Create the spinach layer by first boiling the spinach for 15 minutes to remove oxalates. Combine the spinach with the feta, eggs, and onion in a mixing bowl. Spread the mixture on the bottom of the prepared dish.

4. For the chicken mixture, in a skillet over medium heat, heat the SKINNYFat. Add the chicken, garlic, and oregano, and cook until the chicken is no longer pink.

5. Spoon the chicken layer over the spinach layer.

6. To make the topping, spoon the feta and the tomato sauce over the chicken.

7. Bake for 30 minutes. Let stand for 5 minutes before serving.

Mexican Chicken Wrap

Serves 1

1 Ridiculously Simple Wrap (page 353)

4 oz cooked organic, pasture-raised chicken thighs

1 slice or 1 ounce favorite organic cheese

¼ avocado, sliced, or 2 Tbsp Holy Moly Guacamole (page 327)

2 Tbsp organic salsa

Fill the wrap with all of the ingredients and enjoy.

Optional

· *Try a hot burrito. Fill a wrap with the meat and cheese, wrap in foil, and bake in the oven until hot. Then enjoy with guacamole, sour cream, and salsa.*

· *Try a quesadilla. Layer the cheese and meat on top of the wrap, fold over, and then heat. Top with dollops of guacamole, salsa, and sour cream.*

· *Place any of your favorite salads, such as shrimp salad or curry chicken salad, into the wrap to enjoy a very portable lunch. Always wrap in foil. You can tear back the foil as you eat it so that you don't lose any of the filling!*

Slow-Cooked Beer-Braised Beef

Serves 4

1½ lb organic, grass-fed beef chuck (stew meat)

2 organic onions, diced

2 Tbsp SKINNYFat Original

2 tsp organic fresh thyme

2 Tbsp arrowroot flour

1 tsp unrefined sea salt

½ tsp organic pepper

1 Tbsp organic tomato paste

1 cup beef broth (homemade or an organic, sugar-free, store-bought version)

1 cup dark gluten-free beer

1. Place all of the ingredients in a slow cooker or in a large heavy-bottom pot on the stove over low to medium heat.

2. Allow to simmer, stirring occasionally, for 3½ hours.

3. Using a slotted spoon, remove the beef to a small bowl and set aside.

4. Turn the heat up and allow the liquid to boil, and then reduce the heat and simmer for 10 minutes, until thickened further.

5. Place the beef back into the broth and remove from the heat.

6. Serve over Cauliflower Mash (page 352).

Miracle Chinese Fried "Rice"

Serves 4

4 organic, pasture-raised eggs

1 head cauliflower

2 Tbsp SKINNYFat Original

2 Tbsp sesame oil

1 onion, chopped

2 carrots, cut into small cubes

5 Tbsp coconut aminos

1 can water chestnuts

1 can bamboo shoots

½ cup frozen peas

1½ lb cooked protein (you can use leftovers or quickly broil chicken thighs or shrimp)

1 Tbsp fish sauce (sugar-free)

1. Place a small skillet coated with SKINNYFat or butter over medium heat, scramble the eggs, and set aside.

2. To create the cauliflower "rice," use either a cheese grater or a food processor to chop the cauliflower into pieces the size of a grain of white rice.

3. In an extra-large skillet or wok, warm the SKINNYFat and sesame oil over medium heat. Add the onion and carrots and cook for 4 minutes.

4. Add in the cauliflower, coconut aminos, water chestnuts, bamboo shoots, frozen peas, and fish sauce and mix to coat all the vegetables. Cook for 4 minutes.

5. Add in the cooked protein and scrambled eggs and stir well to coat evenly.

6. Cook for an additional 5 to 10 minutes, covered, on low heat.

Buffalo Chicken Chili

What does a girl from upstate New York (Rochester, near Buffalo) miss most about the area? Buffalo chicken wings, of course. This chili totally hits the spot by combining all of the wing flavors, including the blue cheese dip, in one delicious bowl.

Serves 4

4 Tbsp SKINNYFat Original

1½ lb ground organic, pasture-raised chicken (can sub organic, grass-fed ground beef if you prefer or sprouted black beans to make this vegetarian/ vegan)

1 large organic onion, chopped

2 stalks organic celery, chopped

2 large organic carrots, chopped

4 cloves garlic, diced

1 can (28 oz) organic fire-roasted diced tomatoes (BPA-free can)

2 Tbsp organic chili powder

1 tsp organic ground cumin

1 tsp organic dried oregano

½ tsp organic ground red cayenne pepper

Unrefined sea salt to taste

Organic pepper to taste

½ cup organic crumbled blue cheese (gluten-free!)

3 Tbsp organic white vinegar

1. Heat the SKINNYFat in a large ceramic pot over medium-high heat.

2. Add in the chicken and brown.

3. Stir in the onion, celery, carrots, garlic, diced tomato, and all the spices.

4. Cover and cook on low for approximately 4 hours. *Option:* After browning the chicken in the pot, place all of the ingredients in a slow cooker for 4 hours.

5. Mix in the cheese and vinegar just before serving.

Note: To reduce/eliminate the lectin content of the tomatoes, cook them in a pressure cooker before adding them to the recipe.

Greek Lamb Kabobs

Serves 4

Zest of 1 lemon

Unrefined sea salt to taste

Organic pepper to taste

2 Tbsp chopped fresh organic oregano

2 organic onions, each chopped into quarters

2 organic green zucchini, sliced into thick chunks

2 organic yellow squash, sliced into thick chunks

2 organic tomatoes, each chopped into quarters

1½–2 lb organic lamb loin, cut into 1–2-inch squares

4 oz organic feta cheese (optional)

1. Preheat the oven to 350°F.

2. In a large mixing bowl, combine the lemon zest, salt, pepper, and oregano.

3. Place the onions, zucchini, and squash on a baking sheet and cook for 5 to 10 minutes, or until softened. Do not cook all the way through.

4. Place the softened vegetables, tomatoes, and the lamb in the mixing bowl with the lemony mixture and toss to coat well.

5. Heat the grill to medium-high.

6. Thread a combination of the spice-coated lamb and the vegetables onto 8 skewers.

7. Grill the skewers until lightly charred.

8. Optional: Serve sprinkled with the cheese, if using.

Peppercorn-Crusted Beef Tenderloin

This is lovely served with our 4-Ingredient Blender Hollandaise Sauce (page 323).

Serves 4

1 organic, grass-fed beef tenderloin (2 lb) or 4 tenderloin steaks

1 Tbsp SKINNYFat Original

3 Tbsp organic peppercorn (try and find a good tricolor mix for variety in flavors)

4 tsp unrefined sea salt

1. Bring the meat to room temperature at least 30 minutes prior to cooking.

2. Preheat the oven to 400°F.

3. Pat the meat dry and coat with the SKINNYFat.

4. Crush the pepper, either using a cleaned coffee grinder or a mill. Combine the crushed peppercorns with the salt and pat evenly all over the tenderloin.

5. Cook for 45 minutes (for the loin) or 15 minutes (for the steaks). Use a meat thermometer to check the temperature. Medium rare (145°F) is the goal.

6. Let rest for 10 minutes prior to serving.

Grilled Tandoori Skewers

These skewers can be accompanied by the Cooling Cucumber Raita (page 320) and Indian Garlic-Butter Cheese Non-Naan (page 354).

Serves 4

1¼ cups organic plain Greek yogurt

2 Tbsp fresh lemon juice

2 Tbsp SKINNYFat Olive

3 Tbsp freshly grated ginger

1 tsp unrefined sea salt

1 tsp organic turmeric

1 tsp organic garam masala (Indian spice; we use Frontier brand)

1 tsp organic ground red cayenne pepper (or more for extra spiciness)

1 tsp organic paprika

2 cloves garlic, minced

½ head organic broccoli, cut into large florets

½ head organic cauliflower, cut into large florets

1 large organic yellow onion, cut into about 8 pieces

1 organic zucchini or summer squash, cut into ¾-inch slices

2 medium organic tomatoes, cut into 8 parts each

1½ lb of protein, cut into 1–2-inch squares (choose one protein or a combination of the highest-quality chicken, shrimp, and beef)

1. In a large mixing bowl, combine the yogurt, lemon juice, SKINNYFat, ginger, salt, turmeric, garam masala, cayenne, paprika, and garlic.

2. Place the broccoli, cauliflower, and onion in a steamer on the stove or in a microwave oven to lightly steam. Do not cook all the way through. Simply soften.

3. Place the softened vegetables along with the zucchini or summer squash, tomatoes, and protein in the mixing bowl and coat well with the yogurt mixture.

4. Cover and refrigerate for at least 30 minutes.

5. Heat the grill to medium-high.

6. Create 8 skewers. Thread a combination of the yogurt-coated proteins and the vegetables onto 8 skewers.

7. Grill the skewers until lightly charred.

Moqueca (aka Brazilian Fish Stew)

Bom apetite! That is how you say "enjoy your meal" in Brazil. And if you ordered moqueca, you would be enjoying it for sure. This fish stew, traditionally from Bahia, Brazil, is incredibly delicious, and even individuals who don't love fish will be humming through the bowl.

Serves 4

6 Tbsp SKINNYFat Original

1 organic onion, diced

1 clove garlic, minced

1 organic red bell pepper (roasted, if you have time), diced

1 can (28 oz) organic diced tomatoes (BPA-free can)

1 organic green chile pepper, chopped

1½ lb of wild-caught white fish (grouper, mahimahi, flounder, and snapper all work well), cut into 1-inch cubes

¼ Tbsp organic ground red cayenne pepper (We use 1 Tbsp, but we like it hot!)

¼ cup fresh organic cilantro, chopped

1 cup coconut milk (or whole cream, if you don't want it as sweet)

2 Tbsp fresh lime juice

Unrefined sea salt to taste (for us, ½ tsp)

Organic pepper to taste (for us, ½ tsp)

1. Heat the SKINNYFat in a saucepan over medium heat.

2. Cook the onion for several minutes, or until translucent.

3. Add the garlic and bell pepper and cook for several minutes.

4. Add the tomatoes, chile pepper, fish, cayenne, and cilantro, and simmer gently until the fish begins to flake.

5. Pour in the coconut milk and cook just until heated through; do not boil.

6. Add the lime juice and season with the salt and black pepper.

Rustic Portobello Pizza Caps

Serves 2

4 large portobello mushroom caps, stems and gills removed

4 Tbsp SKINNYFat Pizza in a Bottle Italian-Infused Oil (page 318)

Unrefined sea salt to taste

Organic pepper to taste

4–8 Tbsp organic pizza sauce of your choice (sugar-free); we recommend using Mom's Organic Roasted Pepper Pasta Sauce or using our Mom's Beef Bolognese recipe (page 324)

4–8 organic black olives, sliced

2 anchovy fillets, chopped (optional, but preferred for flavor and omega-3 content)

8–16 slices organic pepperoni

¼ lb cooked organic Italian sausage (optional)

4–8 cloves garlic, roasted and smashed

1–2 cups shredded organic mozzarella cheese (buy a block and shred it yourself to avoid added cellulose powder)

Organic red-pepper flakes (optional)

1. Preheat the oven to 425°F.

2. Brush each mushroom cap with 1 Tbsp of the SKINNYFat and sprinkle with a pinch of salt and a grind of black pepper.

3. Roast for 15 to 20 minutes (depending on the size of the mushrooms), or until the mushroom caps are nicely roasted but still holding their general shape.

4. Let the caps cool until they can be handled.

5. Drain or pat dry the caps to remove any excess moisture.

6. Spoon 1 to 2 tablespoons of the sauce into each one.

7. Top with the olives, anchovy pieces (if using), pepperoni, Italian sausage (if using), garlic, cheese, red-pepper flakes (if using), and another small grind of the black pepper.

8. Place the mushrooms back in the oven until the cheese is melted and beginning to brown, like on pizza.

9. Serve immediately. *Buon appetito!*

Zughetti—or Zucchini Spaghetti

Serves 2 to 4

4 large organic zucchini　　　　　　　**1 Tbsp SKINNYFat Olive**

1 Tbsp unrefined sea salt

1. Make zucchini noodles using either an inexpensive julienne peeler or a vegetable mandolin/spiral slicer. (You can find our favorite picks in the resource center on caltonnutrition.com. We love the long zughetti ribbons that the slicer forms. You can even wrap them around a fork like the real thing. A small investment with a ton of great uses.)

2. Put the zughetti ribbons in a colander and toss with the salt. The salt with help pull the water out of the zucchini and make the ribbons even more noodlelike. Place the colander over a bowl to catch the released water. Let stand for 20 minutes.

3. Rinse the zughetti well, and pat it dry.

4. When you are ready to eat the zughetti, add it to a large skillet with the SKINNYFat and heat for about 1 minute. Then add your choice of a Miracle Pesto (pages 315 to 318), Bolognese (page 324), Alfredo (page 319), or any other sauce you are making.

5. Heat thoroughly and serve.

Rustic Flatbread

This recipe can also be made into breadsticks for appetizers or mini pizzas for parties.

Serves 2

1 head organic cauliflower

1 cup shredded organic mozzarella cheese (do not use the moist "fresh")

1 organic, pasture-raised egg

½ tsp organic dried basil

½ tsp organic dried oregano

½ tsp organic garlic powder

½ tsp organic onion powder

½ tsp unrefined sea salt

½ tsp organic red-pepper flakes

1. Preheat the oven to 400°F. Line a baking sheet with parchment paper or a silicone pad.

2. To create the cauliflower "rice," use either a cheese grater or a food processor to chop the cauliflower into pieces the size of a grain of white rice.

3. Steam the "rice." This can be done either in a pan and steamer basket or in a microwave, for quicker preparation. You want the cauliflower pieces to become soft and almost translucent.

4. Allow to cool.

5. Using a strainer, cheesecloth, or a clean kitchen towel, wring the cauliflower to get it really dry. Even when you think you are done, do it again. It cannot be too dry.

6. Stir the dry cauliflower rice with the cheese, egg, basil, oregano, garlic powder, onion powder, salt, and pepper flakes until well combined.

7. Using a spoon and a spatula, shape the cauliflower crust mixture into a thin rectangle on the baking sheet.

8. Bake for approximately 35 minutes, or until golden brown.

9. Remove from the oven and top the crust with the desired toppings (see below).

10. Place the topped flatbread back into the oven and bake for 10 minutes.

11. Serve with a side salad.

Optional

For toppings, choose what you have available.

· *Traditional pizza: Tomato sauce, mozzarella cheese, and pepperoni*

· *Perfect pesto pizza: Pesto and cooked shrimp*

· *Greek flatbread: Chicken, tomato sauce, and feta cheese*

· *"French onion tart" bread: Caramelized onions and Gruyère cheese*

· *Moroccan style: Sausage, mozzarella cheese, and tomato sauce seasoned with cumin, coriander, and paprika*

Coq Au Vin

On one trip to Paris we were lucky enough to spend a day studying privately with Chef Marie-Blanche de Broglie. We made a traditional coq au vin, and she taught us about French cooking methods and much more about French culinary traditions, with valuable tips on entertaining *à la Française*. While we say *au revoir* to the flour in her traditional coq au vin, we have miraculously altered it so that we can still enjoy this hearty chicken stew.

Serves 4

4 slices organic, pasture-raised bacon

5 organic, pasture-raised chicken legs or 1 whole chicken, cut into pieces

1 package (10 oz) mushrooms, each cut in half

2 large or 3 medium organic onions, chopped

Unrefined sea salt to taste

Organic pepper to taste

1 Tbsp arrowroot flour

2 large organic carrots, chopped

4 cloves garlic, chopped

1 cup organic dry red wine

2 Tbsp organic tomato paste

2 organic bay leaves

¾ cup chicken broth (homemade or an organic, sugar-free, store-bought version)

1. In a skillet over medium-high heat, cook the bacon. When it is crunchy, remove it from the skillet, crumble it, and set it aside for later.

2. In the skillet with the bacon grease, brown the chicken on all sides.

3. Place the browned chicken in a slow cooker with the rest of the ingredients.

4. Cook on low for 7 hours.

5. Remove the bay leaves and sprinkle with the crispy bacon before serving.

Thai-Style Chopped Pork

Serves 4

½ cup coconut milk

⅓ cup coconut aminos

½ cup fresh organic cilantro, chopped

¼ cup fresh lime juice (or the juice of 1 lime)

2 Tbsp freshly grated ginger

1½ lb boneless organic, pasture-raised pork loin, chopped into bite-size pieces

1 Tbsp SKINNYFat Original

2 cups organic green beans

2 organic carrots, chopped into long strips

1. Combine the coconut milk, coconut aminos, cilantro, lime, and ginger in a mixing bowl.

2. Add in the pork and toss to coat well.

3. In a wok or large skillet, heat the SKINNYFat over medium heat. Add the pork mixture and cook for 3 to 5 minutes.

4. Add in the green beans and cook for 5 minutes.

5. Toss the carrots into the wok and cook for 1 minute only, to keep crisp.

Optional

· Serve alongside lettuce or cabbage as a wrap filling.

· Use to top salads or enjoy it cold as a grab-and-go lunch.

Micronutrient-Packed "Offaly" Tasty Meatloaf

You don't have to be afraid of liver any longer. You can hide it in this "offaly" tasty meal. If you get farm-fresh liver from grass-fed cows, like we do, the rich, silky texture really adds to the beef in this loaf.

Serves 4

¼ lb organic liver

1 lb organic grass-fed ground beef

1 cup mushrooms (we like reconstituted dried wild porcini mushrooms), chopped

½ cup organic crumbled blue cheese (gluten-free!)

1 Tbsp organic garlic powder

1 Tbsp organic onion powder

2 tsp organic red-pepper flakes

1 Tbsp unrefined sea salt

1 Tbsp organic pepper

1 Tbsp organic chipotle powder

¾ cup organic tomato sauce

¼ cup freshly grated or finely sliced organic cheese (Optional, but we love Port du Salut for this!)

1. Preheat the oven to 350°F.

2. Liquefy the liver in a blender or food processor.

3. Place the ground beef and mushrooms into a baking pan or a glass baking dish and pour in the liquefied liver. Add the blue cheese, garlic powder, onion powder, red-pepper flakes, salt, pepper, and chipotle.

4. Use your hands to combine the ingredients and shape the mixture into a loaf. Bake for 30 minutes.

5. Remove from the oven and cover with the tomato sauce and grated cheese. Return to the oven for an additional 10 minutes to allow the cheese to melt.

Fabulous Fajitas

Serves 4

4 Tbsp SKINNYFat Olive, divided

1 tsp organic chili powder

1½ tsp organic dried oregano

1 tsp unrefined sea salt

1 tsp organic paprika

1 tsp organic onion powder

1 tsp organic garlic powder

½–1 tsp organic ground red cayenne pepper (optional for heat preference)

1½ tsp organic ground cumin

1½ lb organic, pasture-raised chicken thighs, cut into strips (you can also swap for shrimp or beef)

2 organic red bell peppers, sliced into strips

2 organic yellow bell peppers, sliced into strips

2 organic onions, thinly sliced into strips

1. Create a marinade by combining 2 Tbsp of the SKINNYFat with the chili powder, oregano, salt, paprika, onion powder, garlic powder, cayenne (if using), and cumin in a large mixing bowl.

2. Add the chicken and toss to coat well.

3. Cover and let sit in the refrigerator for 1 to 5 hours.

4. In a large skillet over medium heat, heat the remaining SKINNYFat.

5. Add the red peppers, yellow peppers, and onions and cook covered, stirring frequently, until they begin to soften.

6. Add the chicken. Stir so the seasonings coat the vegetables, as well.

7. Remove from the heat after the chicken is thoroughly cooked.

8. Serve with the Holy Moly Guacamole (page 324), organic salsa, shredded organic cheese (Manchego), organic sour cream, and Ridiculously Simple Wraps (optional, page 353).

Fish and Chips

On a trip through England we decided to find the perfect recipe for fish and chips. In every city we visited, we would ask locals which restaurant served the best plate and then we would test it ourselves. We visited a lot of cities on that trip, and our favorite was in Dartmouth. (We went back a few times, just to be sure.) It was the haddock and the rice flour combination in their gluten-free batter that did it for us. So we brought the recipe home and now use it as a starchy treat every now and again.

Serves 4

SKINNYFat Original

½ Tbsp aluminum-free baking powder

1½ tsp unrefined sea salt

½ tsp freshly ground organic pepper

1¼ cups organic rice flour, divided

1 large organic, pasture-raised egg, lightly beaten

6 oz sparkling or soda water

2 large organic russet potatoes or 2 organic sweet potatoes, cut into chips (what we call french fries in the United States) about the size of your index finger

4 wild-caught haddock fillets, 4 oz each (can be purchased frozen and thawed; cod also works well)

1. Fill a deep fryer to the fill line with the SKINNYFat and heat to 325°F, or use a deep skillet and thermometer if you don't have a fryer.

2. In a mixing bowl, combine the baking powder, salt, pepper, and 1 cup of the rice flour. Mix the egg with the soda water and add it to the bowl. Mix well to make a smooth batter.

3. Pour the remaining ¼ cup of rice flour on to a plate, for dredging.

4. Fry the potatoes for 6 to 8 minutes, or until golden brown and crisped to your preference.

5. Remove the chips and blot on a paper towel–lined plate to remove the excess oil.

6. Move the chips to a baking sheet and keep in a warmed oven to keep heated while frying the fish.

7. Lightly coat (dredge) a fish fillet with the rice flour, and then coat in the batter. A thin coating is best. Do this for all the fillets and fry for approximately 5 minutes, turning once.

8. Serve with organic vinegar (to be more traditional) or SKINNYFat Tartar Sauce (page 322).

Shepherd's Pie

While traveling in London, it became immediately evident to us that this city is the best place to get great Indian food. So, that is why we decided to give one of Great Britain's most traditional comfort foods a spicy new makeover. It was such a huge hit at our Sunday extended family dinners that we included it here for you.

Serves 4

TOP LAYER

> 1 full recipe for Cauliflower Mash (page 352)

BOTTOM LAYER

> 2 Tbsp SKINNYFat Olive
>
> 2 organic onions, chopped
>
> 2 cloves garlic, minced
>
> 1½ lb organic, grass-fed ground beef
>
> 2 Tbsp organic curry powder
>
> 2 Tbsp organic turmeric
>
> 1 Tbsp organic ground cumin

> ½ tsp organic ground ginger
>
> ½ Tbsp organic cinnamon
>
> ½–1 tsp organic ground red cayenne pepper
>
> 1 bag organic frozen peas
>
> 2 organic carrots, cut into small cubes

1. Prepare the Cauliflower Mash and set it aside. Preheat the oven to 350°F.

2. In a large skillet over medium heat, heat the SKINNYFat. Cook the onions and garlic until the onions just begin to become translucent.

3. Add the ground beef and cook until browned.

4. Add in all the spices, peas, and carrots. Reduce the heat to medium-low and cook for 15 minutes.

5. Spread the meat mixture across the bottom of a 9 x 13 baking dish. Create a second layer on top with the Cauliflower Mash. You can refrigerate until needed or pop it in an oven at 350°F until piping hot.

SENSATIONAL SIDE DISHES AND RAD WRAPS

Oven-Roasted Brussels Sprouts
Serves 4

4 cups organic Brussels sprouts

2 Tbsp SKINNYFat Olive (bacon fat and butter can be substituted, as well)

Coarse unrefined sea salt

Organic pepper

1. Preheat the oven to 325°F.

2. Cut the Brussels sprouts in half if they are big and remove the ends and any browned outer leaves.

3. On a baking sheet, coat the sprouts with the SKINNYFat and season with a healthy amount of the salt and pepper.

4. Bake for 25 to 30 minutes.

5. Do not discard the burnt leaves that fall off; they are delicious!

Optional

· *Spice it up with organic ground red cayenne pepper and SKINNYFat Hot Pepper–Infused Oil (page 319)*

· *Complement an Italian dish by using SKINNYFat Pizza in a Bottle Italian-Infused Oil (page 318) and finish with a sprinkle of Parmesan cheese.*

Cauliflower Mash
Serves 4

1 head organic cauliflower, chopped

2 Tbsp organic, grass-fed salted butter

2 Tbsp organic cream cheese

½ tsp organic garlic powder

¼ tsp organic onion powder

Unrefined sea salt to taste

Organic pepper to taste

1. Steam the cauliflower until soft.

2. Place the cauliflower and the remaining ingredients in a blender or food processor and process until smooth. We like to keep it a bit chunky, as the texture more resembles potato.

Sweet Potato, Yam, and Apple Casserole
Serves 4

1 organic yam, sliced

2 large organic sweet potatoes, sliced

3 medium organic apples, sliced

8 Tbsp organic, grass-fed salted butter, cut into chunks

1 Tbsp organic cinnamon

1. Preheat the oven to 350°F.

2. Place the yam, sweet potatoes, and apples in layers in a 9 x 13 baking dish.

3. Cover with the butter and cinnamon.

4. Bake for 40 minutes or until the ingredients are softened.

Ridiculously Simple Wraps

These can be made fresh, or make a larger batch and keep them in the refrigerator for grab-and-go meals.

Makes 1 large or 2 small wraps (eat only 1 recipe per person per seating)

1 organic, pasture-raised egg

1 Tbsp SKINNYFat Original

1 Tbsp freshly grated organic Parmesan cheese

1 Tbsp water

1 Tbsp IN.POWER protein

½ Tbsp buckwheat flour

½ Tbsp coconut flour

1. Mix all of the ingredients together in a bowl to form the batter.

2. Heat a small ceramic skillet lightly coated with SKINNYFat or another fat over medium heat.

3. Pour in the batter so it forms a thin layer across the bottom of the skillet.

4. Cover and cook until bubbles form; don't hurry this.

5. Flip and cook for 1 minute.

Indian Garlic-Butter Cheese Non-Naan

These are amazing with any Indian-spiced meal, such as Quick Tandoori Shrimp (page 336) and Grilled Tandoori Skewers (page 342). If making more "non-naan"—say for a family dinner—keep them warm in the oven as you make them. Place shavings of butter in between each piece of naan. Then watch them disappear at the dinner table.

Makes 1 wrap—perfect for 1 person (If following a weight-loss protocol, enjoy these sparingly.)

1 organic, pasture-raised egg

1 Tbsp SKINNYFat Original

1 Tbsp freshly grated organic Parmesan cheese

1 Tbsp water

1 Tbsp IN.POWER protein

½ Tbsp buckwheat flour

½ Tbsp coconut flour

½ tsp organic garlic powder

1 tsp minced garlic

1 oz organic mozzarella cheese, finely chopped

Organic, grass-fed salted butter

1. Mix all of the ingredients together in a bowl to form the batter.

2. Heat a small ceramic skillet lightly coated with butter over medium heat.

3. Pour in the batter so it forms a thin layer across the bottom of the skillet.

4. Cover and cook until bubbles form.

5. Flip and cook for 30 to 60 seconds.

DESSERTS

You might notice that there are no desserts listed on your menu plans. That is because your plans supply a very satisfying amount of nutrient-dense foods each and every day, so you don't need to eat any more food. We included these desserts here so that you can use them to celebrate special occasions, like birthdays and holidays. Other times, we make these treats and freeze them into small, personal-size portions. That way, on the rare occasion we find ourselves wanting dessert, we can defrost them in the refrigerator. Use these delicious, high-quality desserts sparingly, especially if your goal is weight loss. For everyday treats, use the Triple Threat puddings and ice cream as meal replacements. They satisfy the protocol as well as your sweet tooth.

Cream Cheese Swirl Brownies

Makes 12

1 full recipe for Chocolate Brownies batter (page 357)

4 oz organic cream cheese, softened at room temperature

1 organic, pasture-raised egg

3 Tbsp Lakanto sweetener

¼ tsp organic vanilla extract

1. Preheat the oven to 350°F. Coat a 6 x 9-inch baking dish with SKINNYFat or coconut oil.

2. Prepare the Chocolate Brownies but do not cook.

3. Combine all the other ingredients in a bowl to make the cream cheese filling.

4. Place ¾ of the brownie mix in the prepared baking dish.

5. Place the cream cheese filling in a layer on top, and then cover with the remaining ¼ of the brownie mix.

6. Use a knife to slice through the brownies to create swirls.

7. Bake for approximately 35 minutes. Store in the refrigerator.

Creamy Dreamy Cheesecake with Chocolate Cookie Crust

Makes 12 to 16 slices

CRUST (OPTIONAL)

¼ cup coconut flour

½ cup almond flour

3 Tbsp SKINNYFat Original

1 organic, pasture-raised egg

½ cup Stevita Delight chocolate drink mix

½ tsp unrefined sea salt

FILLING

5 packages organic cream cheese (8 oz each), softened at room temperature

1 cup organic full-fat sour cream

3 organic, pasture-raised eggs

¾ cup Lakanto sweetener or stevia to taste

1 Tbsp organic vanilla extract

1 tsp. lemon zest

1. Grease a springform pan and wrap the bottom with foil. This will allow the cream to cook more evenly in the cheesecake. The foil should be wrapped at least 2 inches high around the entire pan.

2. Fill a very large baking pan (with sides) with about 1 inch of water to create a water bath that your springform pan will cook in. Place in the oven and preheat to 350°F.

3. If making the crust: Mix all of the crust ingredients in a bowl. Press the crust down by hand to form a thin layer at the bottom of the springform pan.

4. Mix all of the filling ingredients in a bowl and blend until super smooth.

5. Fill the springform pan with the filling. Place in the heated water bath in the oven.

6. Bake for 1 hour or until the center appears solid.

7. Remove and let sit until cool. Make sure to run a knife around the cooled cheesecake before removing it from the springform pan.

Chocolate Brownies (Dairy-Free)

Makes 12

1 block dark Baker's Chocolate
(4 oz sugar-free)

1 Tbsp SKINNYFat Original

2 very ripe avocados, halved, pitted,
and peeled

¼ cup Stevita Delight chocolate
drink mix

1 Tbsp coconut flour

1 Tbsp organic vanilla extract

1 tsp aluminum-free baking powder

5 Tbsp Lakanto sweetener

1 pinch of unrefined sea salt

CHOCOLATE CREAM CHEESE FROSTING
(OPTIONAL)

8 oz organic cream cheese

8 Tbsp (1 stick) organic, grass-fed
salted butter

2 cups Lakanto sweetener

⅓ cup chocolate Stevita Delight

1. Preheat the oven to 350°F.

2. Coat a 6 x 9-inch baking dish with SKINNYFat or coconut oil.

3. Melt the chocolate and SKINNYFat in a small pot on the stove or in the microwave;
do not burn.

4. Place the avocados in a blender and process until smooth.

5. In a large mixing bowl, combine the melted chocolate and blended avocados.

6. Add in the remaining ingredients and use a hand mixer or large wooden spoon to
completely combine into a luxuriously dark batter.

7. Pour into the prepared baking dish and bake for 35 minutes.

8. Store in the refrigerator to keep them extra fudgy!

9. Optional: To create the frosting, beat all ingredients together and spread evenly
on the cooled brownies.

Chia Seed Chocolate Pudding

Serves 1 to 2

3 Tbsp chia seeds

1 cup organic milk (coconut, almond,
heavy cream, or full-fat milk)

2 tsp Stevita Delight chocolate drink
mix or 2 tsp unsweetened cocoa and
stevia to taste

1 tsp organic vanilla extract

1. In a small bowl, combine all of the ingredients.

2. Refrigerate overnight.

Optional: If you prefer a smooth texture over that of tapioca, then pour everything
into a blender or food processor and process until smooth. Refrigerate.

Conclusion

Living the Micronutrient Miracle for Life

IT'S NOW TIME FOR you to put all of your new knowledge to work and experience your own Micronutrient Miracle. When you think about it, we really have covered a lot of information and discovered some pretty incredible things along the way. You now have a step-by-step 28-day plan that truly has the power to transform your health and your life. The information we have shared with you throughout this book puts the health-producing power of micronutrient sufficiency in your hands. Now it is up to you to put those small but mighty micronutrients to work and start living the extraordinary life you have always dreamed of.

While our time is almost over here, you can bring us with you on your 28-day journey by visiting our Micronutrient Miracle Motivation and Resource Center and signing up for our personally guided 28-day plan. And the best part is, it's absolutely free, so you have nothing to lose. When you sign up, you get valuable Rich Food coupons, discounts on Calton Nutrition products, helpful quick-start and personal evaluation sheets, video recipes, workout routines and advice, and even daily tips and motivation from, you guessed it, us! The truth is, nothing worthwhile is ever easy, but when you sign up for our personally guided program, we will be with you every step of the way to make sure you stay on track.

As you have seen, the 28-day Micronutrient Miracle plan isn't some variation on those ever-popular eat-less-and-exercise-more diets that have been around for the last 50 years. Nor does it ask you to change your core nutritional philosophy or adhere to strict calorie restrictions. The Micronutrient Miracle is a completely different kind of plan; it requires that you work toward a state of micronutrient sufficiency by making real changes in just about every area of your life—from the food you put into your shopping cart to your lifestyle habits to your choice of multivitamin and even the soap you wash your dishes with. It all adds up in the end, and each and every positive step you make along the way will bring you one step closer to the optimal health you desire. The Micronutrient Miracle plan requires something else of you, too—it requires faith. Faith in the scientific research pointing to the fact that your health conditions, extra weight, or low energy really stem from a deficiency in essential micronutrients. Faith that making all the required changes will reverse those deficiencies. And, finally, faith that when you have done the hard work, your health will truly improve.

As with any act of faith, the hardest part is that no one can offer you any real guarantee. However, what we can tell you with complete certainty is that the steps we have outlined within the Micronutrient Miracle plan, when followed correctly, will improve your health. We have personally witnessed it with thousands upon thousands of our personal clients—people just like you, who came to us suffering from a wide range of health conditions and diseases and were able to dramatically improve their health. The Micronutrient Miracle plan works because it focuses on reversing the condition that has been shown to be a causative factor in nearly every major health condition and disease plaguing the world today—micronutrient deficiency. When the deficiencies causing the body to manifest the health condition or disease are eliminated, the body can heal itself and the health condition or disease improves or is eliminated completely. This is the embodiment of our *micronutrient sufficiency hypothesis of health* first mentioned back in Chapter 1. While this can look and feel like a miracle, the fact is, it is really nutritional science at work. Over the years, we have come to believe strongly that *nutrition is the new medicine*! You now have the nutritional knowledge you need to heal your body and bring your health to a level you may never have dreamed of achieving.

This is your time to reverse the damage of the past, reclaim your health, and start living an extraordinary life. Perhaps, like Jeff in Chapter 1, you will finally lose the weight that has been negatively affecting your health and holding you back from truly experiencing life. Or maybe, like Mabel from Chapter 2 and Craig from the Introduction, you will find your eyesight or your blood pressure improved. Or like Evelyn, whose story we shared in Chapter 3, you will finally conquer food cravings that have been a lifelong struggle. Whatever your miraculous transformation will be, we want you to know that we are proud of you for making a commitment to improve your health and sticking to it! We know the amount of sacrifice and effort it takes to complete the 28-day program. And while you may stumble a time or two when ordering at a restaurant or purchasing food at the grocery store, or you may miss a workout now and again, we are sure that, in the end, you will be surprised by just how easy all of the changes actually were to implement and follow. The fact is, implementing our simple three-step plan to micronutrient sufficiency by eliminating toxic micronutrient-depleting

Poor Foods, improving your lifestyle habits, and supplementing smart becomes second nature when you make up your mind to put your health first.

One sure way to know you are really making positive changes is when friends, relatives, and coworkers start coming up to you, out of the blue, to tell you that they notice a difference. Pay attention when this starts to happen and use that positive reinforcement as motivation to continue your journey and make the Micronutrient Miracle plan the foundation of your healthy lifestyle. Some of you may decide to keep on cutting out the sugar, wheat, soy, GMOs, and other micronutrient-depleting and health-robbing foods and lifestyle habits after finishing the 28-day plan. You might think that these permanent changes fit your lifestyle perfectly. Others might feel that adding in some of the eliminated foods once in a while, for special occasions, is the right path. And that is okay, too. The Micronutrient Miracle plan gives you the power of choice. As long as you stick to its core philosophies the majority of the time, it can help to protect you from micronutrient deficiency conditions for years to come. However, if you choose to allow Poor Foods and detrimental lifestyle habits back in, just beware: Many of these foods and lifestyle habits can be addictive and cause you to backslide rather quickly.

Remember, the further you stray from our Signature and condition-specific protocols, the more likely you are to suffer from a micronutrient deficiency and potentially a related health condition or disease. But don't worry, regardless of the path you take from this point on, we know that the principles and lessons you have learned thus far, and will be implementing during your 28-day plan, have the power to improve your health in truly miraculous ways.

What will your micronutrient miracle look like? No one knows for sure, but one thing we do know is that you are about to embark on one of the greatest journeys any human can undertake—the journey to becoming the best possible you, to discovering extraordinary health. Now get out there and live your optimal life.

To get started, come visit us at the Micronutrient Miracle Motivation and Resource Center at mymiracleplan.com and sign up for your personally guided 28-day Micronutrient Miracle plan; we can't wait to work with you. While you're there, you can read about other Micronutrient Miracle success stories, and don't forget to write us and tell us about your Micronutrient Miracle—we'll be looking for your e-mail.

M. Calton

Acknowledgments

WE WOULD LIKE TO acknowledge a few individuals who made the process of writing *The Power Nutrient Solution* seamless and thoroughly enjoyable. First, to Lora, our editor, who initially contacted us because she really liked our earlier books and believed that we had more to share. Thank you for putting the wheels in motion. Without you, we would have never put our 28-day plan on paper to share with the world. Your belief in our message made this whole journey possible. Next, to Celeste, who is our friend above and beyond being our literary agent. You have taught us the business of book selling and your personal involvement and professional touch on every aspect of the book has been invaluable.

We could not create a successful plan without successful clients, so to all of the people who have put their faith and their health in our hands and in the power of micronutrient therapy, we thank you. We would especially like to thank Craig, Kym, Jeff, Mabel, Winona, Rock, and Evelyn, as well as our Inner Circle, whose journeys will help motivate and inspire others for years to come. Thank you for sharing your stories and your successes so honestly and selflessly.

Thank you to the amazing companies that joined the Calton Global Health Initiative. You gave your amazing products generously and proved that you truly care about the health of America. To our Diamond Mastermind Group: Brent, Brett, Cassie, Izabella, Michael, Tami, and Trevor, thank you for all you do to help others with your messages—you are making real changes in the world. We also want to thank our Certified Micronutrient Specialists (CMS) for educating their clients and patients as to the role micronutrient sufficiency can play in the prevention and reversal of disease. Finally, to our core Calton Nutrition team that makes it all possible: Camper, Jeanne, Gina, Brandon, Vaine, Stacie, Mike, and Sarah. We count on you more than you know. You always have our backs and you never let us down. Thank you for joining us in this fight and helping others to live their optimal lives.

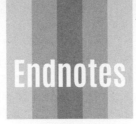

Endnotes

INTRODUCTION

1 cdc.gov/bloodpressure/faqs.htm

2 P. Anand, A. B. Kunnumakara, C. Sundaram et al., "Cancer is a Preventable Disease that Requires Major Lifestyle Changes," *Pharmaceutical Research* 25, no. 9 (September 2008); 2097–16.

3 Q. Xu, C. G Parks, L. A. DeRoo et al., "Multivitamin Use and Telomere Length in Women," American Journal of Clinical Nutrition 89, no. 6 (June 2009): 1857–63.

4 crnusa.org/CRNfoundation/HCCS/chapters/CRNFrostSullivan-fullreport0913.pdf.

CHAPTER 1

1 NHANES 1999–2004 * Vitamin D data from NHANES 2003–2006.

2 theheartfoundation.org/heart-disease-facts/heart-disease-statistics/.

3 seer.cancer.gov/statfacts/html/all.html.

4 niams.nih.gov/Health_Info/Bone/Osteoporosis/osteoporosis_ff.asp.

5 diabetes.org/diabetes-basics/statistics/.

6 drhyman.com/blog/2011/04/08/
how-dietary-supplements-reduce-health-care-costs/.

7 "Dr. Oz's Ultimate Supplement Checklist," Retrieved 2011, from *The Dr. Oz Show:* doctoroz.com/videos/dr-ozs-ultimate-supplement-checklist.

8 World Health Organization, World Health Report, 2000 (Geneva: World Health Organization, 2000).

9 T. H. Tulchinsky. "Micronutrient Deficiency Conditions: Global Health Issues," *Public Health Reviews* 32 (2010): 243–55.

10 D. Ruston et al., "The National Diet & Nutrition Survey: Adults Aged 19 to 64 Years, Volume 4," Retrieved 2011 from the Food Standards Agency: food.gov.uk /multimedia/pdfs/ ndnsv3.pdf.

11 H. K. Lu et al., "High Prevalence of Vitamin D Insufficiency in China: Relationship with the Levels of Parathyroid Hormone and Markers of Bone Turnover," *PLoS ONE* 7, no. 11 (2012): e47264. doi:10.1371/journal.pone.0047264.

12 wam.ae/en/news/emirates/1395274836939.html.

13 Vitamin and Mineral Nutrition Information System (VMNIS): "Global Prevalence of Vitamin A Deficiency in Population at Risk: 1995–2005," Retrieved 2010, from the World Health Organization (WHO): who.int/vmnis/database/vitamina/x/en/.

14 dailymail.co.uk/news/article-2543724/Rickets-soar-children-stay-indoors
    -Number-diagnosed-disease-quadruples-ten-years.html#ixzz3AYczNJLL.

15 worldhistoryforusall.sdsu.edu/themes/keytheme1.htm.

16 world.time.com/2012/12/14/what-if-the-worlds-soil-runs-out/.

17 J. Marler, J. Wallin, "Human Health, The Nutritional Quality of Harvested Food and
    Sustainable Farming Systems," Retrieved 2010, from the Nutrition Security
    Institute: nutritionsecurity.org/PDF/NSI_White%20Paper_Web.pdf.

18 senate.gov/reference/resources/pdf/modernmiraclemen.pdf

19 J. Marler, J. Wallin, "Food Nutrition Has Been Declining! Minerals Go Down,
    Disease Goes Up!" Retrieved 2010, from the Nutrition Security Institute:
    nutritionsecurity.org/PDF/Food%20Nutrition%20Decline.pdf.

20 I. Loladze, "Hidden Shift of the Ionome of Plants Exposed to Elevated CO_2 Depletes
    Minerals at the Base of Human Nutrition," Ed. Ian T Baldwin. *eLife* 3 (2014): e02245.
    PMC. Web. 18 Mar. 2015.

21 online.wsj.com/news/articles/SB10001424052970203400604578073182907123760.

22 nongmoproject.org/learn-more/what-is-gmo/.

23 non-gmoreport.com/articles/may10/consequenceso_widespread_glyphosate_use
    .php.

24 yesmagazine.org/issues/can-animals-save-us/joel-salatin-how-to-eat-meat-and
    -respect-it-too.

25 R. Pirog, A Benjamin. "Checking the Food Odometer: Comparing Food Miles for
    Local versus Conventional Produce Sales to Iowa Institutions 2003," Retrieved 2011,
    from the Leopold Center for Sustainable Agriculture: leopold.iastate.edu/pubs
    /staff/files/food_travel072103.pdf.

26 ers.usda.gov/media/157859/fau125_1_.pdf.

27 organicconsumers.org/corp/foodtravel112202.cfm.

28 chgeharvard.org/sites/default/files/resources/local_nutrition.pdf.

29 R. D. Shaver. "By-product Feedstuffs in Dairy Cattle Diets in the Upper Midwest,"
    Retrieved 2011, from University of Wisconsin-Extension: uwex.edu/ces
    /dairynutrition/documents/byproductfeedsrevised2008.pdf.

30 A. Tolan, J. Robertson, C. R. Orton, M. J. Head, A. A. Christie, and B. A. Millburn,
    "Studies on the Composition of Food," *British Journal of Nutrition* 31 (1974), 185–200.
    doi:10.1079/BJN19740024.

31 fda.gov/AdvisoryCommittees/CommitteesMeetingMaterials
    /VeterinaryMedicineAdvisoryCommittee/ucm222635.htm.

32 Farmed salmon and human health. Retrieved 2011, from the Pure Salmon
    Campaign: puresalmon.org/human_health.html

33 "Food Irradiation and Vitamin Loss 2007," Retrieved 2010, from Food and Water
    Watch: foodandwaterwatch.org/factsheet/food-irradiation-and-vitamin-loss/.

34 Food Irradiation Q&As. Retrieved 2011, from Mercola: mercola.com/article
    /irradiated/irradiation.htm.

35 Food Irradiation—The Problems and Concerns: Position Statement of The Food Commission–July 2002. Retrieved 2010, from The Food Commission: foodmagazine. org.uk/campaigns/irradiation_concerns/.

36 cdc.gov/mmwr/preview/mmwrhtml/mm4840a1.htm.

37 K. M. Fairfield and R. H. Fletcher, "Vitamins for Chronic Disease Prevention in Adults: Scientific Review," *Journal of the American Medical Association* 2002. 287, no. 23(June 19, 2002):3116–26. doi:10.1001/jama.287 .23.3116 PMID:12069675.

38 P. H. Langsjoen, S. Vadhanavikit, K. Folkers, "Response of Patients in Classes III and IV of Cardiomyopathy to Therapy in a Blind and Crossover Trial with Coenzyme Q10," *Proceedings of the National Academy Sciences of the United States of America* 82, no. 12 (June 1985), 4240–44. PMID: 3858877.

39 M. F. Holick, "Vitamin D and Sunlight: Strategies for Cancer Prevention and Other Health Benefits," *Clinical Journal of the American Society of Nephrology* 3, no.5 (September 2008):1548–54. PMID: 18550652

40 P. J. Goodwin, M. Ennis, K. I. Pritchard, J. Koo, N. Hood, "Frequency of Vitamin D (Vit D) Deficiency a Breast Cancer (BC) Diagnosis and Association with Risk of Distant Recurrence and Death in a Prospective Cohort Study of T1-3, N0-1, M0 BC," *Journal of Clinical Oncology 20, no. 26 (*May 2008):511. Retrieved 2011, from American Society of Clinical Oncology: Asco.org/ASCOv2/Meetings/Abstracts?&vmview =abst_detail_view&confID=55&abstractID=31397.

41 M . Kivipelto et al., "Homocysteine and Holo-trans-cobalamin and the Risk of Dementia and Alzheimer's Disease: A Prospective Study," *European Journal of Neurology* 16, no. 7 (July 2009): 808–13. PMID: 19453410.

42 webmd.com/alzheimers/news/20140806/low-vitamin-d-levels-may-boost -alzheimers-risk-study-finds.

43 L. C. Clark, "Decreased Incidence of Prostate Cancer with Selenium Supplementation: Results of a Double-Blind Cancer Prevention Trial," *British Journal Urology* 81, no. 5 (May 1998): 730–34. PMID: 9634050.

44 N. G. Stephens, "Randomised Controlled Trial of Vitamin E in Patients with Coronary Disease: Cambridge Heart Antioxidant Study (CHAOS)," *Lancet* 23, no. 347 (9004) (March 1996): 781–86.

45 M. G. Showell et al., "Antioxidants for Male Subfertility," *Cochrane Database System Review* 19, no. 1, (January 2011): CD007411. doi: 10.1002/14651858.CD007411.pub2.

46 Ibid.

47 J. M. Howard. "Red Cell Magnesium and Glutathione Peroxidase in Infertile Women—Effects of Oral Supplementation with Magnesium and Selenium," *Magnesium Research* 7, no. 1 (March 1994): 49–57.

48 J. M. Geleijnse et al., "Dietary Intake of Menaquinone Is Associated with a Reduced Risk of Coronary Heart Disease: The Rotterdam Study," *Journal of Nutrition* 134, no. 11 (November 2004): 3100–3105. Retrieved 2014 from cardient.com/reference-library/rotterdam-vitamin-k2-study

49 S. Kanellakis et al., "Changes in Parameters of Bone Metabolism in Postmenopausal Women Following a 12-Month Intervention Period Using Dairy Products Enriched with Calcium, Vitamin D, and Phylloquinone (Vitamin K_1) or Menaquinone-7

(Vitamin K$_2$): The Postmenopausal Health Study II," *Calcified Tissue International* 90, no. 4 (April 2012): 251–62. doi: 10.1007/s00223-012-9571-z. Epub 2012 Mar 4. Retrieved 2013, from the National Center for Biotechnology Information: ncbi.nlm.nih.gov /pubmed/22392526.

50   crnusa.org/CRNfoundation/HCCS/chapters/CRNFrostSullivan-fullreport0913.pdf.

51   "How Dietary Supplements Reduce Health Care Costs," Retrieved 2011, from Dr. Mark Hyman: drhyman.com/how-dietary-supplements-reduce-health-care-costs-3250/.

52   M. Hyman, "Paradigm Shift. The End of 'Normal Science' in Medicine Understanding Function in Nutrition, Health, and Disease," *Alternative Therapies in Health and Medicine* 10, no. 5 (Sept–Oct 2004), Retrieved 2011, from Dr. Hyman: drhyman.com/downloads/Paradigm-Shift.pdf.

CHAPTER 2

1   M. R. Turner and K. Talbot, "Functional Vitamin B$_{12}$ Deficiency," *Practical Neurology* 9, no. 1 (February 2009): 37–41.

2   A. Duncan et al.. "Quantitative Data on the Magnitude of the Systemic Inflammatory Response and Its Effect on Micronutrient Status Based on Plasma Measurements," *American Journal Clinical Nutrition*. 95, no. 1 (January 2012): 64–71.

CHAPTER 3

1   https://credit-suisse.com/us/en/news-and-expertise/topics/health-care.article .html/article/pwp/news-and-expertise/2013/09/en/is-sugar-turning-the-economy-sour.html.

2   forbes.com/sites/alicegwalton/2012/08/30/how-much-sugar-are-americans -eating-infographic/.

3   http://articles.mercola.com/sites/articles/archive/2011/05/02/is-sugar-toxic.aspx.

4   spectracell.com/media/uploaded/3/0e2747083_1388158470_303nutrientchart1013 -pdf.pdf.

5   M. L. Pelchat, A. Johnson, R. Chan, J. Valdez, and J. D. Ragland, "Images of Desire: Food-Craving Activation During fMRI,": NeuroImage 23 (2004): 1486–93.

6   M. G. Tordoff, "Adrenalectomy Decreases NaCl Intake of Rats Fed Low-Calcium Diets," *American Journal of Physiology* 270 (1996): R11–R21.

7   card.iastate.edu/iowa_ag_review/winter_05/article5.aspx.

8   accessdata.fda.gov/scripts/cdrh/cfdocs/cfcfr/CFRSearch.cfm?fr=184.1866.

9   goranlab.com/pdf/Ventura%20Obesity%202010-sugary%20beverages.pdf.

10   ers.usda.gov/topics/crops/sugar-sweeteners/background.aspx#.U-uhvFYVrwI.

11   non-gmoreport.com/articles/jun08/sugar_beet_industry_converts_to_gmo.php.

12   articles.chicagotribune.com/2011-05-24/health/ct-met-gmo-food-labeling —20110524_1_gmos-food-safety-foods-market/2

13   M. Lenoir et al., "Intense Sweetness Surpasses Cocaine Reward," *PLoS ONE* 2, no. 8 (2007): e698. doi:10.1371/journal.pone.0000698

14   N. M. Avena et al., "Evidence for Sugar Addiction: Behavioral and Neurochemical Effects of Intermittent, Excessive Sugar Intake," *Neuroscience and Biobehavioral Reviews* 32, no. 1 (2008):20–39. doi:10.1016/j.neubiorev.2007.04.019.

15   S. M. Grundy, "Hypertriglyceridemia, Insulin Resistance, and the Metabolic Syndrome," *American Journal of Cardiology* 83, no. 9: 25–29

16   health.harvard.edu/fhg/updates/update1204b.shtml.

17   nytimes.com/2011/04/17/magazine/mag-17Sugar-t.html?pagewanted=9&_r=3.

18   D. B. Boyd, "Insulin and Cancer," *Integrative Cancer Therapy* 2, no. 4 (December 2003): 315–29

19   B. Arcidiacono et al., "Insulin Resistance and Cancer Risk: An Overview of the Pathogenetic Mechanisms," *Experimental Diabetes Research* 2012 (2012), article ID 789174, 12 pages. doi:10.1155/2012/789174.

20   Y. Onodera, J-M. Nam, M. J. Bissell, "Increased Sugar Uptake Promotes Oncogenesis via EPAC/RAP1 and O-GlcNAc Pathways," *Journal of Clinical Investigation* 124, no. 1 (2014): 367–84. doi:10.1172/JCI63146.

21   heart.org/HEARTORG/GettingHealthy/NutritionCenter/HealthyEating/Added -Sugars-Add-to-Your-Risk-of-Dying-from-Heart-Disease_UCM_460319_Article.jsp.

22   theguardian.com/lifeandstyle/2014/oct/16/sugar-soft-drinks-dna-ageing-study.

23   K. A. Page et al., "Effects of Fructose vs Glucose on Regional Cerebral Blood Flow in Brain Regions Involved with Appetite and Reward Pathways," *Journal of the American Medical Association* 309, no..1 (2013): 63–70. *PMC*. Web. 18 Mar. 2015.

24   K. Teff et al., "Dietary Fructose Reduces Circulating Insulin and Leptin, Attenuates Postprandial Suppression of Ghrelin, and Increases Triglycerides in Women," *Journal of Clinical Endocrinology & Metabolism* 89, no. 6 (2004): 2963-72.

25   wheatbellyblog.com/2014/09/lose-grains-save-green-excerpt-wheat-belly-total -health/.

26   S. Drago et al., "Gliadin, zonulin, and gut permeability: Effects on celiac and non-celiac intestinal mucosa and intestinal cell lines," *Scandinavian Journal of Gastroenterology* 41, no. 4 (April 2006): 408–19.

27   health.harvard.edu/newsweek/Glycemic_index_and_glycemic_load_for_100_foods .htm.

28   ars.usda.gov/SP2UserFiles/Place/80400525/Data/isoflav/Isoflav_R2.pdf.

29   M. Behr et al., "Estrogens in the Daily Diet: In Vitro Analysis Indicates That Estrogenic Activity Is Omnipresent in Foodstuff and Infant Formula," *Food and Chemical Toxicology* 49, no. 10 (October 2011): 2681–88.

30   A. Cassidy et al., "Biological Effects of a Diet of Soy Protein Rich in Isoflavones on the Menstrual Cycle of Premenopausal Women," *American Journal of Clinical Nutrition* 60, no. 3 (September 1994): 333–40.

31   washingtonpost.com/wp-dyn/content/article/2004/05/04/AR2005033109963.html.

32   V. de Graff, K. M. Fox, and S. Ira, *Concepts of Human Anatomy and Physiology* (Boston, MA: Wm C. Brown Publishers, 1995).

33   preventdisease.com/news/13/122013_Soy-Causes-Insulin-Resistance-Reduction -Hormones-Involved-In-Blood-Sugar-Fat.shtml.

34 worldwildlife.org/industries/soy.

35 ers.usda.gov/data-products/adoption-of-genetically-engineered-crops-in-the-us /recent-trends-in-ge-adoption.aspx#.U-5wDksVrwI.

36 euroresidentes.com/Blogs/2005/12/scientists-in-spain-link-additive-to.htm.

37 holisticmed.com/aspartame2/aspart.p10a.

38 dorway.com/doctors-speak-out/dr-blaylock/excitotoxins-neurodegeneration -neurodevelopment/.

39 niehs.nih.gov/health/topics/agents/sya-bpa/.

40 S. M. Duty et al., "Personal care product use predicts urinary concentrations of some phthalate monoesters," *Environmental Health Perspectives* 113, no. 11 (2005): 1530–35. *PMC*. Web. 18 Mar. 2015.

41 S. Perrine and H. Hurlock, *The New American Diet.* (Emmaus, PA: Rodale, 2009).

42 S. Soriano et al., "Rapid insulinotropic action of low doses of bisphenol-A on mouse and human islets of langerhans: role of estrogen receptor," *PLoS ONE* 7, no. 2 (2012): e31109. doi:10.1371/journal.pone.0031109.

43 R. W. Stahlhut et al., "Concentrations of Urinary Phthalate Metabolites Are Associated with Increased Waist Circumference and Insulin Resistance in Adult U.S. Males," *Environmental Health Perspectives* 115, no. 6 (June 2007): 876–82. Epub 2007 Mar 14.

44 A. Deutschmann et al., "Bisphenol A Inhibits Voltage-Activated Ca2 Channels In Vitro: Mechanisms and Structural Requirements," *Molecular Pharmacology* (November 2012); DOI: 10.1124/mol.112.081372.

45 P. S. Liu, F. W. Tseng, and J. H. Liu, "Comparative Suppression of Phthalate Monoesters and Phthalate Diesters on Calcium Signalling Coupled to Nicotinic Acetylcholine Receptors," *Journal of Toxicological Sciences* 34, no. 3 (2009): 255-263; Web. europepmc.org/abstract/MED/19483380/reload=0;jsessionid= rZdodFtvtcBr5cQMNAqD.12

46 M. R. Wills et al., "Phytic Acid and Nutritional Rickets in Immigrants. *Lancet* 1, no. 7754 (April 8, 1972): 771–73.

47 R. Nagel, "Living with Phytic Acid," *Wise Traditions* (March 2010). Retrieved 2010, from The Weston A. Price Foundation: westonaprice.org/food-features /living-with-phytic-acid.

48 W.Chai, "Effect of different cooking methods on vegetable oxalate content," *Journal of Agricultural and Food Chemistry 53*, no. 8 (2005): 3027–30. DOI: 10.1021/jf048128d

49 pubs.acs.org/doi/pdf/10.1021/jf048128d.

50 J. Shemer and D.LeRoith, "The Interaction of Brain Insulin Receptors with Wheat Germ Agglutinin," *Neuropeptides* 9, no. 1 (January 1987): 1–8.

51 G. Ponzio, A. Debant, J. O. Contreras, and B. Rossi, "Wheat Germ Agglutinin Mimics Metabolic Effects of Insulin without Increasing Receptor Autophosphorylation," *Cell Signal* 2, no. 4 (1990):377–86.

52 N. Kitano et al., "Detection of antibodies against wheat germ agglutinin bound glycoproteins on the islet-cell membrane," *Diabetes Medicine* 5, no. 2 (March 1988):139–44.

53   J. L. Messina, J. Hamlin, and J. Larner, "Insulin-mimetic actions of wheat germ agglutinin and concanavalin A on specific mRNA levels," *Archives of Biochemistry and Biophysics* 254, no. 1 (April 1987):110–5.

54   I. J. Goldstein and R. D. Poretz, *The Lectins.* (Orlando, FL: Academic Press, 1986), 529–52.

55   Y. Shechter, "Bound Lectins That Mimic Insulin Produce Persistent Insulin-Like Activities," *Endocriology* 113, no. 6 (December 1983): 1921–26.

56   P. J. D'Adamo, *Live Right for Your Type.* 1st edition (New York: Penguin Putnam Inc. 2001), 168.

57   A. Pusztai, "Dietary Lectins Are Metabolic Signals for the Gut and Modulate Immune and Hormonal Functions," *European Journal of Clinical Nutrition* 47, no. 10 (October 1993): 691–99 (A. Pusztai, Rowett Research Institute, Bucksburn, Aberdeen, UK).

58   vrp.com/digestive-health/digestive-health/lectins-their-damaging-role-in -intestinal-health.

59   B. A. Myers, J. Hathcock, et al., "Effects of Dietary Soya Bean Trypsin Inhibitor Concentrate on Initiation and Growth of Putative Preneoplastic Lesions in the Pancreas of the Rat," *Food and Chemical Toxicology* 29, no. 7 (July 1991): 437–43.

60   J. J. Rackis and M. R. Gumbmann. "Protease Inhibitors Physiological Properties and Nutritional Significance," *Antinutrients and Natural Toxicants in Foods,* Robert L. Ory, ed. (Westport, CT: Food and Nutrition Press, 1981), 203–38.

61   cancer.net/cancer-types/pancreatic-cancer/statistics.

62   westonaprice.org/health-topics/plants-bite-back/.

63   K. S. Kiran et al., "Inactivation of Trypsin Inhibitors in Sweet Potato and Taro Tubers During Processing." *Plant Foods for Human Nutrition* 58, no. 2 (Spring 2003): 153–63.

64   medicaldaily.com/daily-glass-wine-protects-against-thinning-bones-well-drugs -241737.

65   I. Sommer et al., "Alcohol Consumption and Bone Mineral Density in Elderly Women." *Public Health Nursing* 16, no. 4 (Apr 2013): 704–12. DOI: 10.1017 /S136898001200331X. Epub 2012 Jul 17.

66   C. A.,Camargo et al., "Prospective Study of Moderate Alcohol Consumption and Mortality in US Male Physicians." *Archives of Internal Medicine* 159, no. 79 (1997): 79–85.

67   C. S. Fuchs et al. "Alcohol Consumption and Mortality Among Women," *The New England Journal of Medicine* 332, no. 19, (1995): 1245–50.

68   M. J. Barger-Lux et al., "Caffeine and the Calcium Economy Revisited," *Osteoporosis International* 5, no. 2 (March 1995): 97–102.

69   T. A. Morck, S. R. Lynch, and J. D. Cook. "Inhibition of Food Iron Absorption by Coffee," *American Journal of Clinical Nutrition* 37, no. 3 (1983): 416–20.

70   L. Hallberg and L. Rossander, "Effect of Different Drinks on the Absorption of Non-Heme Iron from Composite Meals," *Human Nutrition—Applied Nutrition* 36, no. 2 (1982):116-23.

71   sciencedaily.com/releases/2012/06/120629120445.htm.

72   M. Nelson et al., "Impact of Tea Drinking on Iron Status in the UK: A Review," *Journal of Human Nutrition & Dietetics* 17, no. 1 (February 2004): 43–54.

CHAPTER 4

1   J. Dollahite, D. Franklin, and R. McNew, "Problems Encountered in Meeting the Recommended Dietary Allowances for Menus Designed According to the Dietary Guidelines for Americans," *Journal of the American Dietetic Association* 95, no. 3, (March 1995): 341–44, 347; quiz 345–46. PMID: 7860947

2   J. C. Winston, "Health Effects of Vegan Diets," *American Journal of Clinical Nutrition* 89, no. 5 (2009): 1627S–3S; First published online March 11, 2009. DOI: 10.3945 /ajcn.2009.26736N.

3   P. Mariani et al., "The Gluten-Free Diet: A Nutritional Risk Factor for Adolescents with Celiac Disease?" *Journal of Pediatric Gastroenterolgy Nutrition* 27, no. 5 (November 1998):519–23. PMID: 9822315.

4   ajcn.nutrition.org/content/89/5/1627S.full.

5   G. K. Davey et al., "EPIC-Oxford: Lifestyle Characteristics and Nutrient Intakes in a Cohort of 33,883 Meat-eaters and 31,546 Non-meat-eaters in the UK," *Public Health Nutrition* 6, no. 3 (2003): 259.

6   B. D. Hokin, "Cyanocobalamin (Vitamin B-12) Status in Seventh-Day Adventist Ministers in Australia," *American Journal of Clinical Nutrition* 70, no. 3 (1999): 576S–578S.

7   H. Truby et al., "Commercial Weight Loss Diets Meet Nutrient Requirements in Free Living Adults Over 8 Weeks: A Randomized Controlled Weight Loss Trial," *Nutrition Journal* 7, no. 25 (2008). DOI: 10.1186/1475-2891-7-25.

8   L. Pachocka and L. Klosiewicz-Latoszek. "Changes in Vitamins Intake in Overweight and Obese Adults after Low-Energy Diets," *Rocz. Panstw. Zakl. Hig.* 53(3 (2002): 243–52. PMID: 12621879. Retrieved 2011, from National Center for Biotechnology Information: ncbi.nlm.nih.gov/pubmed/12621879.

9   medicine.virginia.edu/clinical/departments/medicine/divisions/digestive-health /nutrition-support-team/nutrition-articles/ODonnellArticle.pdf.

10. cnn.com/2009/HEALTH/conditions/03/20/economic.stress/index.html?_s=PM :HEALTH.

11   M. Hamer G. Owen, and J. Kloek, "The Role of Functional Foods in the Psychobiology of Health and Disease," *Nutrition Research Reviews* 18, no. 1 (June 2005): 7

12   K. A. Matthews and B. B. Gump, "Chronic Work Stress and Marital Dissolution Increase Risk of Posttrial Mortality in Men from the Multiple Risk Factor Intervention Trial," *Archives of Internal Medicine* 162, no. 3 (February 2002): 309–15.

13   G. Veen et al., "Salivary Cortisol, Serum Lipids, and Adiposity in Patients with Depressive and Anxiety Disorders." *Metabolism* 58, no. 6 (June 2009): 821–27.

14   J. F. Thayer, S. S. Yamamoto, and J. F. Brosschot. "The relationship of autonomic imbalance, heart rate variability and cardiovascular disease risk factors," *International Journal of Cardiology* 141, no. 2 (May 28, 2010): 122–31.

15   A. Heraclides, T. Chandola, D. R. Witte, and E. J. Brunner. "Psychosocial Stress at Work Doubles the Risk of Type 2 Diabetes in Middle-Aged Women: Evidence from the Whitehall II Study," *Diabetes Care* 32, no. 12 (December 2009): 2230–35.

16   J. Kruk, "Self-Reported Psychological Stress and the Risk of Breast Cancer: A Case-Control Study," *Stress* 15, no. 2 (March 2012):162–71. DOI: 10.3109/10253890.2011.606340 . Epub 2011 Aug 29.

17   R. Ballentine, MD. *Diet and Nutrition* (Honesdale, PA: Himalayan Institute Press, 1978).

18   psychologytoday.com/articles/200304/vitamin-c-stress-buster.

19   Dr. Oz's Cure for Stubborn Belly Fat, First for Women (March 14, 2011): 32–37.

20   D. S. Taylor, "Stress Can Cause Nutrient Deficiencies; Enough of the Right Nutrients Can Prevent Stress, and Controlling Stress Can, in Turn, Prevent Nutrient Deficiencies" *Better Nutrition* 1989–90.

21   menshealth.com/nutrition/multivitamin-stress.

22   T. Hamazaki, "The effect of docosahexaenoic acid on aggression in young adults. A placebo-controlled double-blind study," *Journal of Clinical Investigation* 97, no. 4 (February 15, 1996)::1129–33.

23   J. Delarue et al., "Fish Oil Prevents the Adrenal Activation Elicited by Mental Stress in Healthy Men," *Diabetes & Metabolism* 29, no. 3 (June 2003):289–95.

24   E. Noreen et al., "Effects of Supplemental Fish Oil on Resting Metabolic Rate, Body Composition, and Salivary Cortisol in Healthy Adults," *Journal of the International Society of Sports Nutrition* 7, no. 31 (2010). DOI:10.1186/1550-2783-7-31.

25   R. J. Maughan, "Role of Micronutrients in Sport and Physical Activity," *British Medical Bulletin* 55, no. 3 (1999): 683–90.

26   E. R. Eichner, "Sports Anemia, Iron Supplements, and Blood Doping," *Medicine & Science in Sports & Exercise* 24, supp. 9 (September 1992): S315–18.

27   mensfitness.com/nutrition/supplements/can-calcium-supplements-protect-against -exercise-related-bone-loss.

28   A. Cordova et al., "Effect of Training on Zinc Metabolism: Changes in Serum and Sweat Zinc Concentrations in Sportsmen," *Annals of Nutrition and Metabolism* 42, no. 5 (1998): 274–82.

29   H. Forrest, N. Henry, and C. Lukaski, "Update on the Relationship between Magnesium and Exercise," Magnesium Research 19, no. 3 (2006): 180–89.

30   A. J. Alberg et al., "Household Exposure to Passive Cigarette Smoking and Serum Micronutrient Concentrations, *American Journal of Clinical Nutrition* 72, no. 6 (December 2000): 1576–82.

31   National Research Council, *Hidden Costs of Energy: Unpriced Consequences of Energy Production and Use.* (Washington, DC: The National Academies Press, 2010).

32   Q. Gu, C. F. Dillion, and V. L. Burt, "Prescription Drug Use Continues to Increase: US Prescription Drug Data for 2007–2008," *NCHS Data Brief* 42 (September 2010). Retrieved 2011, from Centers for Disease Control and Prevention: cdc.gov/nchs/ data/databriefs/db42.htm

33 newsnetwork.mayoclinic.org/discussion/nearly-7-in-10-americans-take
-prescription-drugs-mayo-clinic-olmsted-medical-center-find/.

34 hscic.gov.uk/catalogue/PUB11291.

35 jppr.shpa.org.au/lib/pdf/gt/gt0603.pdf.

36 lef.org/magazine/mag2006/mar2006_report_drugs_01.htm.

37 D. Benton et al., "The Impact of Selenium Supplementation on Mood." *Biological Psychiatry* 29, no. 11 (1991): 1092–98.

38 N. Mokhber et al., "Effect of Supplementation with Selenium on Postpartum Depression: A Randomized Double-Blind Placebo-Controlled Trial," *Journal Maternal-Fetal & Neonatal Medicine* 24, no. 1 (2011):104–8.

39 H. C. Corbett, "Natural Alternatives to the Top 10 Most Prescribed Drugs," prevention.com/mind-body/natural-remedies/top-10-prescription-drugs-and -natural-remedies.

40 S. Billioti de Gage et al., "Benzodiazepine Use and Risk of Alzheimer's Disease: Case-Control Study," *BMJ* 349 (2014): g5205

41 m.medicalxpress.com/news/2014-09-long-term-pills-anxiety-problems-linked.html.

42 forbes.com/sites/melaniehaiken/2012/02/29/the-latest-statin-scare-are-you-at-risk/.

43 cbsnews.com/news/13-million-more-americans-would-take-statins-if-new -guidelines-followed-study/.

44 smh.com.au/national/health/oecd-says-australians-take-too.many-pills-and-must -tackle-nations-obesity-problem-20131121-2xyqn.html.

45 H. Cederberg et al., "Increased Risk of Diabetes with Statin Treatment Is Associated with Impaired Insulin Sensitivity and Insulin Secretion: A 6-Year Follow-up Study of the METSIM cOhort," *Diabetologia* (March 2015).

46 X. Huang et al., "Statins, Plasma Cholesterol, and Risk of Parkinson's Disease: A Prospective Study," Movement Disorders (January 14, 2015). doi: 10.1002/mds.26152.

47 L. Eleanor, "The Lipitor Dilemma," *Smart Money: The Wall Street Journal Magazine of Personal Business*, November 2003.

48 "Antacids—Aluminum, Calcium, and Magnesium-Containing Preparations," Retrieved 2011 from the University of Maryland Medical Center: umm.edu/health /medical-reference-guide/complementary-and-alternative-medicine-guide /depletion/antacids-aluminum-calcium-and-magnesiumcontaining-preparations.

49 lef.org/magazine/mag2006/mar2006_report_drugs_01.htm.

50 M. Calton and J. Calton, *Naked Calories* (Cleveland, OH: Changing Lives Press, 2010): 124–25.

51 H. Smith, *Diagnosis in Paediatric Haematology.* (New York: Churchill Livingstone, 1996): 6–40.

52 ewg.org/skindeep/top-tips-for-safer-products/.

53 rodalenews.com/nonstick-safe.

54 L. Pelton and K. Hawkins, *Drug-Induced Nutrient Depletion Handbook,* 2nd ed. (Hudson, OH: Lexi-Comp Inc., 2001).

55   R. Pelton and J. B. LaValle. *Drugs and Their Effects on Nutrition In: The Nutritional Cost of Prescription Drugs,* 2nd ed. (Englewood, CO: Morton Publishing Co., 2004).

56   F. Vaglini and B. Fox, *The Side Effects Bible: The Dietary Solution to Unwanted Side Effects of Common Medications* (New York: Broadway Books, 2005).

57   invitehealth.com/Drug-Induced-Nutrient-Depletion.html.

CHAPTER 5

1   S. Pandrangi and L. F. LaBorde, Retention of Folate, Carotenoids, and Other Quality Characteristics in Commercially Packaged Fresh Spinach," Journal of Food Science 69, no. 9 (2004): C702–C707. doi: 10.1111/j.1365-2621.2004.tb09919.x.

2   F. Beltrán-González et al., "Effects of Agricultural Practices on Instrumental Colour, Mineral Content, Carotenoid Composition, and Sensory Quality of Mandarin Orange Juice, cv. Hernandina," *Journal of the Science and of Food and Agriculture* 88 (2008): 1731–38.

3   theguardian.com/environment/2014/jul/11/organic-food-more-antioxidants-study.

4   epa.gov/pesticides/food/risks.htm.

5   sciencemag.org/content/341/6147/740.

6   rmit.edu.au/browse;ID=e3hoqm8befvj1.

7   ncbi.nlm.nih.gov/pmc/articles/PMC1115659/.

8   food.dtu.dk/english/News/2013/07/Most-pesticides-in-foreign-fruit.

9   todaytonightadelaide.com.au/stories/vegetable-chemicals.

10   thehealthyhomeeconomist.com/bone-broth-calcium/.

11   lef.org/protocols/health_concerns/heavy_metal_detoxification_10.htm.

12   en.wikipedia.org/wiki/AquAdvantage_salmon.

13   ncbi.nlm.nih.gov/pubmed/?term=Becker+J+American+Journal+of+Preventive+Medicine.

14   C. R. Markus, B. Oliver, G. E. Panhuysen et al., "The Bovine Protein Alpha-Lactalbumin Increases the Plasma Ratio of Tryptophan to the Other Large Neutral Amino Acids, and in Vulnerable Subjects Raises Brain Serotonin Activity, Reduces Cortisol Concentration, and Improves Mood under Stress," *American Journal of Clinical Nutrition* 71, no. 6 (June 2000): 1536–44.

15   C. R. Markus, B. Oliver, E. H. de Haan, et al.,."Whey Protein Rich in Alpha-Lactalbumin Increases the Ratio of Plasma Tryptophan to the Sum of the Other Large Neutral Amino Acids and Improves Cognitive Performance in Stress-Vulnerable Subjects," *American Journal of Clinical Nutrition* 75, no. 6 (June 2002):1051–56.

16   D. A. Camfield et al., "Dairy Constituents and Neurocognitive Health in Ageing," *British Journal of Nutrition* 106, no. 2 (July 2011):159-74.

17   usdec.files.cms-plus.com/Publications/CardioHealth_English.pdf. Accessed June 14, 2013.

18 X. Zhang and A. C. Beynen, "Lowering Effect of Dietary Milk-Whey Protein v. Casein on Plasma and Liver Cholesterol Concentrations in Rats," *British Journal of Nutrition* 70, no. 1 (July 1993):139–46.

19 H. G. Shertzer et al., "Dietary Whey Protein Lowers the Risk for Metabolic Disease in Mice Fed a High-Fat Diet," *Journal of Nutrition* 141, no. 4 (April 1, 2011): 582–87.

20 X. Lan-Pidhainy and T. M. Wolever, "The Hypoglycemic Effect of Fat and Protein Is Not Attenuated by Insulin Resistance," *American Journal of Clinical Nutrition* 91. no. 1 (January 2010): 98–105.

21 wheyoflife.org/sites/default/files/us-whey-proteins-and-weight-management.pdf

22 H. Matsumoto et al., New Biological Function of Bovine Alpha-Lactalbumin: Protective Effect Against Ethanol- and Stress-Induced Gastric Mucosal Injury in Rats," *Bioscience Biotechnology and Biochemistry* 65, no. 5 (May 2001):1104–11.

23 P. W. Parodi, "A Role for Milk Proteins and Their Peptides in Cancer Prevention," *Current Pharmaceutical Design* 13, no. 8 (2007):813–28.

24 Z. Zhang et al., "Quantitative Analysis of Dietary Protein Intake and Stroke Risk," *Neurology* 83, no. 1 (July 1, 2014): 19–25. doi: 10.1212/WNL.0000000000000551. Epub 2014 Jun 11.

25 news.illinois.edu/news/14/0225cholesterol_FredKummerow.html.

26 C. A. Mierlo et al., "Weight Management Using a Meal Replacement Strategy: Meta and Pooling Analysis from Six Studies," *International Journal of Obesity and Related Metabolic Disorders* 27, no. 5 (May 2003): 537–49.

27 nutritionj.com/content/pdf/1475-2891-11-98.pdf.

28 D. Jakubowicz et al., "Incretin, Insulinotropic and Glucose-Lowering Effects of Whey Protein Pre-load in Type 2 Diabetes: A Randomised Clinical Trial," *Diabetologia* 57, no. 9 (2014): 1807.

29 S. Nuttall, U. Martin, A. Sinclair, and M. Kendall, "Glutathione: In Sickness and in Health," *Lancet* 351, no. 9103 (1998): 645–46.

30 innovatewithdairy.com/SiteCollectionDocuments/Mono_Immunity_0304.pdf.

31 D. E. Chatterton et al., "Anti-inflammatory Mechanisms of Bioactive Milk Proteins in the Intestine of Newborns," *International Journal of Biochemistry & Cell Biology* 45, no. 8 (2013): 1730–47.

32 I. Rahman and W. MacNee, "Oxidative Stress and Regulation of Glutathione in Lung Inflammation," *European Respiratory Journal* 16, no. 3 (September 2000): 534–54.

33 J. Viña et al., "Molecular Bases of the Treatment of Alzheimer's Disease with Antioxidants: Prevention of Oxidative Stress," *Molecular Aspects of Medicine* 25, no. 1–2 (Feb–Apr 2004): 117–23.

34 biosciencetechnology.com/news/2013/11/protein-sets-bodys-response-fight-infection.

35 P. W. Parodi, "A Role for Milk Proteins and Their Peptides in Cancer Prevention," *Current Pharmaceutical Design* 13, no. 8 (2007): 813–28.

36 S. C. De Rosa et al., "N-acetylcysteine Replenishes Glutathione in HIV Infection," *European Journal of Clinical Investigation* 30, no. 10 (October 2000): 915–29.

37 E. O. Farombi, J. O. Nwankwo, and G. O. Emerole, "The Effect of Modulation of Glutathione Levels on Markers for Aflatoxin B1-induced Cell Damage," *African Journal of Medicine and Medical Sciences* 34, no. 1 (March 2005): 37–43.

38 H. Matsumoto, Y. Shimokawa, Y. Ushida, T. Toida, and H. Hayasawa, "New Biological Function of Bovine Alpha-Lactalbumin: Protective Effect against Ethanol- and Stress-Induced Gastric Mucosal Injury in Rats. *Bioscience, Biotechnology, and Biochemistry* 65, no. 5 (May 2001): 1104–11.

39 cdc.gov/features/vitalsigns/cardiovasculardisease/. Accessed June 14, 2013.

40 usdec.files.cms-plus.com/Publications/CardioHealth_English.pdf. Accessed June 14, 2013.

41 X. Zhang and A. C. Beynen, "Lowering Effect of Dietary Milk-Whey Protein v. Casein on Plasma and Liver Cholesterol Concentrations in Rats," *British Journal of Nutrition* 70, no. 1 (July 1993): 139–46.

42 D. S. Willoughby, J. R. Stout, and C. D. Wilborn. "Effects of Resistance Training and Protein Plus Amino Acid Supplementation on Muscle Anabolism, Mass, and Strength. *Amino Acids.* 32, no. 4, (2007): 467–77. Epub 2006 Sep 20.

43 drhyman.com/blog/2010/05/19/glutathione-the-mother-of-all-antioxidants/#close.

44 L. Patrick, "Mercury Toxicity and Antioxidants: Part 1: Role of Glutathione and Alpha-Lipoic Acid in the Treatment of Mercury Toxicity," *Alternative Medical Review*, 7, no. 6 (December 2002):456–71.

45 L. Kromidas, L. D. Trombetta, and I. S. Jamall, "The Protective Effects of Glutathione Against Methylmercury cytotoxicity. *Toxicology Letters* 51, no. 1 (March 1990): 67–80.

46 C. A. Lang et al., "High Blood Glutathione Levels Accompany Excellent Physical and Mental Health in Women Ages 60 to 103 Years," *Journal of Laboratory and Clinical Medicine* 140, no. 6 (December 2002) : 413–17.

47 J. H. Promislow, D. Goodman-Gruen, D. J. Slymen, and E. Barrett-Connor, "Protein Consumption and Bone Mineral Density in the Elderly: The Rancho Bernardo Study," *American Journal of Epidemiology* 155, no. 7 (April 1, 2002): 636–44.

48 H. Kaunitz and C. S. Dayrit, "Coconut Oil Consumption and Coronary Heart Disease," *Philippine Journal of Internal Medicine* 30 (1992): 165–71.

49 heall.com/body/healthupdates/food/coconutoil.html "An Interview with Dr. Raymond Peat, A Renowned Nutritional Counselor Offers His Thoughts about Thyroid Disease."

50 M. Clark, "Once a Villain, Coconut Oil Charms the Health Food World," *New York Times* (March 1, 2011), nytimes.com/2011/03/02/dining/02Appe.html ?pagewanted=all&_r=1&.

51 Dr. Mary G. Enig, PhD., FACN,. Source: "Coconut: In Support of Good Health in the 21st Century."

52 N. Baba, "Enhanced Thermogenesis and Diminished Deposition of Fat in Response to Overfeeding with Diet Containing Medium-Chain Triglycerides, *American Journal of Clinical Nutrition* 35 (1982): 379.

53 J. J. Kabara et al., "Fatty Acids and Derivatives as Antimicrobial Agents," *Antimicrobial Agents and Chemotherapy.* 2, no. 1 (1972): 23–28.

54 A. Ruzin et al., "Equivalence of Lauric Acid and Glycerol Monolaurate as Inhibitors of Signal Transduction in Staphylococcus Aureus," *Journal of Bacteriology* 182, no. 9 (May 2000): 2668–71.

55 D. O. Ogbolu et al., "In Vitro Antimicrobial Properties of Coconut Oil on Candida Species in Ibadan, Nigeria. *Journal of Medicinal Food* 10, no. 2 (June 2007): 384–87.

56 W. Dean and J. English, "Medium-Chain Triglycerides (MCTs): Beneficial Effects on Energy, Atherosclerosis and Aging," Retrieved from: nutritionreview.org/library /mcts.php.

57 M. P. St-Onge and A. Bosarge, "Weight-Loss Diet That Includes Consumption of Medium-Chain Triacylglycerol Oil Leads to a Greater Rate of Weight and Fat Mass Loss Than Does Olive Oil," *American Journal of Clinical Nutrition* 87, no. 3 (March 2008): 621–26. ajcn.org/cgi/content/abstract/87/3/621.

58 R. J. Stubbs and C. G. Harbron, "Covert Manipulation of the Ratio of Medium- to Long-Chain Triglycerides in Isoenergetically Dense Diets: Effect on Food Intake in Ad Libitum Feeding Men," *International Journal of Obesity and Related Metabolic Disorders* 20, no. 5 (May 1996): 435–44.

59 M. A. Regerm et al., "Effects of Beta-hydroxybutyrate on Cognition in Memory-Impaired Adults." *Neurobiology of Aging* 25, no. 3 (March 2004): 311–14.

60 E. H. Kossoff and A. L. Hartman, Ketogenic Diets: New Advances for Metabolism-Based Therapies," *Current Opinion In Neurology* (February 8, 2012).

61 M. Gasior, M. A. Rogawski, A. L. Hartman, "Neuroprotective and Disease-Modifying Effects of the Ketogenic Diet," *Behavioural Pharmacology* 17, no. 5–6 (September 2006):431–39.

62 MP St-Onge and A. Bosarge, "Weight-Loss Diet That Includes Consumption of Medium-Chain Triacylglycerol Oil Leads to a Greater Rate of Weight and Fat Mass Loss Than Does Olive Oil," *American Journal of Clinical Nutrition* 87, no. 3 (March 2008): 621–26. ajcn.org/cgi/content/abstract/87/3/621.

63 A. Mente, M. J. O'Donnell, S. Rangarajan, et al., "Association of Urinary Sodium and Potassium Excretion with Blood Pressure. *New England Journal of Medicine* 371, no. 7 (August 14, 2014): 601–11. doi: 10.1056/NEJMoa1311989.

64 ecowatch.com/2014/08/11/clean-chai-demand-pesticide-free-tea/.

CHAPTER 6

1 ualberta.ca/~csps/JPPS9(1)/Loebenberg.R/tablets.htm.

2 thornefx.com/build-better-multi-multi-ampm-complex/.

3 G. Tang, "Bioconversion of Dietary Provitamin A Carotenoids to Vitamin A in Humans" American Journal of Clinical Nutrition 91, no. 5 (May 2010): 1468S–1473S. doi: 10.3945/ajcn.2010.28674G. Epub 2010 Mar 3.

4 ajcn.nutrition.org/content/91/5/1468S.full.

5   "Most Multivitamin Extras Don't Add Up," Tufts University Health & Nutrition Letter (February 1, 2010). Retrieved 2010, from Goliath: goliath.ecnext.com/coms2 /gi_0199-12432585/Most-multivitamin-extras-don-t.html.

6   E. Serbinova, D. Han, and L. Packer, "Free Radical Recycling and Intramembrane Mobility in the Antioxidant Properties of Alpha-tocopherol and Alpha-tocotrienol," *Free Radical Biology and Medicine* 10, no. 5 (1991): 263–75.

7   J. Iwamoto, T. Takeda, and S. Ichimura, "Combined Treatment with Vitamin K2 and Bisphosphonate in Postmenopausal Women with Osteoporosis," *Yonsei Medical Journal* 44, no. 5 (October 30, 2003): 751–56.

8   lpi.oregonstate.edu/infocenter/vitamins/vitaminK/.

9   nlm.nih.gov/medlineplus/druginfo/natural/924.html.

10   L. D. Botto and Q. Yang. "5,10-Methylenetetrahydrofolate Reductase Gene Variants and Congenital Anomalies: A Huge Review," *American Journal of Epidemiology* 151, no. 9 (May 1, 2000): 862–77.

11   ods.od.nih.gov/factsheets/Magnesium-HealthProfessional/.

12   P. Willner et al., "Depression Increases "Craving" for Sweet Rewards in Animal and Human Models of Depression and Craving," Psychopharmacology 136, no. 3 (April 1998): 272–83.

13   health.walmart.com/Vitamins-Article/us/assets/generic/multiple-vitamin-mineral -supplements/~default.

14   H. van den Berg and T. van Vliet, "Effect of simultaneous, single oral doses of beta-carotene with lutein or lycopene on the beta-carotene and retinyl ester responses in the triacylglycerol-rich lipoprotein fraction of men," *American Journal of Clinical Nutrition* 68, no. 1 (July 1998): 82–89.

15   healio.com/ophthalmology/retina-vitreous/news/print/ocular-surgery-news /%7Ba4218ad9-3ea3-4248-aadc-88ad14c1b5a2%7D/researchers-continue-to-find -nutritions-value-in-preventing—even-treating—amd.

CHAPTER 7

1   fueluptraining.com/free-workouts/daily-hiit/.

2   K. A. Stokes, M. E. Nevill, G. M. Hall, and H. K. Lakomy, "The Time Course of the Human Growth Hormone Response to a 6 S and a 30 S Cycle Ergometer Sprint. *Journal of Sports Sciences* 20, no. 6 (June 2002): 487–94.

3   shape.com/fitness/workouts/8-benefits-high-intensity-interval-training-hiit/slide/6.

4   sciencedaily.com/releases/2012/08/120806161816.htm.

5   news.appstate.edu/2010/11/29/study-shows-resistance-training-benefits -cardiovascular-health/.

Index

Underscored page references indicate sidebars and tables. **Boldface** references indicate illustrations.

T

U

V